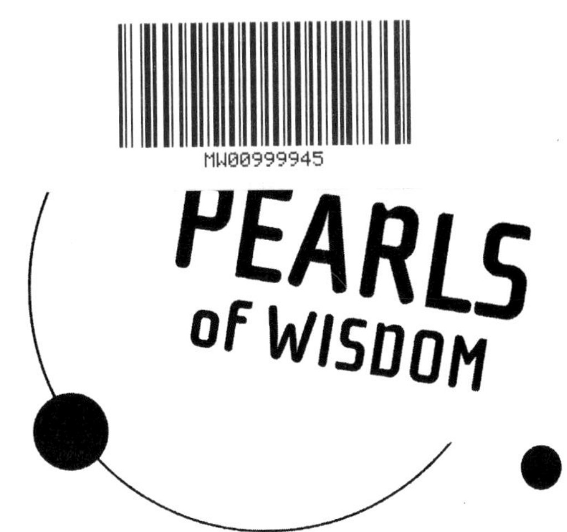

Critical Care

REVIEW

Second Edition

Michael Zevitz
Scott H. Plantz
Richard Lenhardt

McGraw-Hill
Medical Publishing Division

New York Chicago San Francisco Lisbon London
Madrid Mexico City Milan New Delhi
San Juan Seoul Singapore
Sydney Toronto

The McGraw-Hill Companies

Critical Care Review, Second Edition

3 4 5 6 7 8 9 0 IBT/IBT 0 9 8

ISBN 0-07-146424-7

Notice

Medicine is an ever-changing science. As new research and clinical experience broaden our knowledge, changes in treatment and drug therapy are required. The authors and the publisher of this work have checked with sources believed to be reliable in their efforts to provide information that is complete and generally in accord with the standards accepted at the time of publication. However, in view of the possibility of human error or changes in medical sciences, neither the authors nor the publisher nor any other party who has been involved in the preparation or publication of this work warrants that the information contained herein is in every respect accurate or complete, and they disclaim all responsibility for any errors or omissions or for the results obtained from use of the information contained in this work. Readers are encouraged to confirm the information contained herein with other sources. For example and in particular, readers are advised to check the product information sheet included in the package of each drug they plan to administer to be certain that the information contained in this work is accurate and that changes have not been made in the recommended dose or in the contraindications for administration. This recommendation is of particular importance in connection with new or infrequently used drugs.

The editors were Catherine A. Johnson and Marsha Loeb.
The production supervisor was Phil Galea.
The cover designer was Handel Low.
IBT Global was printer and binder.

This book is printed on acid-free paper.

Cataloging-in-Publication data for this title is on file at the Library of Congress.

DEDICATION

For Y.

Mike

For my father, Alan Huntly Plantz, whose love, support and brilliance has always been my guiding light.

Scott

For my Parents, for their constant love.

Richard

EDITORS

Mike Zevitz, M.D.
Assistant Professor
Chicago Medical School
Chicago, IL

Scott H. Plantz, M.D.
Associate Professor
Chicago Medical School
Sinai Medical Center
Chicago, IL

Richard Lenhardt, M.D.
Harvard Medical School
Boston, MA

CONTRIBUTING AUTHORS

Bobby Abrams, M.D.
Attending Physician
Macomb Hospital
Macomb, MI

Jonathan Adler, M.D.
Assistant in Emergency Medicine, Massachusetts General Hospital
Instructor in Medicine,
Harvard Medical School
Boston, MA

Ishtiaq Ahmad, Ph.D., M.B.B.S.
Research Associate
Laboratory of Cellular and Molecular Cerebral Ischemia
Departments of Neurology and Anatomy & Cell Biology
Center of Molecular Medicine and Genetics
Center of Molecular and Cellular Toxicology
Wayne State University School of Medicine
Detroit, MI

James W. Albers, M.D., Ph.D.
Department of Neurology
University of Michigan
Ann Arbor, MI

W. Michael Alberts, M.D.
Professor and Associate Chair
Department of Internal Medicine
H. Lee Moffitt Cancer Center & Research Institute
University of South Florida
Tampa, FL

Pranav Amin, M.D.
Department of Neurology
Duke University Medical Center
Durham, NC

Linda Anderson, M.D.
Department of Internal Medicine
Pulmonary and Critical Care Medicine Section
University of Nebraska Medical Center
Omaha, NE

Michael L. Ault, M.D.
Instructor in Anesthesiology
Section of Critical Care Medicine
Department of Anesthesiology
Northwestern University Medical School
Chicago, IL

Howard Belzberg, M.D.
Los Angeles County and University of Southern California Medical Center
Los Angeles, CA

Brian Bonanni, M.D.
Duke University Medical Center
Durham, NC

Jon M. Braverman, M.D.
Denver Health Medical Center
University of Colorado School of Medicine
Denver, CO

Gwenda Lyn Breckler, D.O.
Dept. of Surgery
Mt. Sinai Hospital
Chicago, IL

David F. M. Brown, M.D.
Instructor in Medicine
Harvard Medical School
Massachusetts General Hospital
Boston, MA

Edward Buckley, M.D.
Department of Neurology
Duke University Medical Center
Durham, NC

Leslie S. Carroll, M.D.
Assistant Professor
Chicago Medical School
Toxicology Director
Mt. Sinai Medical Center
Chicago, IL

Eduardo Castro, M.D.
Instructor in Medicine
Harvard Medical School
Massachusetts General Hospital
Boston, MA

Seemant Chatruvedi, M.D.
Assistant Professor of Neurology
Wayne State University School of medicine
Co-Director, Harper Hospital Acute Stroke Unit
Detroit, MI

Willie Chen, M.D.
Louisville, KY

Ronald D. Chervin, M.D., MS
Sleep Disorders Center
Department of Neurology
University of Michigan Health System
Ann Arbor, MI

David Chiu, M.D.
Assistant Professor of Neurology
Director, Stroke Center
Baylor College of Medicine
The Methodist Hospital
Houston, TX

Charles H. Cook, M.D.
Assistant Professor of Surgery and Critical Care
The Ohio State University Hospitals
Columbus, OH

Joseph T. Cooke, M.D., FACCP
Associate Professor of Clinical Medicine
Associate Director, Medical Critical Care
The New York Hospital-Cornell Medical Center
New York, NY

William M. Coplin, M.D.
Assistant Professor
Neurology and Neurological Surgery
Wayne State University
Detroit, MI

C. James Corrall, M.D., MPH
Clinical Associate Professor of Pediatrics
Clinical Associate Professor of Emergency Medicine
Indiana University School of Medicine
Indianapolis, IN

Douglas B. Coursin, M.D.
Professor of Anesthesiology and Internal Medicine
Associate Director of the Trauma and Life Support Center
University of Wisconsin School of Medicine
Madison, WI

Ruben Vargas-Cuba, M.D.
Instructor in Medicine
Chief Medical Resident
Department of Medicine
Tulane University School of Medicine
New Orleans, LA

G. Paul Dabrowski, M.D.
Assistant Professor of Surgery
University of Pennsylvania
Philadelphia, PA

Brian J. Daley, M.D.
Assistant Professor
Division of Trauma and Critical Care
The University of Tennessee Medical Center
Knoxville, TN

Carl W. Decker, M.D.
Madigan Army Medical Center
Fort Lewis, WA

Joshua De Leon, M.D.
Assistant Professor of Medicine
Mount Sinai School of Medicine
New York, NY
Director, Cardiac Catherization and Invasive Cardiology
Elmhurst Hospital Center
Elmhurst, NY

Peter Emblad, M.D.
Boston City Hospital
Boston, MA

Phillip Fairweather, M.D.
Clinical Assistant Professor
Mount Sinai School of Medicine
New York, NY
Department of Emergency Medicine
Elmhurst Hospital Center
Elmhurst, NY

Craig Feied, M.D.
Clinical Associate Professor
George Washington University
Washington Hospital Center
Washington, D.C.

Eva L. Feldman, M.D., Ph.D.
Department of Neurology
University of Michigan
Ann Arbor, MI

Louis Flancbaum, M.D., FACS, FCCM, FCCP
Associate Professor of Surgery, Anesthesiology, and Human Nutrition
The Ohio State University Hospitals
Columbus, OH

Mark Franklin, M.D.
Department of Anesthesiology
Northwestern University Medical School
Chicago, IL

Rajesh R. Gandhi, M.D.
Critical Care/Trauma Fellow
University of Pennsylvania
Philadelphia, PA

Judith L. Geidebring, M.D.
Lecturer
University of Michigan
Ann Arbor, MI

Sheree Givre, M.D.
Clinical Assistant Professor
Department of Emergency Medicine
Mount Sinai School of Medicine
New York, NY
Associate Director
Department of Emergency Medicine
Elmhurst Hospital Center
Elmhurst, NY

Bill Gossman, M.D.
Chicago Medical School
Mt. Sinai Medical Center
Chicago, IL

Vicente H. Gracias, M.D.
Instructor of Surgery and Trauma
Surgical Critical Care Fellow
University of Pennsylvania
Philadelphia, PA

L. John Greenfield, Jr., M.D., Ph.D.
Assistant Professor
Department of Neurology
University of Michigan
Ann Arbor, MI

Rajan Gupta, M.D.
Instructor of Surgery and Trauma
Surgical Critical Care Fellow
University of Pennsylvania
Philadelphia, PA

Susan M. Harding, M.D.
Assistant Professor of Medicine
Pulmonary and Critical Care Medicine
University of Alabama
Birmingham, AL

Marilyn T. Haupt, M.D.
Professor, Department of Medicine
Wayne State University School of Medicine
Detroit, MI

Jeffrey W. Hawkins, M.D.
Co-Director, Pulmonary and Critical Care Medicine
Norwood Clinic
Birmingham, AL

Thomas W. Hejkal, M.D.
Department of Ophthalmology
University of Nebraska Medical Center
Omaha, NE

James F. Holmes, M.D.
University of California, Davis
School of Medicine
Sacramento, CA

Eddie Hooker, M.D.
Assistant Professor
University of Louisville
Louisville, KY

Shyam Ivaturi, M.D.
Ridgeland, MS

Cameron Javid, M.D.
Department of Ophthalmology
Tulane University
New Orleans, LA

Mishith Joshi, M.D.
Stroke Fellow
Department of Neurology
Wayne State University
Detroit, MI

Marc J. Kahn, M.D.
Assistant Professor of Medicine
Internal Medicine Residency Program Director
Associate Director for Student Programs
Department of Medicine
Section of Hematology/Medical Oncology
Tulane University School of Medicine
New Orleans, LA

Henry J. Kaminski, M.D.
Case Western Reserve University School of Medicine
Department of Veterans Affairs Medical Center
University Hospitals of Cleveland
Cleveland, OH

Stuart Kessler, M.D.
Vice Chairman, Department of Emergency Medicine
Mount Sinai School of Medicine
New York, NY
Director, Department of Emergency Medicine
Elmhurst Hospital Center
Elmhurst, NY

Ali M. Khorrami, M.D., Ph.D.
University Eye Institute
Syracuse, NY

Albert S. Khouri, M.D.
Kentucky Lions Eye Center
Louisville, KY

Lance W. Kreplick, M.D.
Assistant Professor
University of Illinois
EHS Christ Hospital
Oak Lawn, IL

Andrew Lee, M.D.
Department of Ophthalmology
Baylor College of Medicine
Houston, TX

Deborah Anne Lee, M.D., Ph.D.
Assistant Professor
Department of Psychiatry and Neurology
Section of Child Neurology
Clinical Assistant Professor
Department of Pediatrics
Director of the Child Neurology Training Program
Tulane University Medical Center
New Orleans, LA

Kevin R. Lee, M.D.
Chief Resident
Neurological Surgery
Wayne State University
Detroit, MI

Klaus-Dieter K.L. Lessnau, M.D.
New York, NY

Gillian Lewke, P.A., CMA
Physician Assistant
Rockford Memorial Hospital
Rockford, IL

Joseph Lieber, M.D.
Associate Attending in Medicine
Chief, Medical Consult Service
Elmhurst Hospital Center
Elmhurst, NY
Clinical Associate Professor of Medicine
Mount Sinai School of Medicine
New York, NY

Mary W. Lieh-Lai, M.D.
Director, ICU
Associate Professor, Department of Pediatrics
Children's Hospital of Michigan
Wayne State University School of Medicine
Detroit, MI

Marijana Ljubanovic, M.D.
Fellow in Critical Care Medicine
Section of Critical Care Medicine
Department of Anesthesiology
Northwestern University Medical School
Chicago, IL

Bernard Lopez, M.D.
Assistant Professor
Thomas Jefferson Medical College
Thomas Jefferson University Hospital
Philadelphia, PA

Kenneth Maiese, M.D.
Associate Professor
Laboratory of Cellular and Molecular Cerebral Ischemia
Departments of Neurology and Anatomy & Cell Biology
Center of Molecular Medicine and Genetics
Center of Molecular and Cellular Toxicology
Wayne State University School of Medicine
Detroit, MI

John T. Malcynski, M.D.
Instructor of Surgery and Trauma
Surgical Critical Care Fellow
University of Pennsylvania
Philadelphia, PA

Mary Nan S. Mallory, M.D.
Instructor
University of Louisville
Louisville, KY

Sanjeev Maniar, M.D.
Department of Neurology
Wayne State University
Detroit, MI

Gregory P. Marelich, M.D., FACP, FCCP
Assistant Professor of Clinical Internal Medicine
Division of Pulmonary and Critical Care Medicine
University of California Davis Medical Center
Sacramento, CA

Joseph Masci, M.D.
Associate Director of Medicine
Mount Sinai Services
Elmhurst Hospital Center
Elmhurst, NY
Associate Professor of Medicine
Mount Sinai School of Medicine
New York, NY

Terence McGarry, M.D.
Pulmonary and Critical Care Medicine
Elmhurst Hospital Center
Elmhurst, NY
Assistant Professor of Medicine
Mount Sinai School of Medicine
New York, NY

Luis Mejico, M.D.
Department of Neurology
Georgetown University Medical Center
Washington, DC

Kevin Miller, M.D.
Jules Stein Eye Institute
Los Angeles, CA

David Morgan, M.D.
University of Texas
Southwestern Medical Center
Parkland Memorial Hospital
Dallas, TX

Gholam K. Motamedi, M.D.
Department of Neurology
Baylor College of Medicine
Houston, TX

Debasish Mridha, M.D.
Department of Neurology
Wayne State University School of Medicine
Detroit, MI

Anthony M. Murro, M.D.
Associate Professor of Neurology
Department of Neurology
Medical College of Georgia
Augusta, GA

Debra Myers, M.D.
Pulmonary/Critical Care Division
Sleep Disorders Medicine
Assistant Professor
Department of Internal Medicine
Wayne State University School of Medicine
Detroit, MI

Sarah T. Nath, M.D.
Sleep Disorders Center
Department of Neurology
University of Michigan Health System
Ann Arbor, MI

Kurt M. Nellhaus, M.D., FCCP
Pulmonary Service, Department of Medicine
Lakes Region General Hospital
Laconia, NH

N. K. Nikhar, M.D., MRCP
Chief Resident
Department of Neurology
University Health Center
Detroit, MI

Scott Olitsky, M.D.
Children's Hospital of Buffalo
Buffalo, NY

Lavi Oud, M.D.
Department of Critical Care Medicine
Wayne State University School of Medicine
Detroit, MI

Igor Ougorets, M.D.
Chief Resident
Department of Neurology
Department of Veterans Affairs Medical Center
University Hospitals of Cleveland
Cleveland, OH

Edward A. Panacek, M.D.
Associate Professor
University of California, Davis
School of Medicine
Sacramento, CA

Deric M. Park, M.D.
Department of Neurology
The University of Chicago
Chicago, IL
Professor and Chairman
Department of Anesthesiology
Fletcher Allen Health Care
University of Vermont College of Medicine
Burlington, VT

Anthony T. Reder, M.D.
Associate Professor of Neurology
Department of Neurology
The University of Chicago
Chicago, IL

Juan Carlos Restrepo, M.D.
Diplomat of the American Board of Anesthesiology
Board Certified in Critical Care Medicine
VA Medical Center – Jackson Memorial Hospital
University of Miami
Miami, FL

Perry Richardson, M.D.
Department of Neurology
George Washington University Medical Center
Washington, DC

Karen Rhodes, M.D.
University of Chicago Medical Center
Chicago, IL

Luis R. Rodriquez, M.D., F.A.A.P.
Assistant Professor of Pediatrics
Mount Sinai School of Medicine
New York, NY
Elmhurst Hospital Center
Elmhurst, NY

Lisa Rogers, D.O.
Associate Professor of Neurology
Wayne State University School of Medicine
Detroit, MI

Carlo Rosen, M.D.
Instructor in Medicine
Harvard Medical School
Massachusetts General Hospital
Boston, MA

Jeffrey Rosenfeld, Ph.D., M.D.
Director Neuromuscular Program
Carolinas Medical Center-Internal Medicine
Charlotte, NC

James A. Rowley, M.D.
Assistant Professor of Medicine
Division of Pulmonary/Critical Care Medicine
Wayne State University School of Medicine
Medical Director
per Hospital Sleep Disorders Center
Detroit, MI

Bruce K. Rubin, M.D.
Professor of Pediatrics, Physiology and Pharmacology
Brenner Children's Hospital
Winston-Salem, NC

David Rubenstein, M.D.
Division of Cardiology
Elmhurst Hospital Center
Elmhurst, NY

Robert L. Ruff, M.D., Ph.D.
Departments of Neurology and Neurosciences
Case Western Reserve University School of Medicine
Department of Veterans Affairs Medical Center
University Hospitals of Cleveland
Cleveland, OH

James W. Russell, M.D.
Department of Neurology
University of Michigan
Ann Arbor, MI

Nelson R. Sabates, M.D.
Eye Foundation of Kansas City
University of Missouri, Kansas City School of Medicine
Kansas City, MO

Carla Siegfried, M.D.
Department of Ophthalmology and Visual Sciences
Washington University
St. Louis, MO

Harvey M. Shanies, Ph.D., M.D.
Clinical Associate Professor of Medicine
Mount Sinai School of Medicine
New York, NY
Associate Director of Medicine for Clinical and
Academic Pulmonary and Critical Care Medicine
Elmhurst Hospital Center
Elmhurst, NY

Arunabh Sharma, M.D.
Fellow in Pulmonary and Critical Care Medicine
Brigham and Women's Hospital
Harvard Medical School
Boston, MA

Anders A.F. Sima, M.D., Ph.D.
Professor of Pathology and Neurology
Wayne State University School of Medicine
Detroit, MI
Visiting Professor of Pathology
University of Michigan
Ann Arbor, MI
Staff Neuropathologist
Harper Hospital and Detroit Medical Center
Detroit, MI

Sabine Sobek, M.D.
Department of Critical Care Medicine
Wayne State University School of Medicine
Detroit, MI

Dana Stearns, M.D.
Instructor in Medicine
Harvard Medical School
Massachusetts General Hospital

Girish D. Sharma, M.D., FCCP
Assistant Professor of Pediatrics
Section of Pediatric Pulmonology
The University of Chicago Children's Hospital
Chicago, IL

Jack Stump, M.D.
Attending Physician
Rogue Valley Medical Center
Medford, OR

Joan Surdukowski, M.D.
Assistant Professor
Chicago Medical School
Mt. Sinai Hospital
Chicago, IL

Michael J. Taravella, M.D.
University of Colorado
Denver, CO

William O. Tatum, IV, M.D.
Clinical Assistant Professor
Tampa General Hospital Epilepsy Center
Tampa, FL

Menno Terriet, M.D.
Department of Anesthesia
Veterans Affairs Medical Center
Miami, FL

Carlo Tornatore, M.D.
Assistant Professor of Neurology
Department of Neurology
Georgetown University Medical Center
Washington, DC

R. Scott Turner, M.D., Ph.D.
Assistant Professor Department of Neurology
University of Michigan
Ann Arbor, MI

Mythili Venkataraman, M.D.
Attending, Pulmonary Medicine
Director, Bronchology and Invasive Procedures
Elmhurst Hospital Center
Elmhurst, NY
Assistant Professor of Medicine
Mount Sinai School of Medicine
New York, NY

Mladen Vidovich, M.D.
Department of Anesthesiology
Northwestern University Medical School
Chicago, IL

John J. Wald, M.D.
Department of Neurology
University of Michigan
Ann Arbor, MI

Martin Warshawsky, M.D., FACP, FCCP
Director, Respiratory Intensive Care Unit
Elmhurst Hospital Center
Elmhurst, NY
Assistant Professor of Medicine
Mount Sinai School of Medicine
New York, NY

Thais Weibel, M.D.
Department of Neurology
George Washington University Medical Center
Washington, DC

Maria-Carmen B. Wilson, M.D.
Assistant Professor
Department of Neurology
Director, Headache and Pain Program
University of South Florida
School of Medicine
Tampa, FL
Assistant Professor of Medicine
Director of the Trauma and Life Support Center
University of Wisconsin School of Medicine
Madison, WI

A. Zacharias, M.D.
Department of Neurology
Emory University School of Medicine
Atlanta, GA

Jingwu Zhang, M.D., Ph.D.
Associate Professor of Neurology
Department of Neurology
Baylor College of Medicine
Houston, TX

Kristin Zeller, M.D.
Norfolk, VA

INTRODUCTION

Congratulations! *Critical Care Review: Pearls of Wisdom* will help you learn about critical care medicine as well as prepare for the critical care board examination. This book is structured in a question and answer format. Such a format is most useful in certain situations. It is useful as a self-assessment before starting a rotation in critical care medicine or a board exam review. This permits the reader to concentrate on areas of interest or weakness. Some readers will find answering questions the preferred way to study for a board exam. After completing a *Critical Care Review* chapter, these readers are encouraged to examine the corresponding textbook chapter entirely, for comprehensiveness.

Most readers will probably use this book in a post-textbook review mode. One such method involves reading a chapter in a textbook then proceeding to answer the questions posed in this book. Other readers will prefer to comprehensively study the contents of critical care medicine entirely and use this book afterwards. The purpose of the last two methods is to permit the reader to uncover areas of weakness and to become familiarized with the process of answering questions. Answering questions during a board exam is a cognitive task that is optimized by preparing a specific set of cognitive skills.

It must be emphasized that a question and answer book is most useful as a learning tool when used in conjunction with a textbook of critical care medicine. This is because the question/answer format is an active learning process that is at its best when the questioning process continues farther along than ending with answering the *Critical Care Review* question. The more active the learning process, the better the understanding. When the reader approaches a question that he/she cannot recall the answer to or uncovers a topic of interest, he/she is encouraged to read in the textbook at hand.

Most of the questions are short with short answers. This facilitates moving through a large body of knowledge. Some of the questions have longer answers. In these situations, the questions were not altered because of the clinically interesting question posed.

The chapters are organized to include all aspects of critical care medicine. The questions within each chapter are randomly presented, to simulate board exams and the way questions arise in real life. An exception to this is that the pulmonary pearls chapter is arranged in a deliberate manner. Questions pertaining to ARDS, PE/DVT, aspiration and hemoptysis, obstructive airway diseases, pre-operative evaluation, PFTs, pleural conditions and inhaled toxins are sequentially presented in part one of the chapter. The purpose of this was to divide the chapter into two parts, the first corresponding to topics of interest to all practitioners of critical care medicine while the second relates to topics more of interest to pulmonologists who practice critical care medicine.

The entirety of this book is not directed at one specialty group of physicians. Some chapters are most useful to certain readers. For example, the pediatric pearls chapter has the greatest utility to those who care for children. The reader is encouraged to study this book selectively based on their needs.

Certain topics have been repeated in a single chapter and across chapters. This was intentional. Some topics are so important to a practitioner of critical care medicine (as the electrocardiographic changes of hyperkalemia) that repetition was utilized as a learning tool.

Each question is preceded by a hollow bullet, to permit the reader to check off areas of interest, weakness or simply noting that it had been read. This allows for re-reading without having uncertainty of what was reviewed earlier.

Great effort has been made to verify that the questions and answers are accurate. Some answers may not be the answer you would prefer. Most often this is attributable to variance between original sources. Please make us aware of any errors you find. We hope to make continuous improvements and would greatly appreciate any input with regard to format, organization, content, presentation or about specific questions.

Study hard and good luck!

M.Z, S.P, & R. L.

TABLE OF CONTENTS

AIRWAY, RESUSCITATION AND VENTILATOR PEARLS

"The king shall drink to Hamlet's better breath"
Hamlet, Shakespeare

❍ **What is the Mallampati classification?**

Class I: full view
Class II: soft palate, uvula and fauces visible
Class III: soft palate and base of uvula visible
Class IV: hard palate only visible

❍ **Speaking of rapid sequence induction, discuss some agents that may be used to induce unconsciousness.**

Thiopental, etomidate, fentanyl and midazolam. Thiopental and etomidate are preferred in most situations of rapid sequence induction.

❍ **What is the benefit to rapid sequence induction in the emergency setting?**

The use of a paralytic agent, as succinylcholine, enhances the ease of intubation and prevents aspiration by paralyzing the muscles. Paralytic agents should not be used without agents that induce unconsciousness.

❍ **In a trauma patient with multiple fractures, internal injuries and an unstable airway, emergent endotracheal intubation in the emergency department is considered prior to definitive surgical therapy. What are the most likely hemodynamic consequences of intubation and initiation of mechanical ventilation in this subject?**

Hypotension may occur during or following endotracheal intubation and the institution of positive pressure ventilation. This cardiovascular decompensation is due to a decrease in venous return associated with both the use of sympatholytic agents for induction and the positive pressure induced increase in intrathoracic pressure.

❍ **What is the average distance from the external nares to the carina in males and females?**

32 cm and 27 cm, respectively.

❍ **The involvement of which laryngeal joint produces hoarseness in rheumatoid arthritis?**

The cricoarytenoid synovial joint.

❍ **Which of the physiologic functions involving the larynx can occur even in the absence of the epiglottis?**

Phonation and deglutition.

❍ **What is the only abductor muscle of the vocal cords?**

The posterior cricoarytenoid muscle.

❍ **At what thoracic vertebral level is the carina situated during full inspiration and full expiration?**

At the sixth and fourth thoracic vertebral level, respectively.

❍ **How long should a patient be preoxygenated to achieve a denitrogenation level such that apnea for 3 to 5 minutes maintains the oxygen saturation above 90%?**

5 minutes in the normal individual.

❍ **What is the mean average rise of carbon dioxide in apneic oxygenation?**

3 mmHg/min.

❍ **What are the optimal angles of flexion of the neck and extension of the atlanto-occipital joint to achieve axial alignment before intubation ("sniffing" position)?**

30° and 15°, respectively.

❍ **How difficult is conventional endotracheal intubation in a patient with rheumatoid arthritis who presents with a stiff neck and limited mouth opening?**

Impossible

❍ **What is the reason for elective pre-operative tracheostomy in some acromegalic patients?**

Bilateral recurrent laryngeal nerve palsy.

❍ **What is the failure rate at first attempt and the final failure rate with blind nasal intubation?**

70% and 20%, respectively.

❍ **In which clinical situation is retrograde and lightwand intubation considered better choices than fiberoptic assisted intubation?**

Bleeding in the oral cavity.

❍ **What is the maximum safe dose of lidocaine for topical anesthesia of the airway?**

3 mg/kg.

❍ **T/F: Too much lidocaine may cause seizures.**

True.

❍ **In a scenario of failed intubation and impossible mask ventilation, is the use of a laryngeal mask airway contraindicated in a patient with an increased risk for aspiration of gastric contents (e.g., hiatus hernia)?**

No, it is not contraindicated. In fact the use of LMA in this situation may be life saving. Hypoxemia and not aspiration kills most patients after failed intubation and ventilation.

❍ **What are the most frequent causes of failure of fiberoptic laryngoscopy?**

Excessive secretions or blood, fiberoptic tip against mucosa, and inadequate topical anesthesia.

❍ **Which are the only "fail safe" ways to verify correct placement of an endotracheal tube?**

Fiberoptic confirmation and adequate visualization with direct laryngoscopy.

❍ **What is the safest technique to intubate a child with epiglottitis?**

Intubation in the operating room after induction of anesthesia with an inhaled anesthetic (halothane or sevoflurane) in the semi-sitting position.

❍ **Are there any differences between endotracheal and Combitube intubation with regard to oxygenation and ventilation?**

Yes. The $PaCO_2$ is higher with the Combitube. The PaO_2 is also higher due to the physiologic PEEP maintained by the vocal cords.

❍ **What is the incidence of failed intubation in the general surgical population?**

1 in 2230 anesthetics.

❍ **What is the incidence of impossible mask ventilation?**

1 in 5000 anesthetics.

❍ **What should be done immediately after a failed intubation and impossible mask ventilation?**

A laryngeal mask airway should be inserted.

❍ **What is the most effective external laryngeal manipulation to achieve a better laryngoscopic view?**

BURP. Backward, upward and rightward pressure on the thyroid cartilage.

❍ **What is the incidence of malposition of double lumen tubes revealed by fiberoptic bronchoscopy?**

40%.

❍ **At what peak inspiratory pressure should an air leak be detected in pediatric patients intubated with an appropriate sized endotracheal tube?**

25 to 30 cm H_2O.

❍ **What are the initial ATLS steps of resuscitation?**

A - Airway maintenance with cervical spine control
B - Breathing – oxygenation and ventilation
C - Circulation with hemorrhage control

D - Disability - neurologic assessment
E - Exposure/Environmental control - completely undress the patient and prevent hypothermia

❍ **In what circumstances should the above order be modified?**

When a patient in a monitored setting arrests with sudden pulseless ventricular fibrillation. This requires immediate defibrillation.

❍ **What is the most common cause of upper airway obstruction?**

The tongue occluding the posterior oropharynx.

❍ **Name some important adjuncts often needed to help establish basic airway control.**

Suction equipment to remove secretions from mouth and throat, chin lift-jaw thrust maneuver, oral/nasal airway and bag-valve-mask device.

❍ **What are some advanced techniques for airway management?**

Orotracheal intubation, nasotracheal intubation, esophageal obturator airway (EOA), esophageal gastric tube airway (EGTA), pharyngotracheal airway, combination esophageal-tracheal tube, cricothyroidotomy and tracheostomy.

❍ **What are some indications for intubation?**

Apnea, burns, acute airway obstruction, expanding neck hematomas, hemodynamic instability, severe head injuries, poor oxygenation, poor ventilation, prevention of aspiration, inability to maintain a patent airway and impending or potential compromise of the airway.

❍ **What must be kept in mind when performing endotracheal intubation in a trauma patient?**

The potential for cervical spine injury.

❍ **What is a potential problem with bag-valve-mask ventilation?**

Air can enter the stomach via the esophagus causing gastric distention and aspiration.

❍ **How many people does it take to effectively ventilate a patient via the bag-valve-mask technique?**

Two. One to hold the mask securely to the face and a second to squeeze the bag with two hands.

❍ **Does tracheal intubation prevent aspiration?**

No. Microaspiration can still occur.

❍ **What characteristic of gastric contents causes the greatest harm following aspiration?**

Although particulate matter can clog the airways leading to atelectasis, it is the acidity of the gastric contents that leads to the greatest injury.

❍ **Name some factors that place a patient at risk for aspiration.**

Full stomach, trauma, intra-abdominal pathology (obstruction, inflammation, gastric paresis), esophageal disease (symptomatic reflux, motility disorders), pregnancy and obesity.

❍ **Are esophageal obturator, combination esophageal-tracheal tube or pharyngotracheal airways better than orotracheal intubation?**

No. These are substitutes when no trained personnel are available for orotracheal intubation.

❍ **What properties of succinylcholine make it particularly useful as an aid for intubation?**

Succinylcholine, a depolarizing paralytic agent, has a brief duration of action (3 to 5 minutes) and a rapid onset of action (within 60 seconds).

❍ **T/F: Succinylcholine has sedative and amnestic effects as well as muscle relaxant properties.**

False.

❍ **What are the possible deleterious effects of succinylcholine?**

Increased intragastric, intraocular and intracranial pressure.
Hyperkalemia, particularly in neurologic and burn injuries.
Increased duration of action in the rare patient with pseudocholinesterase deficiency.

❍ **What maneuver should be performed during any tracheal intubation?**

The Sellick maneuver (occlusion of the esophagus by pressure on the cricoid cartilage). It can help prevent aspiration during tracheal intubation.

❍ **What equipment is needed to assist with endotracheal intubation?**

Suction for the mouth and pharynx, bag-valve-mask system for oxygenation, functioning laryngoscope, stylet and endotracheal tubes.

❍ **What type of endotracheal tube is used in children?**

Uncuffed.

❍ **Why are uncuffed tubes used in children?**

Young children have a narrow subglottic area. Uncuffed tubes help avoid subglottic edema and ulceration.

❍ **What is the correct tube size for the typical adult male and female?**

Male 8.0 mm ± 1.0 and female 7.0 mm ± 1.0.

❍ **T/F: Female patients have larger airways compared to males but actually need smaller sized tubes.**

False. Female patients have smaller airways necessitating smaller tubes.

❍ **What three axes should be aligned when attempting to perform endotracheal intubation on a patient when motion of the cervical spine is not contraindicated?**

Pharyngeal, oral and laryngeal.

❍ **Where is the tip of the curved blade placed during orotracheal intubation?**

Into the vallecula just anterior to the epiglottis.

❍ **Where is the tip of the straight blade placed during orotracheal intubation?**

Beneath the epiglottis to directly lift the epiglottis anteriorly.

❍ **T/F: To use the laryngoscope correctly, the back of the blade is placed against the upper front teeth and the handle is rotated posteriorly, thus lifting the epiglottis anteriorly.**

False. Once positioned correctly, the handle and blade are lifted anteriorly and inferiorly (relative to the patient) without rotation to lift the epiglottis and expose the cords.

❍ **In the typical male patient, what length of ET tube should lay distal to the lips?**

23 cm.

❍ **In the typical female patient, what length of ET tube should lay distal to the lips?**

21 cm.

❍ **What is the consequence of an ET tube placed too far distally?**

Respiratory insufficiency secondary to right mainstem bronchus intubation.

❍ **How is right mainstem intubation diagnosed?**

Decreased breath sounds on the left that corrects with repositioning of the ET tube.

❍ **What type of endotracheal tube cuff is presently used?**

High-volume, low pressure cuffs. (Pressure = 20 to 25 mmHg.)

❍ **When does tracheal ischemia occur?**

When the pressure in the endotracheal tube cuff exceeds capillary perfusion pressure (typically 25 to 35 mmHg).

❍ **Immediately after inserting an ET tube, what is the next most appropriate step?**

Confirm tube placement.

❍ **How is proper endotracheal tube placement confirmed?**

Symmetric chest expansion, breath sounds in axillae but not over the epigastrium, tube fogs with respirations, end-tidal CO_2, monitoring of oxygen saturation and visualizing the tube passing through the vocal cords.

❍ **Does a chest x-ray guarantee correct endotracheal tube placement?**

No. Clinical signs (see last question) are needed for confirmation of endotracheal tube placement.

❍ **What is the correct position of the tip of the endotracheal tube?**

Approximately 4 cm above the carina.

❍ **What are two contraindications to nasotracheal intubation?**

Maxillofacial trauma (with suspected fracture of the cribriform plate) and apnea.

❍ **What is the most common complication of nasotracheal intubation?**

Epistaxis.

❍ **How is transtracheal needle jet insufflation performed?**

A #12 or #14 gauge plastic cannula is placed through the cricothyroid membrane into the trachea. The cannula should be connected to oxygen at 15 liter/minute (40 to 50 psi). The oxygen is given intermittently, one second on and four seconds off.

❍ **How long can a patient be adequately temporized with needle jet insufflation?**

Approximately 45 to 60 minutes.

❍ **What limits this form of surgical airway?**

Hypercapnia, due to inadequate ventilation.

❍ **When is an emergent cricothyroidotomy indicated?**

When a patient cannot be adequately oxygenated or ventilated, orotracheal intubation and bag ventilation cannot be performedand alternate airway devices have failed (or there is insufficient time to attempt these).

❍ **T/F: Cricothyroidotomy is generally contraindicated in children.**

True. Needle jet insufflation is considered a better choice to avoid injuring the cricoid cartilage

❍ **Why is emergent tracheostomy usually not recommended?**

The trachea lies deeper in the neck than the cricothyroid membrane. The trachea is surrounded by a number of veins and the isthmus of the thyroid gland. Complications such as recurrent laryngeal nerve injury, pneumothorax and esophageal perforation can occur.

❍ **When may emergent tracheostomy be performed instead of emergent cricothyroidotomy?**

In pediatric patients. Cricothyroidotomy is generally contraindicated in the pediatric population. Because of the smaller size and greater soft tissue compliance of the pediatric airway, the cricoid cartilage plays a major role in maintaining patency of the tracheal lumen. An injury to this structure could be disastrous.

❍ **What are the three divisions of the airway?**

1. Extrathoracic - nose to the trachea before it enters the thoracic inlet
2. Intrathoracic, extrapulmonary - trachea at the thoracic inlet to the right and left mainstem bronchi before they enter the lungs
3. Intrapulmonary - bronchi within the lungs

❍ **According to Poiseuille's law, if the airway radius of the conducting airway is reduced from 4 mm to 2 mm, how much will resistance to airflow increase?**

Sixteen-fold.

❍ **What is the narrowest part of the adult airway?**

The glottic opening.

❍ **What is the most common offender in foreign body aspiration?**

Organic substances such as nuts and corn.

❍ **Which site is used to evacuate a tension pneumothorax by using needle thoracentesis?**

The second intercostal space at the midclavicular line or the fifth intercostal space at the midaxillary line.

❍ **What are the signs of tension pneumothorax on physical exam?**

Tachypnea, unilateral absent breath sounds, tachycardia, pallor, diaphoresis, cyanosis, tracheal deviation, hypotension and neck vein distention.

❍ **What is the directional change in intrathoracic pressure in a ventilated patient versus a spontaneously breathing patient?**

It decreases during spontaneous inspiration and increases during positive-pressure inspiration.

❍ **What determines the relationship between changes in airway pressure and lung volume during positive pressure ventilation?**

Lung and chest wall compliance combine to define the relation between airway pressure and lung volume. Increased stiffness of the lungs (pulmonary fibrosis or overdistention) or the chest wall (obesity) will decrease the amount to which lung volume will increase for a given increase in airway pressure.

❍ **Can one assume a constant proportion of the increase in airway pressure induced by positive pressure ventilation will be transmitted to the pleural surface?**

Definitely not. Differences in lung or chest wall compliance can profoundly alter the degree to which increases in airway pressure are felt within the chest and thus the degree to which they alter hemodynamics.

❍ **A young male patient awaiting general anesthesia is found to have a heart rate of 60 beats per minute which increases up to about 80 beats per minute with each spontaneous inspiration. What is this patient's condition?**

He is normal. Healthy young adults normally have a relative bradycardia and normal inspiration induces an in-phase vagal withdrawal that causes heart rate to increase during inspiration and decrease during expiration. This phenomenon is referred to as respiratory sinus arrhythmia.

❍ **In a diabetic patient breathing spontaneously prior to induction of general anesthesia, the physician noted that the baseline heart rate was 88 beats per minute but that there was no discernible heart rate variability on the cardiac monitor, suggesting the absence of respiratory sinus arrhythmia. Is this a problem?**

Potentially yes. Absence of normal respiratory sinus arrhythmia infers dysautonomia. The patient is at increased risk of systemic hypotension following induction of general anesthesia because the normal adaptive autonomic responses may also be absent.

❍ **Acute elevations in pulmonary arterial pressure do what to left ventricular diastolic compliance?**

It is decreased because of interventricular dependence of the left and right ventricles.

❍ **How does spontaneous ventilation, by inducing negative swings in intrathoracic pressure, affect myocardial oxygen demand?**

It is increased becauses of increased left ventricular afterload.

❍ **Under normal conditions at rest, what percentage of the cardiac output goes to the respiratory muscles?**

Less than 3%.

❍ **In patients with COPD, what percentage of the total cardiac output may be directed to the muscles of respiration?**

25 to 30%.

❍ **Positive end-expiratory pressure (PEEP) primarily impairs cardiac output by what mechanism?**

Decrease in LV preload.

❍ **To the extent that LV preload is maintained, positive pressure ventilation has what effect on cardiac output in patients with normal cardiovascular function?**

No measurable effect as compared to spontaneous ventilation.

❍ **When two different modes of ventilation, such as pressure support and inverse ratio ventilation, have similar changes in intrathoracic pressure and ventilatory effort, how do their hemodynamic effects compare?**

Similar.

❍ **Can the hemodynamic effects of mechanical ventilation be seen in non-intubated patients during non-invasive ventilatory support?**

Yes. Identical effects should be seen for the same changes in lung volume and intrathoracic pressure.

❍ **Is there any hemodynamic difference between increasing airway pressure to generate a breath and decreasing extrathoracic pressure (iron lung negative pressure ventilation) to generate a similar tidal volume?**

None, if the iron lung encompasses the entire body. However, if it surrounds only the chest and abdomen, it may have less detrimental effects due to the sparing of venous return.

❍ **Weaning from mechanical ventilation is associated with what effect on myocardial oxygen demand?**

Increased MVO_2. Consider weaning to be a cardiac stress test.

❍ **In patients with congestive heart failure, cardiovascular insufficiency and respiratory distress, the initiation of positive pressure ventilation is often associated with what hemodynamic response?**

Improvement in overall cardiovascular status due to the combined effects of the associated reduced work of breathing and reduced LV afterload.

❍ **In patients with unilateral lung injury, is the effect of positive end-expiratory pressure applied at the trachea the same as in patients with bilateral lung injury?**

No. PEEP may overdistend the healthy lung in subjects with unilateral lung injury causing an increase in the amount of intrapulmonary shunt and pulmonary vascular resistance.

❍ **An intubated patient with ischemic heart disease develops mild inspiratory stridor upon extubation associated with severe chest pain and marked ST segment elevations across the precordium. The immediate treatment of this condition should include what ventilatory therapy?**

Eliminate the markedly negative swings in intrathoracic pressure by re-intubation.

❍ **In a patient with impaired right ventricular dysfunction following anterior chest trauma, excessive positive end-expiratory pressure (PEEP) therapy may induce cardiovascular decompensation by any of three mechanisms, name one.**

1) Hyperinflation will increase pulmonary vascular resistance impeding right ventricular ejection.
2) Hyperinflation will increase intrathoracic pressure reducing venous return and limiting right ventricular filling.
3) Hyperinflation that compresses the heart is similar to tamponade restricting right ventricular filling.

❍ **In a patient with acute lung injury breathing spontaneously, intubation and the application of both an enriched FIO_2 and PEEP sufficient to recruit collapsed alveolar units should do what to pulmonary vascular resistance?**

Decrease it by reversing hypoxic pulmonary vasoconstriction.

❍ **A mechanically ventilated patient with chronic obstructive lung disease is breathing spontaneously on assist-control mode with a measured intrinsic PEEP of 12 cm H_2O. What will the application of 8 cm H_2O extrinsic PEEP (from the ventilatory circuit) do to the patient's work of breathing?**

In general it will decrease the work of breathing by reducing the amount of airway pressure drop needed to trigger the positive pressure breath. Some patients with intrinsic PEEP may have deleterious effect when adding PEEP to the ventilator circuit. Careful monitoring of the patient is mandatory. The level of added PEEP should be less than the amount of intrinsic PEEP.

❍ **What is peripheral cyanosis?**

Peripheral cyanosis is due to shunting or increased O_2 extraction.

❍ **Name the two primary causes (groups) of peripheral cyanosis.**

Cyanosis with a normal SaO_2 can be due to:

Decreased cardiac output.

Redistribution - may be 2° to shock, DIC, hypothermia, vascular obstruction.

❍ **What is heliox and when is it used?**

Helium has less density than oxygen and is thought to decrease the turbulence of flow past sites of obstruction. Heliox is a combination of helium and oxygen that is used when patients have an upper airway obstruction to decrease stridor, increase tidal volume and improve ventilation.

❍ **Is succinylcholine a depolarizing or a non-depolarizing neuromuscular blocking agent?**

It is the only commonly used depolarizing agent. It binds to post-synaptic acetylcholine receptors causing depolarization. It is enzymatically degraded by pseudocholinesterase. Onset is within 1 minute with duration of paralysis of 7 to 10 min.

❍ **What is the rationale for pre-treating a patient with a subpolarizing ("defasciculating") dose of a non-depolarizing agent prior to administration of succinylcholine?**

The pre-treatment agent attenuates fasciculations from succinylcholine induced depolarization. This may decrease subsequent muscle pain. This also blunts increased intragastric and intraocular pressure associated with succinylcholine.

❍ **What disorders are associated with auto-PEEP?**

Asthma, COPD and ARDS.

❍ **What are the pulmonary criteria for extubation?**

Tidal volume of at least 5 ml/kg, vital capacity of 15 ml/kg, negative inspiratory force less than -25 cm H_2O, respiratory rate greater than 10 and less than 30, adequate oxygenation on an inspired oxygen concentration of 40% or less, ratio of spontaneous breathing frequency to tidal volume (in liters) less than 100, ability to protect the airway, and no excessive secretions.

❍ **Which patients are at risk for developing aspiration pneumonia?**

Patients undergoing emergency surgery, pregnant patients, obese patients, those with gastrointestinal obstruction, depressed level of consciousness and laryngeal incompetence.

❍ **What is the appropriate treatment following aspiration?**

Secure the airway, administer oxygen, suction any aspirate, consider bronchoscopy if large particulates are present, ventilatory support and bronchodilators as needed for bronchospasm.

❍ **A patient is admitted to the SICU after surgical debridement for necrotizing pancreatitis. Over the next several hours, the patient's oxygenation deteriorates, with oxygen saturation of 90% on 75% inspired oxygen and 10 of PEEP. What is the most likely diagnosis?**

ARDS.

❍ **T/F: Acute lung injury of the entire lung causes lung compliance to decrease similarly in each region of the lung.**

False. Marked regional differences in the degree of lung consolidation and compliance characterize all forms of acute lung injury.

❍ **How does positive pressure ventilation increase the cardiac output in patients with a low left ventricular ejection fraction?**

Decreased afterload.

❍ **Which lobes of the lung can develop atelectasis from intubation of the right mainstem bronchus?**

Right upper lobe, left upper lobe and left lower lobe.

❍ **What are the determinants of $PaCO_2$?**

Carbon dioxide production and alveolar ventilation.

❍ **What are the components of tidal volume?**

Alveolar volume and dead space volume.

❍ **What is the maximum acceptable endotracheal tube cuff pressure?**

Approximately 25 cm H_2O at the end of expiration.

❍ **What is the potential harm of excess endotracheal tube cuff pressure?**

It can induce ischemia and necrosis of the underlying tissue.

❍ **Adequacy of alveolar ventilation is reflected by which component of arterial blood gas analysis?**

$PaCO_2$.

❍ **$PaCO_2$ is mathematically related to alveolar ventilation in what manner?**

Inverse proportion.

❍ **What factors interfere with the bellows function of the chest?**

Abdominal binding, massive obesity, trauma with flail chest, massive effusion and ascites, pneumothorax, thoracic burn with eschar, neuromuscular blockade and strapping of ribs.

❍ **What is the principal mechanism of increased $PaCO_2$ with increased FIO_2?**

Worsening V/Q mismatch and the Haldane effect.

❍ **How does malnutrition contribute to respiratory failure?**

Respiratory muscle weakness.

❍ **Respiratory failure is worsened in spinal injuries at or above which nerve root?**

C2.

❍ **What infectious syndromes can lead to ventilatory insufficiency?**

Botulism, tetanus, Campylobacter, polio, diphtheria and Guillain-Barré syndrome.

❍ **T/F: Pulmonary capillary wedge pressure (PCWP) is a reflection of left atrial pressure.**

True.

❍ **Deficiency of phosphorus may affect oxygen transfer from erythrocytes as a result of its contribution to what compound?**

2,3-diphosphoglycerate (2,3-DPG).

❍ **T/F: Acute elevations in pulmonary artery pressure increase LV diastolic compliance.**

False.

❍ **What processes cause the work of breathing to increase markedly in patients with COPD?**

Increased dead space ventilation, decreased respiratory muscle efficiency and increased airway resistance.

❍ **What are the most common causes of increased dead space in critically ill patients?**

Decreased cardiac output, pulmonary embolism, pulmonary hypertension, ARDS and excessive PEEP.

❍ **The total work of breathing is divided into what two parts?**

Overcoming lung and chest wall compliance and overcoming airway resistance.

❍ **What are the ventilation and perfusion relationships between Zone 1, Zone 2 and Zone 3 of the lung?**

Zone 1 represents dead space (ventilation occurs without perfusion); zone 2 contains high V/Q mismatch (ventilation occurs in excess of perfusion); zone 3 represents areas of optimal V/Q matching.

❍ **What is the equation for determining a patient's oxygen extraction ratio?**

Oxygen extraction ratio = $(CaO_2 - CvO_2)/CaO_2$ where CaO_2 is arterial blood oxygen content and CvO_2 is the mixed venous blood oxygen content.

❍ **What is a normal oxygen extraction ratio in a healthy adult?**

25%.

❍ **What is the normal whole lung V/Q ratio?**

4 liters of ventilation to 5 liters of blood flow or 0.8.

❍ **Blood drawn from the tip of a pulmonary artery catheter wedged in zone III will reflect PO_2 from what source?**

Pulmonary capillary.

❍ **Which mitral valve abnormalities can lead to large v waves on the pulmonary artery wedge tracing?**

Both mitral stenosis and mitral regurgitation because of overfilling of the left atrium.

❍ **What information regarding flow is obtained from the Reynolds number?**

The Reynolds number is calculated from the equation Re = 2rvd/n, where r = radius, v = average velocity, d = density and n = viscosity. When the Reynolds number exceeds 2000, turbulent flow is probable. Less than 2000 indicates probable laminar flow.

❍ **What property of helium allows less turbulence in a high flow system?**

Density. The low density of helium yields a lower Reynolds number when compared with a gas of higher density (air or oxygen) in the same system.

❍ **What is Boyle's law of gases?**

$P_1V_1=P_2V_2$ where P is pressure, V is volume and temperature is constant.

❍ **What is the hemodynamic response to an acute complete spinal cord injury at the C7 level?**

Initially there is hypertension and tachycardia secondary to increased circulating catecholamines at the time of the injury followed shortly by hypotension due to vasodilatation and bradycardia secondary to loss of cardiac accelerator input.

❍ **During the first minute of apnea, how much would you expect the $PaCO_2$ to rise?**

During apnea, the $PaCO_2$ will increase approximately 6 mmHg during the first minute and then 3 to 4 mmHg each minute thereafter.

❍ **What is the most important factor in control of ventilation under normal conditions?**

Arterial $PaCO_2$.

❍ **What do peripheral chemoreceptors located in the carotid and aortic bodies respond to?**

The peripheral chemoreceptors respond to decreases in arterial PO_2 and pH and increases in arterial PCO_2.

❍ **What is functional residual capacity (FRC)?**

The volume of gas in the lung after a normal expiration is the FRC and is comprised of residual volume and expiratory reserve volume.

❍ **What is the closing capacity of the lungs?**

Closing capacity (closing volume plus residual volume) is the lung volume at which small airways close. Closing capacity is normally well below FRC (functional residual capacity) but rises steadily with age.

❍ **What are the four major forms of cellular hypoxia?**

Anemic, hypoxemic, circulatory and histotoxic hypoxia.

❍ **What are the major causes of arterial hypoxemia?**

Hypoventilation, ventilation/perfusion inequality, shunt, low FIO_2 and diffusion impairment.

❍ **How does one assess oxygenation?**

Skin color, pulse oximetry and blood gas analysis.

❍ **How does one assess ventilation?**

End tidal CO_2 monitoring and blood gas analysis.

❍ **What is a tension pneumothorax?**

An injury to the lung allowing intrapleural air to collect without escaping via the chest wall or trachea. This accumulation of air compresses the lung and shifts the mediastinum, leading to impaired venous return and hypotension.

❍ **What are the physical findings in tension pneumothorax?**

Distended neck veins, hypotension, tracheal deviation and a hyperresonant hemithorax.

❍ **What is the treatment for tension pneumothorax?**

Immediate needle decompression of the hyperresonant hemithorax, based on clinical suspicion. Radiography should not be used to confirm tension pneumothorax.

❍ **What is adequate urinary output to gauge resuscitation in adults?**

0.5 cc/kg or about 50 cc/hr.

❍ **How does one assess for disability in ATLS?**

A rapid assessment to establish level of consciousness (alert, arouses to voice, arouses to pain or unresponsive) and pupillary appearance and reaction constitute the initial assessment. A more detailed examination is performed later.

❍ **What effect does intrinsic PEEP have on the work of breathing in patients receiving mechanical ventilation?**

Increased elastic work and increased work to trigger assisted breaths.

❍ **How can the work of breathing with mechanical ventilation associated with intrinsic PEEP be reduced?**

Add a small amount of PEEP, reduce tidal volume, reduce inspiratory time and increase expiratory time.

❍ **What complications are associated with mask ventilation?**

Skin breakdown, aspiration pneumonia, aerophagia, pneumothorax and barotrauma (volutrauma).

❍ **Through what mechanism does PEEP decrease cardiac output?**

Reduced preload.

❍ **How can static compliance of the lung/chest wall be approximated from airway pressure measurements during mechanical ventilation?**

Tidal volume/(inspiratory plateau pressure - end expiratory (pause) pressure).

❍ **What evidence of barotrauma can be observed on chest x-ray?**

Pneumomediastinum, pneumothorax, pneumopericardium, subcutaneous emphysema and pulmonary interstitial emphysema.

❍ **What are the primary determinants of the work of breathing?**

Minute ventilation, lung/chest wall compliance, airway resistance and presence of intrinsic PEEP.

❍ **What are some conditions under which CO_2 production is increased?**

Lipogenesis, fever and hyperthyroidism.

❍ **What is the preferred FIO_2 for patients with ARDS?**

The lowest that will maintain a hemoglobin oxygen saturation of about 90%.

❍ **How is oxygen delivery calculated?**

Cardiac output x arterial blood oxygen content (x 10 to get units correct).

❍ **What is the primary determinant of the oxygen content of arterial blood?**

The product of hemoglobin concentration and the percent hemoglobin oxygen saturation of arterial blood. The amount of oxygen dissolved in the plasma (a function of the PaO_2) is negligible at one atmosphere of pressure.

❍ **How can adequate tidal volume be delivered to a patient undergoing volume cycled mechanical ventilation whose endotracheal tube cuff is failing to maintain an adequate seal (without changing the tube)?**

Increase the mandatory tidal volume.

❍ **What are indications for stress ulcer prophylaxis in critically ill patients?**

Mechanical ventilation and coagulopathy.

❍ **What combination of medications, often used in the treatment of status asthmaticus requiring mechanical ventilation, may result in prolonged weakness?**

Steroids and neuromuscular blocking agents.

❍ **T/F: Pulse oximetry is a reliable method for estimating oxyhemoglobin saturation in a patient suffering from CO poisoning.**

False. COHb has light absorbance that can lead to a falsely elevated pulse oximeter saturation level. The calculated value from a standard ABG may also be falsely elevated. The oxygen saturation should be determined by using a co-oximeter that measures the amounts of unsaturated O_2Hb, COHb and metHb.

❍ **When may end-tidal carbon dioxide detectors prove inaccurate?**

In patients with very low blood flow to the lungs or in those with a large dead space (e.g., following a pulmonary embolism).

❍ **What is the most common complication of endotracheal intubation?**

Intubation of a bronchus. Other complications include esophageal intubation, lacerations of the lip, tongue and pharyngeal or tracheal mucosa, resulting in bleeding, hematoma or abscess. Tracheal rupture, avulsion of an arytenoid cartilage, vocal cord injury, pharyngeal-esophageal perforation, intubation of the pyriform sinus, gastric content aspiration, hypertension, tachycardia and arrhythmias may also occur.

❍ **What oxygen flow rate is recommended for facemask ventilation?**

At least 5 L/min. Recommended flow is 8 to 10 L/min., which will produce oxygen concentrations as high as 40% to 60%.

❍ **What oxygen concentration can be supplied with a facemask and oxygen reservoir?**

6 L/min. provides approximately 60% oxygen concentration and each liter increases the concentration by 10%. 10 L/min. is almost 100%.

❍ **What are the four commonly used modes of ventilation?**

Intermittent mandatory ventilation (IMV), pressure support (PS), assist control (AC) and pressure control (PC).

❍ **What is the difference between IMV, SIMV and AC? Can you wean a patient using AC?**

IMV provides a given tidal volume at a set respiratory rate. Any breaths initiated by the patient achieve only the tidal volume the patient is able to generate.

In SIMV (synchronized IMV) the ventilator attempts to synchronize the patient's ventilatory effort with an assisted breath. Breaths in excess of the set respiratory rate do not receive assistance from the ventilator.

In AC all tidal volumes whether initiated by the patient or by the ventilator achieve the set tidal volume. Therefore, you cannot wean a patient in the AC mode.

❍ **What is the difference between pressure control ventilation and pressure support ventilation?**

In pressure support ventilation, a breath is spontaneously initiated by the patient. The ventilator delivers a flow of gas to reach a target pressure. This flow is maintained until a flow threshold is reached during the decelerating phase of inspiration. At this time expiration begins.

In pressure control ventilation, a patient receives a mechanical breath at a predetermined rate. Once again the ventilator delivers a flow of gas to reach a certain pressure. Unlike pressure support, the ventilator assists the breath until a predetermined time is reached. This is called time-cycling.

In neither mode is the tidal volume controlled. Instead, the tidal volume is determined by pulmonary compliance, duration of inspiration and synchrony between the ventilator and the patient.

❍ **Describe the events associated with auto-PEEP.**

Also known as air trapping and intrinsic PEEP (positive end-expiratory pressure), auto-PEEP occurs mostly in patients with asthma, chronic obstructive pulmonary disease and acute respiratory distress syndrome. Auto-PEEP occurs when a patient with lung disease is unable to completely exhale each tidal volume. The accumulation of pressure results in a persistent difference between alveolar pressure and external airway pressure at end expiration. The persistent pressure difference results in continued airflow at end exhalation.

❍ **What are the consequences of auto-PEEP?**

Auto-PEEP results in tidal volumes that occur at the upper limit of total lung capacity where compliance is low. Thus higher pressures are required to achieve a given tidal volume and the patient is at increased risk for barotrauma. In a patient who is initiating breaths on the ventilator (e.g., spontaneously breathing with pressure support), auto-PEEP increases the work of breathing. Like extrinsic PEEP, auto-PEEP can compromise cardiac function by decreasing venous return and cardiac output.

❍ **An intubated patient is left on 100% oxygen for 20 hours. Describe changes that can be attributed to oxygen toxicity.**

Tracheobronchial irritation (coughing, substernal discomfort), decreased vital capacity, decreased lung compliance, decreased diffusing capacity, decreased tracheal mucus velocity, increased arteriovenous shunting, absorption atelectasis and increased dead space to tidal volume ratio.

❍ **A patient has been ventilator dependent for almost four weeks. She appears to be making slow progress in weaning from the ventilator. What are the advantages and disadvantages of undergoing a tracheotomy?**

A tracheotomy may help by decreasing dead space, improving clearance of secretions and improving patient comfort. It also partially restores glottic function. Assuming the patient progresses well, a tracheotomy also offers the potential to be able to verbally communicate and to tolerate oral feedings.

However, a tracheotomy requires the patient to undergo another surgical procedure. It is also associated with the risks of stoma granulation, tracheal erosion, tracheal stenosis and tracheo-innominate fistula.

❍ **What ventilator steps can be taken to optimize an ARDS patient's respiratory function?**

Using pressure control to minimize barotrauma, decreasing tidal volume to minimize volutrauma, using inverse ratio ventilation and permissive hypercapnia to maximize inspiration time. None of these strategies have been proven by clinical trials.

❍ **What is nitric oxide?**

Nitric oxide (NO) is a specific pulmonary vasodilator which helps to improve ventilation-perfusion matching and oxygenation. It is useful in treating pulmonary hypertension in pediatric patients and in patients with persistent pulmonary hypertension after cardiac surgery. It increases pO_2 in patients with ARDS. NO is inactivated by rapid binding to hemoglobin.

❍ **What is partial liquid ventilation?**

Partial liquid ventilation is a technique that involves filling the functional residual capacity (FRC) of the lungs with a perfluorocarbon liquid and ventilating the lungs using conventional mechanical ventilation. The perfluorocarbon liquid acts as a liquid PEEP, stenting the lung open. The liquid has a high oxygen carrying capacity facilitating gas exchange, a good spreading coefficient and evaporates fairly quickly.

❍ **What factors shift the oxygen-hemoglobin dissociation curve to the right?**

Acidemia, increased 2,3 DPG and increased temperature.

❍ **What is the equation that relates total pulmonary compliance to lung compliance and chest wall compliance?**

1/total pulmonary compliance = 1/lung compliance + 1/chest wall compliance.

❍ **During sleep what is the normal, expected change in $PaCO_2$ and PaO_2 from the baseline, awake state?**

Normally, $PaCO_2$ increases 4 to 8 mmHg and PaO_2 decreases 3 to 10 mmHg.

❍ **What is Graham's law of gases?**

The rate of diffusion of a gas is inversely proportional to its molecular weight.

❍ **What is the Hering-Breuer inflation reflex?**

Inhibition of inspiratory muscle activity by inflation of the lungs. In newborns overinflation of the lungs during controlled or mechanical ventilation may lead to apnea. This reflex does not appear to be as active in adults.

❍ **What is the Bohr effect?**

Enhanced release of oxygen from hemoglobin in the presence of carbon dioxide.

❍ **What is the Haldane effect?**

Enhanced release of carbon dioxide from hemoglobin in the presence of oxygen.

❍ **What is transpulmonary pressure?**

Transpulmonary pressure is the pressure gradient across the lung measured as the pressure difference between the airway opening and the pleural surface.

❍ **Define compliance.**

The change in volume divided by the change in distending pressure. Elastic recoil is usually measured in terms of compliance. Compliance measurements can be obtained for the chest, the lung or both together.

❍ **What is the predominant stimulus for activation of hypoxic pulmonary vasoconstriction?**

Decreased alveolar oxygen tension.

❍ **What components contribute to physiologic shunting (venous admixture)?**

The bronchial, pleural and thebesian veins and abnormal arterial to venous communications in the lungs.

❍ **What is the respiratory quotient?**

The rate of carbon dioxide production divided by the rate of oxygen consumption.

❍ **What is the primary mechanism responsible for post-operative atelectasis?**

Decreased expiratory reserve volume relative to closing volume.

❍ **Compare the sizes of alveoli at end-exhalation in dependent vs. nondependent lung regions.**

Alveoli in dependent lung regions are smaller than nondependent alveoli at end-exhalation.

❍ **Write a recognized form of the shunt equation.**

$$\frac{CcO_2 - CaO_2}{CcO_2 - CvO_2}$$

CaO_2 = arterial oxygen content
CvO_2 = mixed venous oxygen content
CcO_2 = oxygen content of ideal pulmonary end-capillary blood

Pulmonary end-capillary blood is considered to the have the same concentration of oxygen as alveolar gas.

❍ **Write a recognized form of the Bohr equation.**

$$Vd/Vt = \frac{PaCO_2 - PeCO_2}{PaCO_2}$$

Vd/Vt = Dead space ventilation
$PaCO_2$ = Arterial partial pressure of CO_2
$PeCO_2$ = End-tidal CO_2

❍ **What factors can potentially contribute to the difficulty in weaning critically ill patients from mechanical ventilation?**

Lack of central ventilatory drive due to encephalopathy, primary myopathy, muscle fatigue or weakness and neuropathy of critical illness.

❍ **What is the neuropathy of critical illness?**

Primary axonal degeneration of motor and sensory fibers.

❍ **What is the mechanism of diaphragm dysfunction following open heart surgery?**

Thermal or mechanical injury to the phrenic nerve.

❍ **Which neuromuscular and spinal diseases can lead to ventilatory insufficiency?**

Muscular dystrophy, polymyositis, myotonic dystrophy, polyneuritis, Eaton Lambert syndrome, myasthenia gravis, amyotrophic lateral sclerosis, trauma, Guillain-Barré syndrome, multiple sclerosis, Parkinson's Disease and stroke.

❍ **Inherited abnormalities in which enzyme contribute to respiratory insufficiency after succinylcholine administration?**

Serum cholinesterase.

❍ **Patients on mechanical ventilation can develop hypoventilation based on what pulmonary factors?**

Increased dead space (including length of ventilator circuit proximal to the "Y" piece separating the inspiratory and expiratory limbs), decreased tidal volume, overdistention of lung, air leaks and massive pulmonary embolism.

❍ **What constitutes post polio syndrome?**

Thirty to forty years afterwards, polio survivors experience reduced endurance, reduced ambulation and increased weakness of previously affected limbs.

❍ **Patients with failure of which organs are at increased risk of developing prolonged paralysis following neuromuscular blocker administration?**

Liver and kidney.

❍ **How is the neuropathy of critical illness diagnosed?**

Nerve conduction and electomyography.

❍ **What methods rapidly confirm that an endotracheal tube was not placed in the esophagus?**

Auscultation, capnography and fiberoptic bronchoscopy.

❍ **What are the principal complications of nasal endotracheal intubation (as opposed to oral)?**

Maxillary sinusitis, amputation of turbinates, septal perforation and increased airway resistance associated with a more narrow tube.

❍ **How is the work of breathing affected by patient triggered positive pressure ventilation?**

It can increase, decrease or remain the same.

❍ **What should be done first when tension pneumothorax is suspected?**

Needle thoracostomy followed by tube thoracostomy.

❍ **How can the presence of intrinsic PEEP be confirmed in patients undergoing mechanical ventilation?**

Just prior to the onset of inspiration, one of three may be seen:
1) Expiratory flow has not ceased
2) Positive pressure is measured with an esophageal balloon
3) Positive pressure is measured during an airway occlusion maneuver

❍ **Under what circumstances should dead space be added to the ventilator circuit?**

None.

❍ **What is the FIO_2 at the top of Mount Everest?**

21%.

❍ **What position is preferred for patients suspected of having an air embolism?**

Left lateral decubitus/Trendelenburg position.

❍ **What are the clinical signs of hypercarbia?**

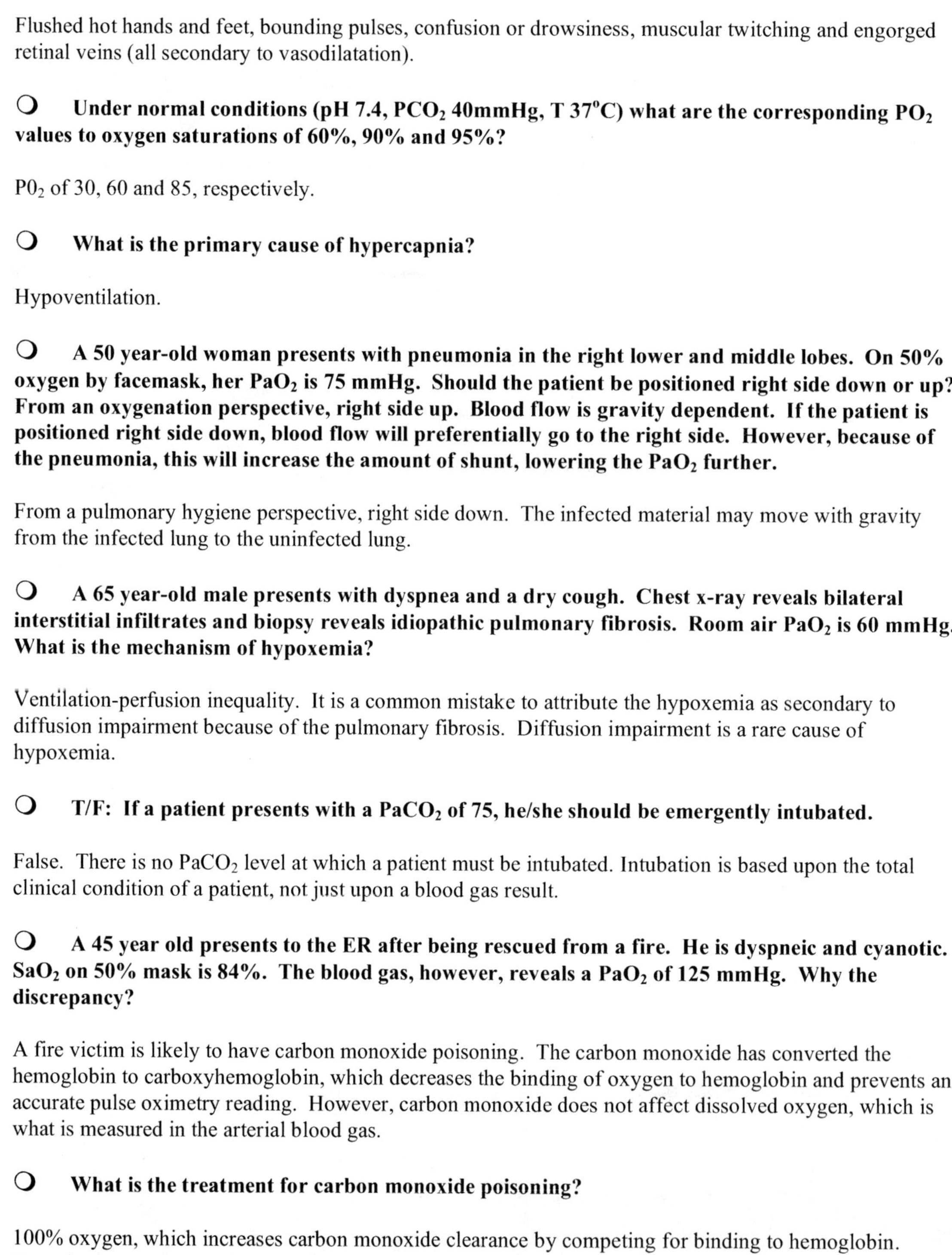

Flushed hot hands and feet, bounding pulses, confusion or drowsiness, muscular twitching and engorged retinal veins (all secondary to vasodilatation).

❍ **Under normal conditions (pH 7.4, PCO_2 40mmHg, T 37°C) what are the corresponding PO_2 values to oxygen saturations of 60%, 90% and 95%?**

$P0_2$ of 30, 60 and 85, respectively.

❍ **What is the primary cause of hypercapnia?**

Hypoventilation.

❍ **A 50 year-old woman presents with pneumonia in the right lower and middle lobes. On 50% oxygen by facemask, her PaO_2 is 75 mmHg. Should the patient be positioned right side down or up? From an oxygenation perspective, right side up. Blood flow is gravity dependent. If the patient is positioned right side down, blood flow will preferentially go to the right side. However, because of the pneumonia, this will increase the amount of shunt, lowering the PaO_2 further.**

From a pulmonary hygiene perspective, right side down. The infected material may move with gravity from the infected lung to the uninfected lung.

❍ **A 65 year-old male presents with dyspnea and a dry cough. Chest x-ray reveals bilateral interstitial infiltrates and biopsy reveals idiopathic pulmonary fibrosis. Room air PaO_2 is 60 mmHg. What is the mechanism of hypoxemia?**

Ventilation-perfusion inequality. It is a common mistake to attribute the hypoxemia as secondary to diffusion impairment because of the pulmonary fibrosis. Diffusion impairment is a rare cause of hypoxemia.

❍ **T/F: If a patient presents with a $PaCO_2$ of 75, he/she should be emergently intubated.**

False. There is no $PaCO_2$ level at which a patient must be intubated. Intubation is based upon the total clinical condition of a patient, not just upon a blood gas result.

❍ **A 45 year old presents to the ER after being rescued from a fire. He is dyspneic and cyanotic. SaO_2 on 50% mask is 84%. The blood gas, however, reveals a PaO_2 of 125 mmHg. Why the discrepancy?**

A fire victim is likely to have carbon monoxide poisoning. The carbon monoxide has converted the hemoglobin to carboxyhemoglobin, which decreases the binding of oxygen to hemoglobin and prevents an accurate pulse oximetry reading. However, carbon monoxide does not affect dissolved oxygen, which is what is measured in the arterial blood gas.

❍ **What is the treatment for carbon monoxide poisoning?**

100% oxygen, which increases carbon monoxide clearance by competing for binding to hemoglobin. Hyperbaric oxygen (oxygen provided at higher than atmospheric pressure) is recommended in more severe cases.

❍ **T/F: A normal $PaCO_2$ in a patient with an asthma exacerbation is a good sign.**

Maybe. A normal $PaCO_2$ in an asthmatic is good if the patient is feeling improved and less dyspneic. However, it can be a sign of impending respiratory failure if the patient continues to feel dyspneic and is working hard to breathe.

❍ **T/F: Oxygen should never be given to a hypoxemic patient with COPD who has chronic CO_2 retention.**

False. Oxygen should always be given to a patient who is hypoxemic.

❍ **What considerations should be addressed while giving the above patient oxygen?**

It has been shown that giving oxygen to a chronic CO_2 retainer usually does not result in a significant decrease in minute ventilation. The $PaCO_2$ will go up, but the rise is probably a result of changes in the ventilation-perfusion inequalities.

Oxygen should be given judiciously with repeat $PaCO_2$ determinations to ensure that the $PaCO_2$ does not rise precipitously.

❍ **What are the indications for chronic oxygen therapy?**

1. Resting $PaO_2 < 55$ mmHg or $SaO_2 < 88\%$.
2. Resting PaO_2 56-59 mmHg or SaO_2 89% in the presence of evidence of cor pulmonale or polycythemia.
3. During exercise if the PaO_2 falls below 55 mmHg or the SaO_2 below 88% with a low level of exertion.

❍ **What are the major mechanisms of hypoventilation and what clinical conditions are associated with each?**

1. Failure of the central nervous system ventilatory centers - drugs (narcotics, barbiturates) and stroke.
2. Failure of the chest bellows - chest wall diseases (kyphoscoliosis), neuromuscular diseases (amyotrophic lateral sclerosis) and diaphragm weakness.
3. Obstruction of the airways – asthma and chronic obstructive pulmonary disease.

❍ **How can hypoxemia secondary to hypoventilation alone be distinguished from other causes of hypoxemia?**

If the hypoxemia is from hypoventilation alone, the A-a O_2 gradient is normal. It is elevated in all other causes.

❍ **What are the most common clinical conditions in which shunt is the primary mechanism for hypoxemia?**

Alveolar filling with fluid (pulmonary edema) or pus (pneumonia). Any condition that fills or closes the alveoli preventing gas exchange can lead to a shunt.

❍ **How can shunt be distinguished from the other causes of hypoxemia?**

If given 100% oxygen, the hypoxemic patient with a shunt will not have a significant increase in their PaO_2. There will be a significant increase in PaO_2 when 100% oxygen is given to patients with hypoventilation or ventilation-perfusion inequality.

❍ **T/F: A leftward shift in the oxyhemoglobin dissociation curve indicates an increased hemoglobin affinity for oxygen.**

True.

❍ **Changes in temperature, $PaCO_2$ or pH or the level of 2,3-diphosphoglycerate (2,3-DPG) cause a shift in the oxyhemoglobin dissociation curve. To cause a rightward shift, what are the changes that must occur?**

Increased temperature, increased $PaCO_2$, decreased pH and increased 2,3-DPG level. An easy way to remember this is that these conditions are often associated with decreased tissue oxygen levels. By right-shifting the curve, more oxygen is released from hemoglobin to the tissues.

❍ **Which types of hemoglobin are associated with a leftward shift of the oxyhemoglobin dissociation curve?**

Hemoglobin F (fetal hemoglobin), carboxyhemoglobin and methemoglobin.

❍ **What drugs cause methemoglobinemia?**

Oxidant drugs, such as antimalarials, dapsone, nitrites/nitrates (nitroprusside) and local anesthetics (lidocaine). Methemoglobinemia occurs when the iron moiety of hemoglobin is oxidized from the ferrous to the ferric state.

❍ **Which common enzyme deficiency predisposes to the development of methemoglobinemia in the presence of the above drugs?**

G-6-PD deficiency.

❍ **What is the treatment of methemoglobinemia?**

Methylene blue.

❍ **What are the determinants of the oxygen content of blood?**

Hemoglobin concentration, PaO_2 and SaO_2. The equation to determine the oxygen content of blood is: $CaO_2 = (1.34 \times [Hgb] \times SaO_2) + (PaO_2 \times 0.003)$. The first term is the hemoglobin bound oxygen and the second is the dissolved oxygen. Dissolved oxygen content is a minor portion of total oxygen content unless PaO_2 is very high.

❍ **How does the shape of the oxyhemoglobin dissociation curve effect the oxygen content of blood?**

Since SaO_2 does not increase significantly if the $PaO_2 > 60$ mmHg, the oxygen content of blood will increase significantly above this level only by increasing the hemoglobin concentration.

❍ **What are some common causes of respiratory alkalosis?**

Respiratory alkalosis is defined as a pH above 7.45 and a pCO_2 less than 35. Common causes of respiratory alkalosis include any process that may induce hyperventilation: shock, sepsis, trauma, asthma, PE, anemia, hepatic failure, heat stroke, exhaustion, emotion, salicylate poisoning, hypoxemia, pregnancy and inadequate mechanical ventilation.

❍ **Calculate the alveolar-arterial oxygen (A-a O_2) gradient given the following arterial blood gas obtained at sea level: pH 7.24, $PaCO_2$ 60 and PaO_2 45.**

30 mmHg.

To calculate the alveolar-arterial oxygen gradient, you must first calculate the expected alveolar partial pressure of oxygen (PAO_2) using the alveolar gas equation. The alveolar gas equation is commonly written: $PAO_2 = PIO_2 - PaCO_2/R$, where PIO_2 is the partial pressure of oxygen in the inspired gas and R is the respiratory exchange ratio, commonly estimated at 0.8. PIO_2 is calculated as follows: $PIO_2 = FIO_2\ (P_B - P_{H2O})$ where FIO_2 is the inspired concentration of oxygen (0.21 at sea level), P_B is the atmospheric pressure

(760 mmHg at sea level) and P_{H2O} is the partial pressure of water (47 mmHg). At sea level, PIO_2 is equal to 150 mmHg. For this example, PAO_2 = 150 - 60/0.8 or 75 mmHg.

The A-a O_2 gradient is PAO_2 - PaO_2. Therefore, in this example, the A-a O_2 gradient is 75 - 45 or 30 mmHg.

❍ **What is the normal A-a O_2 gradient?**

10 mmHg in a 20 year old.

❍ **What is the age related decline in PaO_2?**

The PaO_2 declines by 2.5 mmHg per decade. Given that a PaO_2 of 95-100 mmHg is normal for a 20 year old, a PaO_2 of 75 to 80 would be normal for an 80 year old. This decline is secondary to an increase in the A-a O_2 gradient, which increases from about 10 mmHg in a 20 year old to 20 to 25 mmHg in an 80 year old.

❍ **What are the principal mechanisms that lead to hypoxemia?**

Hypoventilation, diffusion limitation, shunt, ventilation-perfusion inequality, low inspired oxygen concentration, and low mixed venous oxygen in the presence of V/Q mismatch.

❍ **Which of the above mechanisms is the most common?**

Ventilation-perfusion inequality.

❍ **Why does hypoventilation lead to hypoxemia?**

Hypoventilation results in an increase in $PaCO_2$, which in turn decreases the PAO_2 (see the alveolar gas equation above).

❍ **Can shunt be seen in patients without alveolar abnormalities?**

Yes. Shunt can occur if venous blood enters the left atrium without being oxygenated. This can occur in pulmonary arteriovenous malformations and intracardiac shunts.

❍ **T/F: Diffusion limitation is an important cause of hypoxemia clinically.**

False. Diffusion limitation is rarely a cause of hypoxemia.

❍ **Does oxygen or carbon monoxide bind to hemoglobin with more affinity?**

Carbon monoxide has a 240-fold greater affinity for hemoglobin than oxygen.

❍ **What are the effects of carbon monoxide on hemoglobin?**

Carbon monoxide bound to hemoglobin, carboxyhemoglobin, impairs tissue oxygenation by two mechanisms:

1: It decreases oxygen carrying capacity by decreasing the amount of hemoglobin available for oxygen binding.

2: It shifts the oxyhemoglobin dissociation curve to the left.

❍ **What is platypnea?**

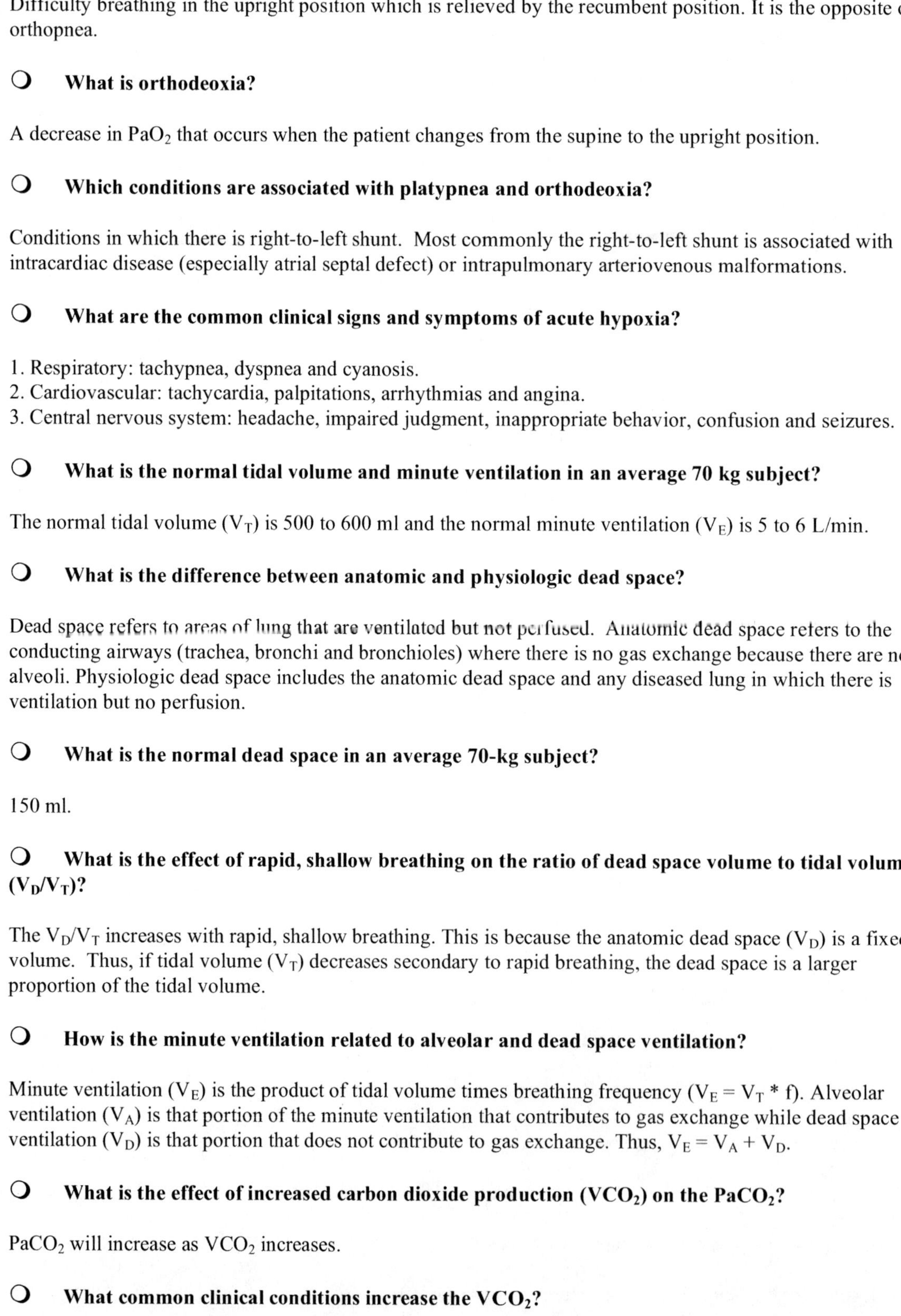

Difficulty breathing in the upright position which is relieved by the recumbent position. It is the opposite of orthopnea.

❍ **What is orthodeoxia?**

A decrease in PaO_2 that occurs when the patient changes from the supine to the upright position.

❍ **Which conditions are associated with platypnea and orthodeoxia?**

Conditions in which there is right-to-left shunt. Most commonly the right-to-left shunt is associated with intracardiac disease (especially atrial septal defect) or intrapulmonary arteriovenous malformations.

❍ **What are the common clinical signs and symptoms of acute hypoxia?**

1. Respiratory: tachypnea, dyspnea and cyanosis.
2. Cardiovascular: tachycardia, palpitations, arrhythmias and angina.
3. Central nervous system: headache, impaired judgment, inappropriate behavior, confusion and seizures.

❍ **What is the normal tidal volume and minute ventilation in an average 70 kg subject?**

The normal tidal volume (V_T) is 500 to 600 ml and the normal minute ventilation (V_E) is 5 to 6 L/min.

❍ **What is the difference between anatomic and physiologic dead space?**

Dead space refers to areas of lung that are ventilated but not perfused. Anatomic dead space refers to the conducting airways (trachea, bronchi and bronchioles) where there is no gas exchange because there are no alveoli. Physiologic dead space includes the anatomic dead space and any diseased lung in which there is ventilation but no perfusion.

❍ **What is the normal dead space in an average 70-kg subject?**

150 ml.

❍ **What is the effect of rapid, shallow breathing on the ratio of dead space volume to tidal volume (V_D/V_T)?**

The V_D/V_T increases with rapid, shallow breathing. This is because the anatomic dead space (V_D) is a fixed volume. Thus, if tidal volume (V_T) decreases secondary to rapid breathing, the dead space is a larger proportion of the tidal volume.

❍ **How is the minute ventilation related to alveolar and dead space ventilation?**

Minute ventilation (V_E) is the product of tidal volume times breathing frequency ($V_E = V_T * f$). Alveolar ventilation (V_A) is that portion of the minute ventilation that contributes to gas exchange while dead space ventilation (V_D) is that portion that does not contribute to gas exchange. Thus, $V_E = V_A + V_D$.

❍ **What is the effect of increased carbon dioxide production (VCO_2) on the $PaCO_2$?**

$PaCO_2$ will increase as VCO_2 increases.

❍ **What common clinical conditions increase the VCO_2?**

Any condition in which there is increased oxygen consumption will increase CO_2 production. Common conditions include exercise, increased work of breathing, fever and shivering.

❍ **What is the effect of increased alveolar ventilation (V_A) on $PaCO_2$?**

$PaCO_2$ will decrease as V_A increases.

❍ **What is relationship between $PaCO_2$ and V_D/V_T?**

$PaCO_2$ is inversely related to the term ($1-V_D/V_T$). Thus, any process that increases the dead space will increase the $PaCO_2$.

❍ **Why do most asthmatics present with a decreased PCO_2?**

First, the increased $PaCO_2$ associated with the increased dead space stimulates the central nervous system chemoreceptors to increase minute ventilation, which in turn decreases $PaCO_2$. Also, the associated hypoxemia and sensation of dyspnea causes the patient to hyperventilate, which lowers the $PaCO_2$.

❍ **Why do asthmatics eventually have an increased $PaCO_2$ if untreated?**

As the asthma attack continues untreated, the work of breathing will continue to increase. Eventually, the diaphragm fatigues and the patient hypoventilates. The hypoventilation, in association with the increased dead space and increased CO_2 production, increases the $PaCO_2$.

❍ **What is the normal $PaCO_2$ and does it vary with age?**

The normal $PaCO_2$ is 35 to 45 mmHg and does not vary with age.

❍ **What is the normal expected change in pH if there is an acute change in the $PaCO_2$?**

The pH will increase or decrease 0.8 units for every 10 mmHg decrease or increase (respectively) in $PaCO_2$.

❍ **In chronic respiratory acidosis or alkalosis, what is the expected change in pH?**

The pH will increase or decrease 0.3 units for every 10 mmHg decrease or increase (respectively) in $PaCO_2$.

❍ **What is the expected change in serum bicarbonate in chronic respiratory acidosis or alkalosis?**

Bicarbonate increases by approximately 3 mEq/L for each 10 mmHg increase in $PaCO_2$ in chronic respiratory acidosis. Bicarbonate decreases by 4 to 5 mEq/L for each 10 mmHg decrease in $PaCO_2$ in chronic respiratory alkalosis.

❍ **What are the consequences of hypercapnia?**

Acute hypercapnia has physiologic consequences due to the increased $PaCO_2$ and to the decreased pH.

Physiologic effects of the $PaCO_2$ increase include:
1. Increase in cerebral blood flow.
2. Confusion, headache ($PaCO_2 > 60$mmHg), obtundation and seizure ($PaCO_2 > 70$mmHg).
3. Depression of diaphragmatic contractility.

The primary consequences of the decreased pH are on the cardiovascular system with in decreased cardiac contractility, decreased fibrillation threshold and vasodilatation.

○ **What are the consequences of hypocapnia?**

Acute hypocapnia has physiologic consequences due to the decreased $PaCO_2$ and to the increased pH.

Physiologic effects of the $PaCO_2$ decrease include:

1. Decreases in cerebral blood flow (this reflex is used in the management of neurologic disorders with high intracranial pressures as a short-term measure to decrease the increased intracranial pressure).
2. Confusion, myoclonus, asterixis, loss of consciousness and seizures.

The primary consequences of the increased pH are again primarily on the cardiovascular system **with** increased cardiac contractility and vasodilatation.

○ **A 32 year old male presents to the emergency room obtunded. Examination is significant for a respiratory rate of 8 and pinpoint pupils. An arterial blood gas reveals pH 7.28, $PaCO_2$ 55 and PaO_2 60. What is the cause of the hypercapnia?**

Acute narcotic overdose leading to hypoventilation.

○ **T/F: A chest x-ray in the above patient would most likely show signs of aspiration pneumonia.**

True. The A-a O_2 gradient is 21 (PAO_2 is 150 - 55/0.8 or 81), which is high, indicating that there are two reasons for the hypoxemia.

○ **A 30 year old female presents with dyspnea and signs of right sided heart failure. The PaO_2 on room air is 55 mmHg and on 100% oxygen is 70 mmHg What is the cause of the hypoxemia?**

Shunt, as there is no significant increase in the PaO_2 on 100% oxygen.

○ **The chest x-ray on the above patient reveals no pulmonary parenchymal lesions but does show prominent hila and an enlarged right ventricle. What diagnostic test should be performed?**

The patient has no pulmonary parenchymal lesions to cause a shunt. She most likely has an intracardiac right-to-left shunt (most likely a previously undiagnosed atrial septal defect). An echocardiogram should be performed.

○ **A 45 year old obese male presents with dyspnea, peripheral edema, snoring and excessive daytime sleepiness. A room air arterial blood gas shows the pH is 7.34, $PaCO_2$ 60 mmHg, PaO_2 58 mmHg and the calculated HCO_3^- is 28 mEq/L. What is the acid-base disturbance?**

Chronic compensated respiratory acidosis. If this were acute, the pH would be 7.28 with a normal HCO_3^-.

○ **What is the cause of the hypoxemia in the above patient?**

Hypoventilation is one cause. However, since the A-a O_2 gradient is elevated, there is another cause in addition to the hypoventilation. In an obese patient, both ventilation-perfusion inequality and shunt (secondary to atelectasis) can contribute to the development of hypoxemia.

○ **What is the cause of the hypoventilation?**

Obesity-hypoventilation syndrome.

❍ **A 25 year old woman with a history of mitral valve prolapse presents with anxiety, chest tightness, hand numbness and mild confusion. Arterial blood gas reveals: pH 7.52, $PaCO_2$ 25 mmHg and PaO_2 108 mmHg. What is the most likely diagnosis?**

An acute anxiety attack.

❍ **Why is the PaO_2 elevated in the above patient?**

Because the lower $PaCO_2$ means a higher PAO_2 (see alveolar gas equation above).

❍ **What is the treatment?**

Having the patient breathe in and out of a bag can terminate the acute hyperventilation. Anxiolytics can also be provided.

❍ **In which pulmonary disease has long term continuous oxygen therapy been proven to be of clinical benefit?**

Studies in both the United States and Great Britain have shown that mortality is reduced in patients with chronic obstructive pulmonary disease and hypoxemia who use long-term oxygen.

❍ **What are the maximal oxygen concentrations that can be achieved by nasal cannula and facemask?**

6 L/min. of nasal cannula oxygen can achieve an FIO_2 of ~44%. A simple facemask can achieve an FIO_2 of ~60%.

❍ **What is a nonrebreather mask?**

A nonrebreather mask has a one-way valve between the mask and a reservoir bag, such that the patient can only inhale from the reservoir bag (which contains 100% oxygen) and exhale through separate valves on the side of the mask.

❍ **What is a Venturi mask?**

An oxygen delivery device in which room air and 100% oxygen are mixed in a fixed ratio allowing for the delivery of an accurate FIO_2 up to 50%.

❍ **Why is a Venturi mask clinically useful?**

The Venturi mask is mostly commonly used for patients with chronic CO_2 retention and acute hypoxemia, where precise titration of the FIO_2 is necessary to prevent a precipitous increase in the $PaCO_2$.

❍ **What should treatment for malignant hyperthermia include?**

A change in the anesthetic agent to remove possible triggers, administration of dantrolene and the procedure should be terminated.

❍ **T/F: Severe auto-PEEP may cause pulseless electrical activity.**

True.

SHOCK PEARLS

"For he was great of heart"
Othello, Shakespeare

❍ **What is a normal oxygen extraction ratio in a healthy adult?**

(20 vol% - 15 vol%)/20 vol% = 5/20 or 25%

❍ **What is the Bowditch effect?**

As heart rate increases myocardial contractility increases.

❍ **How does a cardiac output thermistor resting on a vessel wall alter the cardiac output calculation based on the Stewart-Hamilton equation for thermodilution cardiac output?**

It isolates the thermistor from temperature change causing less of a temperature change in the thermodilution solution thereby overestimating the patient's cardiac output.

❍ **What is Beck's triad for the diagnosis of cardiac tamponade?**

Hypotension, elevated central venous pressure and a quiet precordium on auscultation.

❍ **What is the equation for calculating arterial oxygen content (CaO_2)?**

CaO_2 = (1.39 x Hgb x arterial O_2 Sat) + (.003 x PaO_2) where Hgb is hemoglobin, O_2 sat is oxygen saturation and PaO_2 is arterial partial pressure of oxygen.

❍ **What is the equation for calculating oxygen consumption (VO_2)?**

VO_2 = CO x (CaO_2-CvO_2) x 10 where CO is cardiac output, CaO_2 is arterial oxygen content and CvO_2 is venous oxygen content.

❍ **What hemodynamic changes are associated with sepsis?**

Increased cardiac index, decreased systemic vascular resistance (early stage), increased systemic vascular resistance (late stage), normal to decreased cardiac filling pressures and normal or elevated mixed venous oxygen saturation (early stage).

❍ **What are the indicators of global oxygen transport insufficiency?**

Decrease in mixed venous oxygen saturation, increase in arterial-venous oxygen content difference and development of lactic acidosis.

❍ **What are the clinical manifestations of the systemic inflammatory response syndrome (SIRS)?**

Fever or hypothermia, tachypnea, tachycardia and increased WBCs with a left shift.

❍ **What are the mechanisms of obstructive shock?**

Impedance to filling (e.g., tamponade and restrictive cardiomyopathies) and impedance to outflow (e.g., valvular stenosis and pulmonary embolism).

❍ **What is the classic hemodynamic finding of cardiac tamponade?**

Equalization of the diastolic pressures of the heart chambers.

❍ **Why does removal of very little pericardial fluid in tamponade greatly improve the clinical picture?**

Tamponade occurs at the right side of the pericardial compliance curve where small changes in volume cause large changes in pressure.

❍ **What causes electrical alternans on the ECG of a patient with cardiac tamponade?**

Cyclic motion of the heart in the fluid filled pericardial sac.

❍ **What is pulsus paradoxus?**

A greater than normal decrease in systolic arterial pressure with inspiration.

❍ **What is the differential diagnosis for pulsus paradoxus?**

Cardiac tamponade, status asthmaticus, severe chronic obstructive lung disease, pulmonary embolus, constrictive pericarditis and tension pneumothorax.

❍ **What clinical finding distinguishes cardiac tamponade from constrictive pericarditis?**

Kussmaul's sign (increase in venous pressure during inspiration) is not seen in tamponade.

❍ **What is the most common clinical finding in cardiac tamponade?**

Tachypnea followed by pulsus paradoxus and tachycardia.

❍ **What are the underlying pathogenetic mechanisms of cardiogenic shock?**

Loss of contractile muscle, valvular failure, dysrhythmias and myocardial rupture.

❍ **What is the classic clinical sign of systolic ventricular dysfunction?**

An S3 gallop.

❍ **Can preload and PCWP be used as synonyms?**

No. PCWP is determined by juxtaventricular pressures, ventricular compliance and left ventricular end diastolic volume (LVEDV). LVEDV and preload are synonyms.

❍ **What major conditions are associated with distributive shock?**

Sepsis, anaphylaxis, neurogenic shock and adrenal insufficiency.

❍ **What are the key endogenous molecular mediators of septic shock?**

Cytokines (mainly TNF-α, IL-1, IL-6 and IFN-γ), prostaglandins, complement factors, platelet-activating factor and nitric oxide.

❍ **What is the pathogenesis of anaphylactic shock?**

Anaphylactic shock is an extreme manifestation of an immediate hypersensitivity reaction. It occurs through the interaction of an inciting antigen with mast cells and basophil-bound IgE. These effector cells then release numerous mediators that produce the clinical findings.

❍ **What are the effects of septic shock on cardiac function?**

There is transient dilatation of one or both ventricles, reduced contractility and low ejection fraction. These changes typically last several days and normalize after 7 to 10 days.

❍ **What are the typical clinical findings that distinguish distributive shock from other types of shock?**

Warm, well-perfused skin, wide pulse pressure and reduced diastolic blood pressure.

❍ **What degree of blood loss is required to induce hypotension?**

20 to 25% of the blood volume.

❍ **What are the typical values of mixed venous oxygen saturation in septic shock?**

It is often elevated above normal secondary to inadequate oxygen extraction by tissues.

❍ **T/F: The finding of a hyperdynamic hemodynamic profile confirms or excludes a septic etiology of shock.**

False.

❍ **What are the initial priorities during shock resuscitation?**

Hemodynamic stabilization and cause-specific correction of the systemic and regional circulatory failure.

❍ **What are the metabolic goals of shock resuscitation?**

Correction of oxygen debt, anaerobic metabolism and tissue acidosis.

❍ **What is the importance of the splanchnic circulation during shock and the post-shock phase?**

The splanchnic tissues are preferentially underperfused relative to their metabolic demands during shock. Left uncorrected, this underperfusion is associated with increased morbidity and mortality.

❍ **What is the initial blood pressure goal in shock resuscitation?**

Mean arterial pressure (MAP) of 70 mm Hg.

❍ **What is the significance of blood lactate determination in shock patients?**

Mortality is directly related to the degree of lactic acidosis.

❍ **T/F: Normal cardiac output values exclude cardiac dysfunction.**

False.

❍ **What is the optimal hematocrit in shock patients?**

Approximately 30%.

❍ **What is the role of catecholamines in the resuscitation of shock?**

Inotropic or vasopressor support once effective intravascular volume has been restored.

❍ **What are the major drawbacks of catecholamine use in shock?**

Catecholamines can increase myocardial and systemic oxygen demands, induce arrhythmias and cause excessive vasoconstriction, resulting in ischemia.

❍ **T/F: Normalization of vital signs, such as blood pressure and heart rate indicate complete resuscitation of shock.**

False. Systemic vital signs do not reliably reflect the physiologic end-points of shock resuscitation.

❍ **What is the most common cause of death of shock patients?**

Multiple organ failure (MOF).

❍ **Which parameter obtained on routine vital signs usually indicates a hypodynamic state?**

A narrowed pulse pressure.

❍ **In which lung zone should a pulmonary artery catheter tip be located?**

Zone III.

❍ **How is oxygen consumption (VO_2) calculated?**

$VO_2 = CO \times C(a\text{-}v)O_2 \times 10$.

❍ **What is the normal mixed venous blood oxygen saturation?**

Approximately 75%.

❍ **How is arterial oxygen content (CaO_2) calculated?**

$CaO_2 = (Hgb \times 1.39 \times SaO_2) + (PaO_2 \times 0.0031)$.

❍ **What are the typical PA catheter measurements in early septic shock?**

High cardiac output (CO), low systemic vascular resistance (SVR) and low or normal pulmonary capillary wedge pressure (PCWP). In later stages, CO will drop and SVR may rise.

❍ **What is the treatment of septic shock?**

Volume infusion. Once euvolemia is achieved, vasopressor agents for hypotension or inotropic agents for inadequate tissue delivery of oxygen should be considered.

❍ **How is cardiogenic shock managed?**

Euvolemia first, then inotropic or vasopressor support.

❍ **What are typical PA catheter measurements in neurogenic shock?**

High or low CO, low SVR and low PCWP.

❍ **How is neurogenic shock managed?**

Volume infusion followed by vasopressors, if needed.

❍ **What are the characteristics of dopamine?**

It is primarily a dopaminergic agonist at low doses, a β-1 agonist at moderate doses and an α-agonist at high doses.

❍ **How is oxygen delivery (DO_2) calculated?**

$DO_2 = CO \times CaO_2 \times 10$.

❍ **What is the definition of preload?**

End-diastolic sarcomere length.

❍ **T/F: Colloid solutions are preferred for resuscitation.**

False.

❍ **T/F: Blood products should be given as the initial resuscitation fluid for patients with presumed large blood loss.**

False.

❍ **What parameters indicate successful resuscitation?**

Return of normal vital signs and signs of end organ perfusion (as urine output and clear mentation).

❍ **What are the indications for central venous cannulation?**

As a conduit for PA catheters, lack of peripheral access, CVP monitoring and infusion of vasoactive medications or medications requiring high flow veins.

❍ **What is the preferred site for central venous catheterization?**

Controversial. All three major sites (femoral, internal jugular and subclavian) have advantages and disadvantages that must be weighed.

❍ **T/F: Femoral vein catheters have the highest infection rates and should not be used routinely.**

False.

❍ **What are the most common immediate complications of central venous catheterization?**

Pneumothorax, hemothorax, arrhythmias, arterial puncture, air embolus and malposition.

❍ **What are the common delayed complications from central venous catheterization?**

Infection, thrombus formation, erosion through the SVC or atrium and delayed pneumothorax.

❍ **How is ejection fraction (EF) calculated?**

EF = SV / EDV, where SV = stroke volume and EDV = end diastolic volume.

❍ **What catheter tip culture result is suggestive of catheter sepsis?**

Greater than 15 colonies of the same organism.

❍ **A patient has the following pulmonary artery catheter readings: Cardiac index (CI) of 2.0 L/min., CVP of 2 mm Hg, pulmonary artery occlusion pressure (PAOP) of 7 mmHg and SVR of 1600 dyne/sec/cm^2. What is the most likely diagnosis and what is the appropriate therapy?**

The patient is hypovolemic and would benefit from fluid resuscitation.

❍ **A patient's pulmonary artery catheter readings reveal a CVP of 12 mm Hg, PAOP of 18 mm Hg, CI of 1.7 L/min. and SVR of 1650 dyne/sec/cm^2. What is the most appropriate treatment?**

Inotropic support. However, this must be judiciously balanced against the side effect of increasing myocardial oxygen demand. Depending on the patient's condition, an intrQ:ortic balloon pump may be preferred. Echocardiography is necessary to rule out a structural cause for the decrease in cardiac index.

❍ **How is the optimal filling pressure determined for a patient in cardiogenic shock?**

By obtaining a bedside Starling curve and plotting PCWP against CO after repeated small volume boluses or diuresis.

❍ **What is the average survival rate for patients with septic shock?**

40 to 60%.

❍ **T/F: The circulatory derangements of septic shock precede the metabolic abnormalities.**

False.

❍ **Why has bicarbonate use been de-emphasized?**

Because of its harmful effects, which include hyperosmolarity, alkalemia, hypernatremia, paradoxical CSF acidosis and increased CO_2 production.

❍ **T/F: Vasodilators should be employed early in the management of hemorrhagic shock.**

False.

❍ **Which class of hemorrhagic shock is consistent with a drop in systolic blood pressure?**

Class III.

❍ **What are the CNS symptoms of acute volume loss?**

Lethargy and apathy, progressing to coma.

❍ **What is the best initial fluid management for a patient with hemorrhagic shock?**

Lactated Ringer's.

❍ **What are the signs of volume overload?**

Distended veins, bounding pulse, functional murmurs, peripheral edema and basilar rales.

❍ **What are the characteristics of Class II hemorrhagic shock?**

Loss of 15 to 30% of circulating blood volume, tachycardia and a decrease in the pulse pressure.

❍ **What is the most common volume disorder encountered in surgery?**

Volume deficit. (Loss of isotonic fluid is the most common cause.)

❍ **Which fluids flow faster through IV lines?**

Crystalloid and colloids are faster than red cells

❍ **T/F: Colloid solution is the preferred solution for resuscitation.**

False. In terms of volume required, resuscitation with a colloid solution requires less volume than with a crystalloid solution. However, crystalloid is less expensive and yields no difference in outcome.

❍ **T/F: Blood products should be given as the initial resuscitation fluid for patients with presumed large blood loss.**

False. Non-blood containing fluids can be infused faster and therefore will more quickly support perfusion. Blood, usually in the form of packed red blood cells, should be given early in those patients with presumed large volume blood loss.

❍ **What are the indications for invasive arterial monitoring?**

Need for constant pressure monitoring due to a hemodynamic instability, vasoactive medications and need for frequent arterial blood gas monitoring.

❍ **What are the preferred and acceptable alternative sites for arterial lines?**

The radial artery is preferred due to a very high percentage of collateral flow to hand. Femoral and dorsalis pedis arteries are acceptable.

❍ **T/F: Non-invasive arterial pressure measurements are more accurate than direct arterial measurements.**

False.

❍ **Does the pulmonary artery catheter positively affect patient outcome?**

Not necessarily. Despite its routine use, data are lacking that show conclusively that the PA catheter benefits patients.

❍ **What patient populations are most likely to be helped by the use of the PA catheter?**

Patients with myocardial infarction and shock and those with shock refractory to volume loading, perioperative management of patients undergoing cardiac or vascular surgery and multiple trauma patients.

❍ **What complications are associated with PA catheter usage?**

All possible complications inherent in any central venous access, as well as pulmonary artery rupture, higher incidence of arrhythmias and knotting of the catheter.

❍ **At what points during insertion and use of PA catheters should the balloon be inflated?**

The balloon should be inflated to full volume (to obliterate the tip and avoid vessel puncture) as soon as it is in the SVC. It should remain inflated during any forward movement of the catheter and should be deflated prior to any withdrawal. Once in place, the balloon should be inflated only to the minimum volume necessary to obtain a pulmonary capillary wedge pressure (PCWP).

❍ **What are normal pressures measured by the PA catheter?**

SVC: 1 to 6
PA: 15 to 30 / 5 to 15
PCWP: 6 to 12

❍ **What are we really trying to measure when we measure the wedge pressure?**

Left ventricular end diastolic volume (LVEDV), a measure of the preload on the ventricle.

❍ **What assumptions are made in using PCWP as a substitute for LVEDV?**

Several, most importantly that a stable relationship exists between LVEDP and LVEDV. Also that the PCWP is equal to the left atrial (LA) pressure which is equal to the LVEDP.

❍ **Do these assumptions hold true in a typical critically ill patient?**

No.

❍ **What are sources of error in these assumptions?**

PCWP can be different from LA pressure or LVEDP due to pulmonary venous resistance, valvular abnormalities, positive pressure ventilation, positive end expiratory pressure (PEEP) and catheter placement in lung zones 1 or 2.

❍ **How does PA diastolic pressure compare to PCWP as a measure of left heart filling pressures?**

Under normal conditions, the PCWP is usually within a few mmHg of PA diastolic pressure. Conditions common to critical illness make the two more disparate.

❍ **How does PEEP affect PA catheter measurements?**

PEEP will increase the measured PCWP.

❍ **What is DO_2?**

DO_2 is a measure of the oxygen delivered to the tissues.

❍ **How is it measured?**

DO_2 = CO x [1.36 (ml/gm Hg) x Hg (gm/dl) x SaO_2] + [0.0031 x pO_2] x 10. Units in ml/min.
Where: Hg = hemoglobin, SaO_2 = arterial oxygen saturation and pO_2 = partial pressure of O_2.

❍ **Can increasing the FIO_2 significantly affect DO_2?**

Not much once the pO_2 is high enough to provide high O_2 saturation. The vast majority of delivered oxygen at a physiologic hematocrit is bound to hemoglobin. Therefore, increasing the pO_2 has little effect on total delivered oxygen once hemoglobin is fully saturated.

❍ **What is VO_2?**

VO_2 is the measure of oxygen consumption.

❍ **What is a normal VO_2?**

120 to 160 $mL/m^2/min$.

❍ **What causes changes in VO_2?**

VO_2 decreases in hypothermia and paralysis. It increases during muscular activity, hyperthermia, hyperthyroidism and states of inflammation.

❍ **When is oxygen consumption dependent on oxygen delivery?**

On the low end of the consumption vs. delivery curve, oxygen utilization is supply dependent.

❍ **What does the oxygen saturation of venous blood (SvO_2) tell us in relation to DO_2 and VO_2?**

SvO_2 is a quick way of getting some idea about the adequacy of DO_2 and VO_2. Assuming arterial oxygen saturation of 95 to 100%, the venous saturation should be >70 to 75%. Less than this indicates supply is suboptimal. In some conditions such as sepsis, SvO_2 will actually be higher than normal even with inadequate tissue oxygenation.

❍ **What are typical PA catheter measurements in hypovolemic shock?**

Low cardiac output, high systemic vascular resistance (SVR), low PCWP.

❍ **When should the PA catheter be removed?**

When the information obtained is no longer being used to make clinical decisions. Not all critically ill patients need them.

❍ **Ideally, how does the pulmonary artery catheter aid patient management?**

The usual scenario for placement of the catheter is when one of the parameters is in doubt, most commonly fluid status with unstable hemodynamics. The numbers obtained by the PA catheter may help guide management of fluids, diuretics and inotropic agents.

❍ **How does phenylephrine differ from norepinephrine?**

Phenylephrine is a pure alpha-1 agonist. It can be used to increase SVR and BP. Like norepinephrine it is associated with a reflex bradycardia. Norepinephrine has both alpha-1 and beta-1 effects.

❍ **Compare nitroglycerin and sodium nitroprusside.**

Both are vasodilators. Nitroglycerin is a greater venous vasodilator than an arterial vasodilator. In contrast, nitroprusside is primarily an arterial vasodilator. Unlike nitroprusside which is used primarily to manage hypertension and hypertensive crisis, nitroglycerin is also used to treat angina and congestive heart failure. Prolonged use of nitroprusside may cause thiocyanate toxicity.

❍ **Discuss amrinone and milrinone.**

Both are phosphodiesterase inhibitors which have a relative selectivity for phosphodiesterase III, the predominant cAMP-specific form in cardiac tissue. They have an inotropic as well as a vasodilator effect. A major drawback is the development of thrombocytopenia. Milrinone is at least as effective if not more potent than amrinone. Another benefit of milrinone is that its incidence of thrombocytopenia is much lower than amrinone.

❍ **Name three limitations of pulmonary artery catheter readings.**

PA catheter readings can fluctuate during respiratory variations and should therefore be read at end expiration. High PEEP can falsely elevate PA readings, particularly PAWP. Heart rates exceeding 120 beats/minute can also falsely elevate pulmonary artery diastolic pressure readings. A pressure change should be greater than 4 mmHg is considered clinically significant.

❍ **What is the hallmark hemodynamic finding of constrictive pericarditis?**

Early diastolic dip and late diastolic plateau in the right ventricular pressure curve ("square root sign").

❍ **What is the differential diagnosis if clotting blood is aspirated during a pericardiocentesis attempt?**

Either the ventricle was inadvertently entered or the pericardial hemorrhage was massive, overwhelming the defibrinating mechanism.

❍ **What should be the first intervention in a patient with blunt chest trauma who has engorged neck veins, distant heart sounds, decreased breath sounds and hypotension after unsuccessful attempts to stabilize the patient with aggressive fluid replacement?**

Needle decompression of the chest for possible tension pneumothorax. If the shock state persists, an emergent pericardiocentesis for cardiac tamponade should be performed.

❍ **What is the mortality of patients with acute right ventricular failure due to pulmonary embolism (PE)?**

Approximately 30%.

❍ **How much of the pulmonary vascular bed needs to be occluded to cause shock in the setting of PE?**

More than 60% in patients with no prior cardiopulmonary disease.

❍ **What is the survival benefit of patients with massive PE in shock given thrombolytic therapy compared to heparin alone?**

Faster clot lysis and improvement of right ventricular pressures have clearly been shown with thrombolytic agents. No study has ever been designed to demonstrate a survival advantage with thrombolytic agents.

❍ **What is the treatment for patients with massive PE and hypotension?**

Vasopressors, heparin and thrombolytic agents. Embolectomy is a consideration as well.

❍ **Under which circumstances should a surgical embolectomy be strongly considered?**

In any hemodynamically unstable patient with documented massive PE and absolute contraindications to thrombolytic therapy.

❍ **What are the four Killip classes and how do they relate to mortality?**

Killip 1: no heart failure, mortality 8%; Killip 2: mild to moderate failure (bibasilar rales, S3 gallop), mortality 30%; Killip 3: pulmonary edema, mortality 44%; Killip 4: cardiogenic shock, mortality 80 to 100%.

❍ **What is the classical hemodynamic picture seen in cardiogenic shock?**

Low cardiac index, high systemic vascular resistance and high pulmonary capillary wedge pressure (PCWP). The PCWP may not be elevated in right ventricular infarction.

❍ **What are the Forrester classes?**

Class 1: PCWP <18 mmHg, CI (cardiac index) > 2.2 l/min.; Class 2: PCWP >18mmHg, CI> 2.2 l/min.; Class 3: PCWP <18 mmHg, CI < 2.2 l/min.; Class 4: PCWP > 18 mmHg, CI < 2.2 l/min.

❍ **What is the prognostic significance of the four Forrester classes?**

Mortality increases with increasing Forrester class: Class 1: 3%; Class 2: 9%; Class 3: 23%; Class 4: 51%.

❍ **How much left ventricular muscle needs to be involved in the setting of an acute myocardial infarction (MI) to cause cardiogenic shock?**

40% or more.

❍ **What are the causes of cardiogenic shock in the setting of an acute MI?**

> 40% loss of left ventricular myocardium, ventricular wall rupture, septal rupture, left ventricular aneurysm and acute mitral regurgitation due to papillary muscle rupture/dysfunction.

❍ **What is the suspected diagnosis if a patient's blood pressure drops significantly with administration of nitroglycerin in the setting of an acute MI?**

Inferior wall MI with right ventricular involvement.

❍ **By how much does an intra-aortic balloon pump (IAPB) increase cardiac output?**

10 to 20%.

❍ **Why does an IABP increase cardiac output?**

An IABP decreases left ventricular afterload and increases coronary perfusion.

❍ **What is the survival benefit of patients with an acute MI in Killip class 4 after receiving thrombolytic therapy?**

Probably none. One study found no difference in 30 day mortality in those treated with thrombolytics compared to placebo (subgroup analysis).

❍ **What is the treatment of choice for a patient in cardiogenic shock in the setting of an acute MI?**

Primary angioplasty.

❍ **What seems to be the main predictor of survival of patients with cardiogenic shock due to an acute MI?**

Successful myocardial reperfusion.

❍ **How often does a careful clinical examination fail to correctly predict a patient's cardiac output and left ventricular filling pressure?**

In 30% of cases an experienced clinician incorrectly predicts those parameters.

❍ **How can a septal rupture be distinguished from papillary muscle rupture in the setting of acute cardiogenic shock?**

In both conditions, "V waves" may be seen on the PCWP tracing. However, only with septal rupture will an oxygen saturation step up be seen in blood withdrawn from the right atrium compared to blood withdrawn from the right ventricle and pulmonary artery.

❍ **How often does septal rupture occur in the setting of an acute MI?**

1 to 3% of cases. All occur within one week, with 20 to 30% occurring during the first 24 hours.

❍ **T/F: Septal rupture occurs more commonly in anterior infarcts than in inferior infarcts.**

False. The incidence is approximately the same.

❍ **Why does the posteromedial papillary muscle of the mitral valve rupture most often?**

It is perfused from only one of the coronary arteries, whereas the anterolateral is perfused from the left and right coronary circulation.

❍ **What are predisposing factors for free ventricular wall rupture?**

Age >60, peri-infarct hypertension, a large area of infarcted myocardium, a transmural MI and poor collateral circulation.

❍ **What percentage of deaths in patients with acute MIs are caused by ventricular wall rupture?**

10 to 15%. Mortality approaches 100%. 84% of the ruptures occur within the first week and 33% within the first 24 hours.

❍ **How often is right ventricular (RV) involvement seen in patients with inferior acute MI?**

40% of cases.

❍ **What is the incidence of pure right ventricular MI?**

2%.

❍ **What is a simple way of predicting RV dysfunction in the setting of an acute inferior MI?**

Elevation of the ST segment in lead V3R is seen only in patients with RV dysfunction. One study found that no patient with normal RV ejection fraction had this finding whereas all patients with ST elevation had RV ejection fractions of < 40%.

❍ **What is the first line treatment of a patient in cardiogenic shock due to RV infarction?**

Aggressive volume replacement as the right ventricle is "volume sensitive." Treatment may need to be guided by pulmonary artery catheter measurements.

❍ **What is the myocardial depressant factor (MDS)?**

MDS refers to circulating molecule(s) present in patients in septic shock that induce(s) myocardial dysfunction. Although various candidate substances have been proposed, including TNF-alpha and nitric oxide, the identity of MDS is presently unknown.

❍ **Describe the typical hemodynamic profiles of distributive and hypovolemic shock.**

Distributive shock: normal or low pulmonary capillary wedge pressure (PCWP), low systemic vascular resistance (SVR) and increased cardiac output (CO). Hypovolemic shock: low PCWP, increased SVR and low CO.

❍ **What is the role of anti-mediator therapy in septic shock?**

Anti-mediator therapy has been most extensively studied in septic shock. At this time, none of the studied agents appear to clearly improve patient outcome.

❍ **How should cardiac output (CO) values be interpreted during shock resuscitation?**

CO is the total systemic blood flow. Normal or high values do not exclude cardiac dysfunction and do not assure matching of systemic or regional metabolic demands. Thus, CO determinations should be interpreted in combination with other hemodynamic and metabolic indicators.

❍ **What is a common electrolyte abnormality associated with transfusion of packed red blood cells?**

Hypocalcemia secondary to citrate toxicity. Citrate, when rapidly infused, binds ionized calcium and therefore decreases the calcium level. Hyperkalemia may also develop with rapid packed red blood cell transfusion, especially if the patient is in renal failure or if the blood products are old.

❍ **What is the calculation for mean arterial pressure (MAP) based on systolic (SBP) and diastolic pressure (DBP)?**

MAP = DBP + 1/3(SBP - DBP).

❍ **What are the two most important determinants of coronary perfusion pressure?**

The two most important determinants of coronary perfusion pressure are diastolic blood pressure and left ventricular end-diastolic pressure:

CPP = DBP - LVEDP.

❍ **What are the determinants of stroke volume?**

Preload, contractility and afterload.

❍ **How would you calculate systemic vascular resistance (SVR)?**

$$\frac{\text{MAP - CVP}}{\text{CO}} \times 80 \text{ [dyne x sec/cm}^5\text{]}$$

❍ **How would you calculate pulmonary vascular resistance (PVR)?**

$$\frac{\text{Mean PAP - PCWP}}{\text{CO}} \times 80 \text{ [dyne x sec/cm}^5\text{]}$$

❍ **What is afterload?**

Afterload is either ventricular wall tension during systole or arterial impedance to ejection. Wall tension is usually described as the pressure the ventricle must overcome to reduce cavity size.

❍ **What is the baroreceptor reflex?**

Increase in blood pressure stimulates peripheral baroreceptors located at the bifurcation of the common carotid arteries and the aortic arch. These baroreceptors then send afferent signals to the brainstem circulatory centers via the glossopharyngeal and vagus nerves, allowing an increase in vagal tone and, consequently, vasodilatation and a decrease in heart rate.

CARDIOVASCULAR PEARLS

"I come not, friends, to steal away your hearts"
Anthony in *Julius Caesar*, Shakespeare

❍ **What is the significance of large pulmonary V waves on the pulmonary capillary wedge tracing?**

Abnormally large V waves, greater than 10 mmHg greater than the mean pulmonary wedge pressure, represent filling of the left atrium during systole against an abnormally large left atrial pressure. It is most commonly found in mitral regurgitation, but can also be seen in mitral stenosis, congestive left ventricular failure, ventricular septal defects, Eisenmenger's complex, and, in rare instances, severe aortic regurgitation.

❍ **What is the ateriovenous difference?**

Arteriovenous difference is the extraction of oxygen from the circulation across a given organ or tissue.

❍ **What is the extraction reserve?**

Extraction reserve is the factor by which the AV difference can increase at a constant blood flow.

❍ **What is the arterial oxygen saturation in a normal human? Venous saturation?**

The arterial saturation in a normal human is 95%. The venous saturation in a normal human is around 75%, but differs slightly, depending on where you measure.

❍ **What is the normal AV difference for oxygen in man?**

40 mL per liter of blood.

❍ **What is the normal extraction reserve for oxygen?**

Three. This means that, given adequate metabolic demand, the body's tissues can extract three times the AV difference for oxygen, or 120 mL per liter of blood. This also means that oxygen extraction increases as cardiac output falls until AV oxygen difference has tripled and cardiac output has fallen to one-third of its normal value. Thereafter, further reduction of cardiac output will result in tissue hypoxia, anaerobic metabolism, acidosis, and eventually, circulatory collapse.

❍ **What is the normal cardiac output in an adult human?**

Approximately 4-6 L/min, depending on numerous factors such as body size, metabolic rate, posture, age, body temperature, anxiety, environmental heat and humidity and a host of other factors.

❍ **What is the most accepted method of expressing cardiac output?**

Cardiac index. Cardiac index is the cardiac output divided by the body surface area in square meters.

❍ **What is the Fick method of determining cardiac output?**

Cardiac output = measured oxygen consumption/AV oxygen difference. In actual practice, the rate at which oxygen is taken up from the lungs is not measured, but rather the uptake of oxygen from room air is measured. Furthermore, the AV oxygen difference is not measured directly, but oxygen saturations of blood taken from the pulmonary artery and systemic arterial blood are sampled. The saturations are respectively converted to oxygen contents by multiplying the oxygen saturation percentage and a theoretic oxygen carrying capacity (patient's hemoglobin x 13.6). The difference in arterial oxygen content and pulmonary artery oxygen content is the AV oxygen difference.

❍ **When is the pulmonary venous blood oxygen saturation not approximated accurately by the systemic arterial oxygen saturation?**

When there is a right-to-left intracardiac shunt.

❍ **When do intracardiac shunts become physiologically important?**

When the pulmonary blood flow exceeds 1.5 to 2 times the systemic flow.

❍ **Which method of calculating cardiac output is more accurate and reliable, Fick or thermodilution method?**

Fick. Thermodilution method is easier to perform, but is prone to significant overestimation of cardiac output at low-flow, low cardiac output states.

❍ **What is the formula for estimation of systemic vascular resistance?**

SVR = (mean systemic arterial pressure – mean right atrial pressure) x 80/cardiac output.

❍ **What is the formula for estimation of pulmonary vascular resistance?**

PVR = (mean pulmonary artery pressure – mean left atrial pressure) x 80/pulmonary blood flow. Pulmonary blood flow is assumed to be equal to the cardiac output unless there is a shunt between the pulmonary and systemic circulations or an intracardiac shunt.

❍ **What is the normal value for systemic vascular resistance?**

800-1400 dynes-sec-cm^{-5}.

❍ **A 71 year-old male is admitted with hypotension, tachypnea and tachycardia. His HR is 122, systemic, blood pressure is 83/48 and the respiratory rate is 28. A Swan-Ganz pulmonary artery catheter is inserted and the cardiac output is 9.3 L/min. The pulmonary capillary wedge pressure is 11 mmHg and the SVR is 550 dynes-sec-cm^{-5}. What is this hemodynamic picture consistent with?**

Distributive shock, secondary to sepsis.

❍ **What is the diagnosis of a patient with the following hemodynamic profile on Swan-Ganz hemodynamic monitoring: cardiac output- 3.4 L/min, PCWP- 6 mmHg, SVR- 1990 dynes-sec-cm^{-5}?**

Hypovolemic shock.

❍ **A 71 year-old gentleman presents to the hospital with increasing shortness of breath, orthopnea, PND, and palpitations. He has a long history of recurrent CHF. His physical exam reveals bibasilar rales and he is hypotensive with a BP of 70/40 mmHg. Right heart catheterization**

reveals the following: cardiac output- 2.6 L/min, BSA 1.9 m^2, PCWP 34 mmHg, SVR 2100 dynes-sec-cm^{-5}, PA pressure of 65/36 mmHg, and a right atrial pressure of 37 mmHg. What is the diagnosis?

Cardiogenic shock from left heart failure.

❍ **In the above patient, what is the preferred drug of choice for this problem?**

Dobutamine. This will reduce SVR and PCWP and potentially increase cardiac output. However, it is doubtful this patient will survive, given the profound cardiac depression found in this patient.

❍ **In the above patient, what is the expected pulmonary artery oxygen saturation?**

40-50%. Remember, as cardiac output falls, oxygen extraction increases by the same proportion.

❍ **What is the most widely used hemodynamic measures of myocardial contractility?**

dP/dt, the maximum rate of rise of left ventricular systolic pressure.

❍ **What is left ventricular stroke work?**

Left ventricular stroke work is a reasonably good measure of left ventricular systolic function in the absence of left ventricular volume or pressure overload conditions, both of which may substantially increase calculated LV stroke work. Left ventricular stroke work (LVSW) may be calculated, in the absence of LV pressure tracings, by the following formula: LVSW = (mean aortic systolic mean pressure – mean pulmonary capillary wedge pressure) x stroke volume x .0136. This calculation is a close approximation of LV systolic function in the absence of severe mitral or aortic regurgitation. Since mean systemic arterial pressure closely approximates the mean aortic systolic pressure, one can use the following formula: LVSW = (mean systemic pressure – mean pulmonary capillary wedge pressure) x stroke volume (cardiac output/heart rate) x .0136.

❍ **What is the normal LVSW in adults?**

90 +/- 30 gm-m.

❍ **What is the LVSW in patients with dilated cardiomyopathy? In patients with severe LV failure?**

LVSW is often less than 40 gm-m in patients with dilated cardiomyopathy and often less than 25 gm-m in patients with severe left ventricular failure. When LVSW is less than 20 gm-m, death is expected.

❍ **What is the major drawback to LVSW as a measure of LV systolic function?**

LVSW is a measure of <u>total</u> LV systolic function and can be considered to be a reflection of myocardial contractility only when the ventricle is reasonably homogeneous in its composition, as in most patients with dilated cardiomyopathy. In patients with marked regional wall motion abnormalities, as in coronary artery disease, particularly after myocardial infarction, LVSW may be depressed even though there remain well perfused areas of myocardium with normal contractility.

❍ **What is the formula for LVSW when one has LV pressure tracing measurements?**

LVSW = (mean LV systolic pressure – mean LV diastolic pressure) x stroke volume x .0136.

❍ **What is the LV stroke work index (LVSWI)?**

The LVSW, indexed to body surface area. It normally ranges from 35 gm-m/M^2 to 70 gm-m/M^2.

❍ **What is the point where exercising muscle begins anaerobic metabolism?**

Anaerobic threshold (AT).

❍ **What does the O_2 pulse reflect?**

Stroke volume. Reduced in cardiac disease.

❍ **Why is a peak O_2 consumption less than 10 mls/kg/min an indication for heart transplant?**

When due to cardiac disease, this level shows severe impairment and predicts poor survival without intervention. Levels more than 20 indicate minimal functional impairment.

❍ **What are the negative effects of PEEP on cardiovascular function?**

PEEP may reduce cardiac output by reducing venous return, by increasing pulmonary vascular resistance, and by shifting the interventricular septum to the left, thus reducing the left ventricular end diastolic volume.

❍ **What are three ways that "best" PEEP can be determined?**

Compliance, oxygenation, and cardiac output.

❍ **What is the role of corticosteroids in ARDS?**

Several studies have failed to show any benefit for the use of steroids in ARDS. There is some evidence that there may be a danger in using steroids in ARDS associated with sepsis. There is some evidence to suggest that in certain cases, in the late phases of ARDS steroids may reduce the fibrosis associated with late ARDS.

❍ **What interventions have been shown to reduce the mortality of ARDS?**

Although a great number of studies have been done to reduce the mortality of ARDS, to date the only strong evidence for reduced mortality is in the computerized protocol for management of ventilator support. Other studies on a variety of interventions in the inflammatory cascade including prostaglandins and steroids have failed to show benefit. There is recent interest in the use of prone positioning for patients with ARDS.

❍ **What are the most common presenting findings in ARDS?**

Tachypnea and hypoxemia.

❍ **What are the NIH criteria for the diagnosis of ARDS?**

PaO_2/FiO_2 ratio < 200, bilateral infiltrates, wedge pressure < 18.

❍ **What is the cause of hypoxemia in ARDS?**

An increase in alveolar fluid causes reduced diffusion of oxygen into capillaries, thus increasing the shunt.

❍ **What is the mortality of ARDS?**

Most series show a mortality of 40-60%. Some research protocols have shown a reduction to 25-30%.

❍ **What are the most risk factors for ARDS?**

Sepsis, trauma, aspiration, multiple transfusions, shock, pulmonary contusions. However, many other systemic and local insults may trigger ARDS.

❍ **Why is the pulmonary artery wedge pressure an important feature in the diagnosis of ARDS?**

The presence of a significantly elevated wedge pressure implies that the pulmonary edema may be hydrostatic and therefore due to left ventricular dysfunction rather than alveolar or pulmonary dysfunction and ARDS— that is, noncardiogenic pulmonary edema.

❍ **Does PEEP improve ARDS?**

PEEP commonly improves oxygenation; however, it does not reduce the amount of total lung water, which is the marker for the amount of pulmonary edema present.

❍ **What is the distribution of pulmonary edema in ARDS?**

Routine chest x-ray appears to show a diffuse distribution. However, CAT scan studies reveal an increased involvement in the dependent portions of the lung fields.

❍ **What are the x-ray findings in ARDS?**

Diffuse ground-glass-like infiltrates that do not follow anatomical boundaries, usually bilateral.

❍ **What complications are associated with ARDS?**

Barotrauma leading to pneumothorax, pulmonary infection, pulmonary hypertension, multisystem organ failure.

❍ **What are the three phases of ARDS?**

Acute or exudative (up to 6 days), proliferative phase (4 to 10 days), chronic or fibrotic phase (after 7 days).

❍ **What are the cellular mediators involved in the development of ARDS?**

Macrophages-TNF, monocytes-il1, endothelial cells-arachidonic acid.

❍ **What is the role of PEEP in ARDS?**

Maintain alveolar inflation and functional residual capacity.

❍ **The most feared complication associated with Extra Corporeal Membrane Oxygenation?**

Intracranial hemorrhage.

❍ **The risks and complications of pericardiocentesis include?**

Cardiac tamponade, myocardial infarction, intra-abdominal injuries and pneumothorax.

❍ **Decompensated shock is characterized by?**

Hypotension and low cardiac output.

❍ **Oxygen delivery (DO_2) can be calculated using?**

Arterial oxygen content x cardiac output x 10.

❍ **Arterial oxygen content (ml O_2/dl blood) is calculated by using?**

Hemoglobin concentration (g/dl) x 1.34 ml O_2/gm hemoglobin x oxygen saturation.

❍ **In hypovolemia from hemorrhage, the blood pressure is maintained until?**

The blood volume falls by 25% to 30%.

❍ **The most important action of epinephrine when used during resuscitation is?**

Alpha-adrenergic effect = vasoconstriction.

❍ **The indications for calcium therapy include?**

Documented or suspected hypocalcemia, hyperkalemia, hypermagnesemia, and calcium channel blocker overdose.

❍ **The treatment of choice for patients with supraventricular tachycardia and cardiovascular compromise?**

Adenosine, but in the event that vascular access is not available quickly synchronized cardioversion becomes the treatment of choice.

❍ **When should atropine be used for the treatment of bradycardia?**

Only after adequate ventilation and oxygenation have been established, since hypoxemia is a common cause of bradycardia.

❍ **T/F: Defibrillation is indicated for the treatment of asystole.**

False. Defibrillation is the definitive treatment for ventricular fibrillation or pulseless ventricular tachycardia. The treatment for asystole is epinephrine.

❍ **After a cardiac arrest, the most common reason for poor perfusion is?**

Cardiogenic shock resulting from arrest-associated myocardial ischemia.

❍ **What are the only two pharmacologic agents that have been proven to improve survival in cardiac arrest?**

Epinephrine and atropine.

❍ **Of all of the components of cardiopulmonary resuscitation as outlined by ACLS protocol, which has the greatest impact on survival?**

Adequacy of chest compression to maintain sufficient coronary perfusion pressure to sustain myocardial viability.

❍ **What is the immediate treatment of choice in ventricular fibrillation?**

Immediate defibrillation, starting at 200 Joules. If unsuccessful, repeat at 300 Joules, and if still unsuccessful, repeat a third time at 360 Joules. If still unsuccessful, start CPR and achieve adequate ventillation with immediate intubation.

❍ **What is the treatment of choice for hemodynamically stable ventricular tachycardia?**

Intravenous bolus of lidocaine at 1 mg/kg, followed by an infusion of lidocaine at 2-4 mg/min. A repeat bolus should be given at .5 mg/kg, 15 minutes after the initial bolus.

❍ **In CPR, what is the ventilation to compression ratio for one rescuer? For two rescuers?**

1 rescuer: 2 breaths to 15 compressions
2 rescuers: 1 breath to 5 compressions

❍ **Non-traumatic cardiac arrest patients are most likely to be successfully resuscitated from what abnormal rhythm?**

Ventricular fibrillation. Success is time dependent, generally declining at a rate of 2-10% per minute.

❍ **How many deaths per year in the U.S. are due to cardiovascular disease?**

930,000, 43% of all deaths per year. More than 1/2 of all deaths occur in women. 2/3 of sudden deaths, due to CAD, take place outside the hospital, and most occur within 2 hours of the onset of symptoms.

❍ **In a patient with ventricular fibrillation, what regimen should be used in the administration of IV amiodarone?**

300 mg IV bolus followed by 150 mg IV bolus Q 5 minutes. The maximum dose is 2.2 grams per 24 hours.

❍ **What drug is used in the treatment of verapamil overdose?**

Calcium chloride.

❍ **If a defibrillator is available, what is the immediate treatment of a patient with ventricular fibrillation?**

Unsynchronized countershock at 200J.

❍ **What is the differential diagnosis of pulseless electrical activity?**

Tension pneumothorax, acidosis, MI, PE, OD, cardiac tamponade, hypoxia, hypovolemia, hyperkalemia and hypothermia (TAMPOT plus 4H is the pnemonic).

❍ **What is the differential diagnosis of asystole?**

Drug overdose, acidosis, hyperkalemia, hypothermia, hypokalemia, hypoxia.

❍ **How much myocardial damage from an acute myocardial infarction is necessary to result in congestive heart failure?**

Congestive heart failure is usually evident clinically if more than 25% of the left ventricle is infarcted.

❍ **How much functional loss of left ventricular myocardium is required to result in cardiogenic shock?**

40%.

❍ **What three secondary processes resulting in myocardial deterioration occur following acute myocardial infarction?**

Ventricular remodeling, typically following Q-wave infarctions; infarct expansion, occurring most frequently from anterior-apical infarctions and results in thinning of the left ventricular wall; and ventricular dilatation, an early and progressive response to acute myocardial infarction that is an important predictor of increased mortality following myocardial infarction.

❍ **What factors play a role in the peak incidence of myocardial infarction being from 6 AM to noon?**

Blood pressure, coronary arterial tone, blood viscosity, circulating catecholamines and platelet aggregability increase on awakening and assumption of an erect posture.

❍ **What is the most common cause of death related to acute myocardial infarction?**

Ventricular fibrillation, occurring within the first hour following symptoms.

❍ **What percentage of patients with acute myocardial infarction develop cardiogenic shock?**

10%.

❍ **What percentage of patients who are found to have myocardial infarction by other objective means, such as cardiac enzymes or radionuclide imaging studies, have normal initial ECGs?**

10%.

❍ **What is the mortality among patients with their first myocardial infarction?**

2-3% in patients under 40 years of age, 7-10% in patients between 70-80 years of age and 32% in patients older than 80 years of age.

❍ **A 60 year-old patient suffers an acute inferior myocardial infarction. Three hours after he arrives in the hospital, he develops ventricular fibrillation and is successfully defibrillated back to normal sinus rhythm within 30 seconds. He makes a full recovery and has no further post-MI complications. What does his ventricular fibrillation episode indicate with regard to his subsequent risk of sudden death?**

This episode has no bearing on his subsequent risk of sudden death. Ventricular fibrillation in the immediate setting of an acute myocardial infarction has no prognostic significance.

❍ **A 65 year-old female presents to the hospital with sudden crushing chest discomfort and moderate shortness of breath. Her initial ECG reveals 2mm ST depression in leads V1-V4 with inverted T waves. She has bibasilar rales in the lower half of both lungs on ausculatation. CXR reveals moderate pulmonary edema. Serial ECGs and CPKs confirm a non-Q wave myocardial infarction. With diuretics, her pulmonary edema resolves within 24 hours. What is the most appropriate management strategy at this point?**

Cardiac catheterization with coronary angiography. A non-Q wave MI that results in pulmonary edema signifies a large amount of myocardium at risk for reinfarction within the next year.

❍ **What arrhythmias that occur in patients with acute myocardial infarction require temporary pacing?**

Complete heart block (3° AV block); new LBBB; new bifasicular block; marked sinus bradycardia with ischemic pain, hypotension, CHF, frequent PVC's or syncope despite atropine; and Mobitz II type 2° AV block.

❍ **A 54 year old gentleman admitted two days ago with an acute anterolateral myocardial infarction suddenly develops atrial fibrillation with a ventricular rate of 135/min. He subsquently complains of substernal chest discomfort. His BP is 135/70. What is the most appropriate immediate action to be taken?**

Synchronized DC cardioversion.

❍ **What percentage of patients with acute myocardial infarction develop paroxysmal atrial fibrilllation?**

10-15%.

❍ **T/F: The presence of occasional PVCs is a reliable predictor of ventricular fibrillation following acute myocardial infarction.**

False.

❍ **A 58 year-old gentleman is admitted with an acute anteroseptal myocardial infarction. He is in pulmonary edema clinically, confirmed by CXR. His blood pressure is 122/76, his HR is 122. Despite two doses of 80 mg of intravenous furosemide, he remains in pulmonary edema. A Swan-Ganz pulmonary artery catheter is inserted and his initial hemodynamics reveal a cardiac output of 3.1 L/min and a pulmonary capillary wedge pressure of 27 mmHg. What is the most appropriate pharmacologic agent in this setting?**

Intravenous Dobutamine, at a dose of 5 to 20 mcg/kg/min.

❍ **What is the mortality of cardiogenic shock in acute myocardial infarction?**

>70%.

❍ **What is the incidence of rupture of the free wall of the left ventricle in patients with acute myocardial infarction?**

10%. It is almost always fatal, occurring between 1 and 5 days following infarction.

❍ **What percentage of patients with acute myocardial infarction develop left ventricular aneurysms?**

10%. 80% of LV aneurysms are located in the anterior-apical segment and result from occlusion of the left anterior descending artery.

❍ **What percentage of patients with acute anterior-apical Q wave infarctions develop LV mural thrombi?**

50%. Over half develop mural thrombi within the first 24 hours.

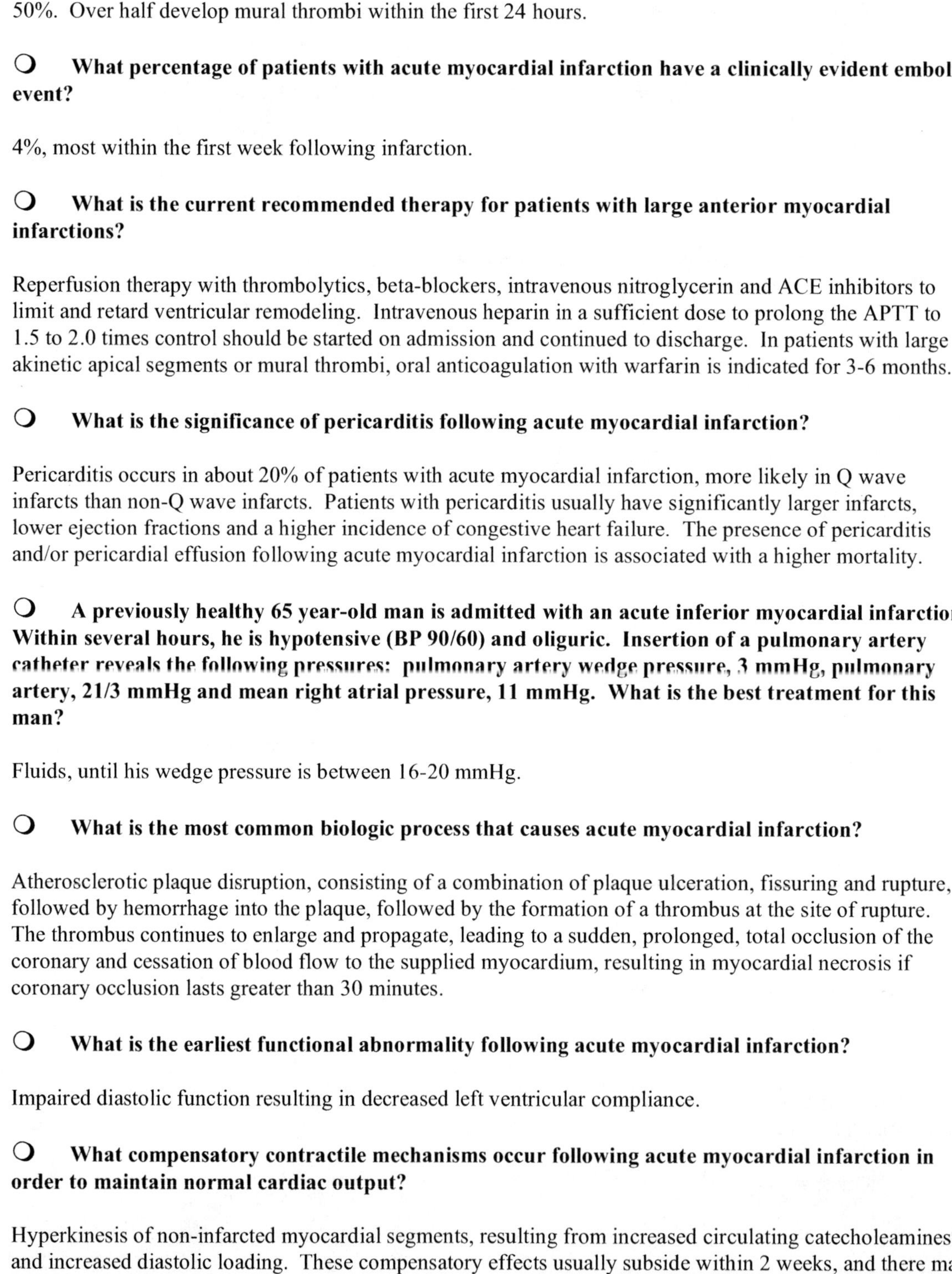

❍ **What percentage of patients with acute myocardial infarction have a clinically evident embolic event?**

4%, most within the first week following infarction.

❍ **What is the current recommended therapy for patients with large anterior myocardial infarctions?**

Reperfusion therapy with thrombolytics, beta-blockers, intravenous nitroglycerin and ACE inhibitors to limit and retard ventricular remodeling. Intravenous heparin in a sufficient dose to prolong the APTT to 1.5 to 2.0 times control should be started on admission and continued to discharge. In patients with large akinetic apical segments or mural thrombi, oral anticoagulation with warfarin is indicated for 3-6 months.

❍ **What is the significance of pericarditis following acute myocardial infarction?**

Pericarditis occurs in about 20% of patients with acute myocardial infarction, more likely in Q wave infarcts than non-Q wave infarcts. Patients with pericarditis usually have significantly larger infarcts, lower ejection fractions and a higher incidence of congestive heart failure. The presence of pericarditis and/or pericardial effusion following acute myocardial infarction is associated with a higher mortality.

❍ **A previously healthy 65 year-old man is admitted with an acute inferior myocardial infarction. Within several hours, he is hypotensive (BP 90/60) and oliguric. Insertion of a pulmonary artery catheter reveals the following pressures: pulmonary artery wedge pressure, 3 mmHg, pulmonary artery, 21/3 mmHg and mean right atrial pressure, 11 mmHg. What is the best treatment for this man?**

Fluids, until his wedge pressure is between 16-20 mmHg.

❍ **What is the most common biologic process that causes acute myocardial infarction?**

Atherosclerotic plaque disruption, consisting of a combination of plaque ulceration, fissuring and rupture, followed by hemorrhage into the plaque, followed by the formation of a thrombus at the site of rupture. The thrombus continues to enlarge and propagate, leading to a sudden, prolonged, total occlusion of the coronary and cessation of blood flow to the supplied myocardium, resulting in myocardial necrosis if coronary occlusion lasts greater than 30 minutes.

❍ **What is the earliest functional abnormality following acute myocardial infarction?**

Impaired diastolic function resulting in decreased left ventricular compliance.

❍ **What compensatory contractile mechanisms occur following acute myocardial infarction in order to maintain normal cardiac output?**

Hyperkinesis of non-infarcted myocardial segments, resulting from increased circulating catecholeamines and increased diastolic loading. These compensatory effects usually subside within 2 weeks, and there may be some recovery of wall motion of the infarcted segment, particularly if there was early reperfusion.

❍ **Infarct expansion occurs most commonly in what type of myocardial infarctions?**

Antero-apical infarction, resulting in thinning of the left ventricular wall. It is associated with a higher incidence of complications such as congestive heart failure, cardiac rupture and left ventricular aneurysm.

❍ **What physiologic changes that are affected by circadian variation play a role in an increased incidence of myocardial infarction from 6 A.M. to noon?**

Increased blood pressure, increased coronary arterial tone, increased circulating catecholamines and increased platelet aggregability.

❍ **What two groups of patients are more likely to present with "silent" myocardial infarction?**

Patients with diabetes mellitus and the elderly.

❍ **Moderate to heavy physical exertion and emotional stress or excitement are temporally related to the onset of symptoms in what percentage of patients with acute myocardial infarction?**

About 50%.

❍ **What is the median time between onset of symptoms and arrival at a hospital in patients with acute myocardial infarction?**

Two to five hours.

❍ **What is the most useful test for the immediate confirmation of the diagnosis of acute myocardial infarction?**

The electrocardiogram. It is diagnostic of acute myocardial infarction in about two-thirds of patients.

❍ **What percentage of patients with confirmed acute myocardial infarction, determined by other objective means, have a normal initial ECG?**

10%.

❍ **What is the normal sequential changes in the electrocardiogram during the first several days following a wave myocardial infarction?**

1) "Hyperacute," symmetrical, peaked T waves, 2) ST-segment elevation, 3) loss of R wave amplitude in the infarct-related leads, 4) development of Q waves in the infarct-related leads, 5) return of the ST-segment to baseline, and 6) progressive inversion of the T wave.

❍ **What is the usual time sequence of the onset, peak and duration of the elevation of CK-MB levels in an acute myocardial infarction?**

CK-MB levels are usually elevated within 4-6 hours following the onset of acute myocardial infarction, peak at approximately 18-24 hours and usually return to normal at 36-48 hours following an uncomplicated infarction.

❍ **At what time frame do LDH levels peak following acute myocardial infarction?**

24-48 hours.

❍ **What isoforms or subforms of CK-MB have been identified, and how are they useful in detecting acute myocardial infarction?**

CK-MB activity is equally divided between a plasma form (MB-1) and a tissue form (MB-2). An increase in the normal 1 to 1 ratio of MB-2 to MB-1 to >1.5 has been shown to correlate highly with acute myocardial infarction. It is also useful in differentiating myocardial necrosis from insignificant elevation of total CK-MB in the presence of a normal total CK. An increase in the ratio of CK-MM3 (tissue form) to CK-MM1 and CK-MM2 (plasma forms) is also useful in the early and reliable diagnosis of acute myocardial infarction. Other biochemical methods of early detection of acute myocardial infarction include myoglobin and cardiac troponin T.

❍ **What is the most reliable and useful method of evaluating the extent of an acute myocardial infarction?**

Two-dimensional echocardiography.

❍ **What is the most important strategy for treating patients with acute myocardial infarction?**

Early reperfusion with either intravenous thrombolytic therapy or immediate primary percutaneous transluminal coronary angioplasty (PTCA).

❍ **How much myocardial necrosis in an acute Q wave myocardial infarction is completed within 1 hour after the onset of symptoms? Within 2 hours? Within 4 hours?**

50%, 75% and 95% percent, respectively.

❍ **What are the absolute contraindications to intravenous thrombolytic therapy?**

Major surgery, organ biopsy or major trauma within 2 weeks; significant GI or GU bleeding within 2 months; known or suspected aortic dissection; known or suspected pericarditis; known intracranial tumor; previous neurosurgery or hemorrhagic cerebrovascular accident at any time; acute severe hypertension (>200 mmHg systolic or >120 mmHg diastolic; head trauma within one month; thrombotic cerebrovascular accident within two months and active internal bleeding, excluding menses.

❍ **What are the relative contraindications to intravenous thrombolytic therapy?**

Mild to moderate hypertension (>180 mmHg systolic and/or >110 mmHg diastolic); cardiopulmonary resuscitation for < 10 minutes; puncture of non-compressible vessel; recent TIAs; thrombotic cerebrovascular accident between 2 to 6 months ago; diabetic retinopathy; active peptic ulcer; known bleeding diathesis or current anticoagulant usage; pregnancy; and exposure to streptokinase or APSAC within the last 6-9 months (does not apply to prospective t-PA administration).

❍ **What is the mortality rate of patients under the age of 40 with their first myocardial infarction?**

2-4%.

❍ **What is the mortality rate of patients over age 80 with their first myocardial infarction?**

25-35%.

❍ **Which age group has the greatest reduction in mortality following the administration of thrombolytic therapy in the presence of an acute myocardial infarction?**

Patients over the age of 65, and more specifically, those patients over age 75.

❍ **Previously, there had been concerns over increased likelihood of intracranial hemorrhage following the administration of thrombolytic therapy in patients over age 75. What are the respective incidences of intracranial hemorrhage following the administration of thrombolytic therapy in patients under age 75 and over age 75?**

The overall incidence of intracranial hemorrhage in patients under age 75 is 1%, slightly higher with t-PA, as opposed to streptokinase or APSAC. The overall incidence of intracranial hemorrhage in patients over age 75 is 1.3%, again slightly higher with t-PA, as opposed to streptokinase or APSAC.

❍ **What are the two most common and serious side effects of streptokinase and APSAC?**

Hypotension and hypersensitivity reaction, which is antigen mediated and manifested by vomiting, itching and swelling.

❍ **What is the rethrombosis rate following the administration of t-PA without the concomitant use of intravenous heparin?**

20-30%.

❍ **What is the rethrombosis rate following the adminstration of streptokinase in the absence of intravenous heparin adminstration following the completion of streptokinase therapy?**

15-20%.

❍ **What is the rethrombosis rate following the adminstration of APSAC in the absence of subsequent intravenous heparin use?**

10%.

❍ **What is the rationale for intravenous heparin administration being started concomitantly with t-PA administration?**

Because the plasma clearance time of t-PA is 4-8 minutes, the coronary rethrombosis rate in the absence of intravenous heparin is significantly increased and ranges between 20-30%. With concomitant heparin administration and continued heparinization for at least 24 hours following t-PA therapy, the coronary rethrombosis rate is reduced to approximately 5-10%.

❍ **What is the 90-minute infarct-related coronary artery patency rate following the adminstration of "front-loaded" or accelerated intravenous t-PA in acute myocardial infarction, assuming concomitant administration of intravenous heparin and oral aspirin?**

80-90%.

❍ **What is the 90-minute infarct-related coronary artery patency rate following the adminstration of intravenous streptokinase in acute myocardial infarction, assuming concomitant aspirin administration?**

55-70%.

❍ **What is the 90-minute infarct-related coronary artery patency rate following the administration of intravenous APSAC in acute myocardial infarction, assuming concomitant aspirin adminstration?**

70-80%.

❍ **In the GUSTO-1 trial, what was the percentage of grade TIMI-3 (normal) flow occurring in infarct-related arteries following the administration of accelerated t-PA with intravenous heparin, compared to streptokinase and intravenous heparin?**

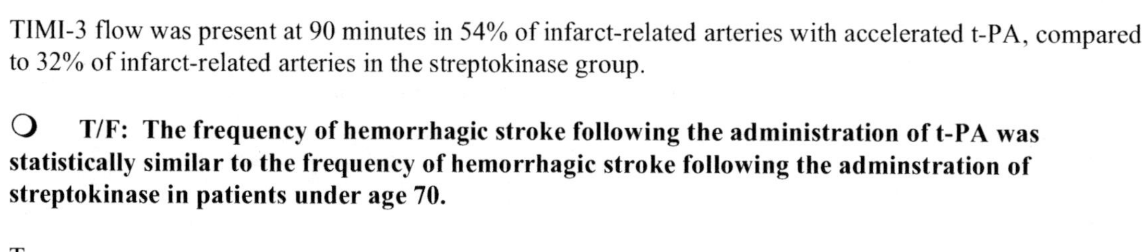

TIMI-3 flow was present at 90 minutes in 54% of infarct-related arteries with accelerated t-PA, compared to 32% of infarct-related arteries in the streptokinase group.

❍ **T/F: The frequency of hemorrhagic stroke following the administration of t-PA was statistically similar to the frequency of hemorrhagic stroke following the adminstration of streptokinase in patients under age 70.**

True.

❍ **T/F: The frequency of hemorrhagic stroke following the adminstration of t-PA was statistically similar to the frequency of hemorrhagic stroke following the adminstration of streptokinase in patients over age 75.**

False. The incidence of hemorrhagic stroke following the adminstration of t-PA was statistically higher than that following the adminstration of streptokinase. The overall incidence of hemorrhagic stroke in patients over age 75 receiving streptokinase is 1.1%, and 1.5% in patients over age 75 receiving t-PA.

❍ **Which of the thrombolytic agents, administered to patients with acute myocardial infarction, preserves left ventricular function the most?**

Except for the GUSTO-1 trial, left ventricular function, measured within the first week, as well as after one month, was similar, regardless of the thrombolytic agent used. In the GUSTO-1 trial, left ventricular function paralleled the patency rates at 90 minutes, and the group that received accelerated t-PA and intravenous heparin had slightly better left ventricular function, post-infarct, than the group that received streptokinase or the combination of streptokinase and standard dose t PA.

❍ **Which adjunctive pharmacologic therapies have been shown to improve both short-term and long-term survival following acute myocadial infarction?**

Aspirin, beta-blockers and ACE inhibitors, when given within the first 24 hours after the onset of symptoms, have all been shown to improve short-term survival following an acute myocardial infarction. Aspirin, beta-blockers and ACE inhibitors, when started between 24 hours and seven days following an acute myocardial infarction, have been shown to improve long-term survival following an acute myocardial infarction. Intravenous heparin, when administered with or immediately after thrombolytic therapy, has been shown to improve short-term survival following an acute myocardial infarction. Calcium channel blockers, nitroglycerin or nitrates, and intravenous or oral magnesium have not been shown to improve either short-term or long-term survival in acute myocardial infarction.

❍ **A 57 year-old gentleman with hypertension and diabetes mellitus presents to your hospital's Emergency Department with abrupt onset of crushing substernal chest pressure radiating to the jaw. His blood pressure is 75/40, his pulse is 132, his respiratory rate is 36. His lung exam reveals bibasilar rales in the lower half of both lungs, and he has both severe JVD and an S3 gallop. His electrocardiogram shows 4 mm ST segment elevation in leads V1 through V6. He has never had a myocardial infarction in the past. His symptoms began 45 minutes ago. What should be the favored treatment regimen for this patient?**

If your hospital has a catheterization laboratory and it is unoccupied, this patient should undergo immediate coronary angiography with immediate PTCA of the culprit vessel. If your hospital does not have a catheterization lab, thombolytic therapy should be immediately administered and hemodynamic support with an intra-aortic balloon counterpulsation should be strongly considered.

❍ **A 63 year-old gentleman presents to your hospital with substernal chest tightness of 45 minutes duration. His electrocardiogram reveals 1.5 mm ST depression in leads I, aVL, and V4-V6. Should you give him thrombolytic therapy if he has no contraindications?**

No. Patients with non-Q wave myocardial infarctions and those with unstable angina, who eventually rule out for myocardial infarction, do not appear to benefit from thrombolytic therapy. These patients should be started on intravenous heparin, given aspirin, and if they do not have pulmonary edema on initial presentation, should be started on Diltiazem.

❍ **What is the acute mortality of patients with non-Q wave myocardial infarction?**

2-3%, as opposed to 10% for Q wave infarction.

❍ **What percentage of patients with acute myocardial infarction will develop transient supraventricular arrhythmias?**

33%.

❍ **What percentage of patients with acute myocardial infarction develop atrial fibrillation?**

10-15%.

❍ **What is the preferred agent of choice in the treatment of atrial fibrillation occurring in the setting of acute myocardial infarction?**

Beta-blockers. Alternative agents, such as procainamide or amiodarone, are particularly useful in converting atrial fibrillation to sinus rhythm.

❍ **A 60 year-old woman presents to your hospital with substernal chest tightness and her electrocardiogram reveals acute ST elevation in the anterior leads, consistent with an acute myocardial infarction. She is given aspirin, t-PA, beta-blockers and heparin. She is hemodynamically stable and not in heart failure. Her cardiac monitor shows 4-6 PVCs per minute with rare couplets. Should she receive lidocaine "prophylactically"?**

No. The risk-benefit ratio is unfavorable in this setting, and occasional PVCs are an unreliable predictor of ventricular fibrillation following an acute myocardial infarction. Lidocaine may also block the "escape" rhythm of accelerated idioventricular rhythm that occurs with coronary reperfusion, thus, creating a potentially life-threatening event.

❍ **What is the percentage of rupture of the free wall of the left ventricle occurring in patients who die as a result of acute myocardial infarction?**

10%. This event occurs between 1 and 5 days following infarction and is almost always fatal.

❍ **A 66 year-old woman has sudden onset of substernal chest pressure and comes to the Emergency Department. Her electrocardiogram and cardiac enzymes confirm an acute anterior myocardial infarction. On admission, she is hemodynamically stable, but on day 3, she develops sudden shortness of breath and she is noted to have a blood pressure of 85/50. On physical exam, she is noted to have an loud apical holosystolic murmur, bibasilar rales and an S3 gallop at the apex. A Swan-Ganz pulmonary artery catheter is placed and the pulmonary capillary wedge pressure tracing shows prominent V waves. What is the diagnosis?**

Partial or total rupture of a papillary muscle with severe mitral insufficiency.

❍ **In the above patient, what is the best way to confirm the diagnosis?**

Two-dimensional and color flow Doppler echocardiography.

❍ **In the above patient, what is the preferred treatment?**

Aggressive vasodilator therapy, insertion of an intra-aortic balloon counterpulsation device and then emergent repair of the papillary muscle and mitral valve apparatus. Mortality with medical treatment alone in this setting is 80-90%.

❍ **Pericarditis occurs in what percentage of patients with acute myocardial infarction?**

10-20%, as defined by the presence of a friction rub.

❍ **What is the significance of infarct-related pericarditis?**

Patients with infarct-related pericarditis usually have larger infarcts, have lower post-MI ejection fractions, and a higher incidence of congestive heart failure and serious ventricular arrhythmias. Patients with infarct-related pericarditis and/or the presence of pericardial effusion have a higher mortality, again related to infarct size.

❍ **What is the most important prognostic determinant following acute myocardial infarction?**

Infarct size.

❍ **What is the most important post-infarct diagnostic strategy following acute myocardial infarction?**

Pre discharge non-invasive testing to risk stratify patients into those low-risk and those who are at high risk to develop non-fatal or fatal reinfarction or sudden death from arrhythmias. Many advocate pre-discharge submaximal treadmill testing, particularly in those who received thrombolytic therapy, so long as the patient did not have post-infarct angina, congestive heart failure, hypotension or serious arrythmias. Those patients with post-infarct angina, congestive heart failure, post-infarct silent ischemia as measured by ST depression and serious arrhythmias, should undergo pre-discharge cardiac catheterization and/or further intervention (e.g., antiarrhythmic therapy, PTCA or CABG). Some advocate symptom-limited treadmill exercise testing, instead of submaximal testing, before discharge, and there is good evidence that this is safe. Symptom-limited stress testing, either on a treadmill, or pharmacologic stress, with supplementary imaging techniques using technetium-99m sestamibi or thallium, or echocardiographgy, should be carried out between 10 days and 6 weeks following acute myocardial infarction in those patients deemed low-risk at discharge. Those patients with abnormal post-infarct stress tests should be referred for cardiac catheterization and, if warranted, revascularization.

❍ **What percentage of patients who received thrombolytic therapy for acute myocardial infarction have single vessel disease and a total occlusion of the infarct-related artery?**

15%.

❍ **What percentage of patients who received thrombolytic therapy for acute myocardial infarction have a patent infarct-related artery with a less than 50% stenosis?**

15%.

❍ **What percentage of patients who received thrombolytic therapy for acute myocardial infarction have single vessel disease and > 50% stenosis in the infarct-related artery?**

35%.

❍ **What percentage of patients who received thrombolytic therapy for acute myocardial**

infarction have a patent infarct related vessel and 2- or 3-vessel disease?

30%.

❍ **What percentage of patients with acute myocardial infarction, who receive thrombolytic therapy, have left main disease and a patent infarct-related artery?**

5%.

❍ **What is the concept of "stunned myocardium"?**

This refers to muscle that is hypocontractile as a result of a brief ischemic insult but is still viable. In this situation, progressive recovery of contractile function following reperfusion may occur several hours to weeks after the ischemic insult. This recovery occurs without revascularization from PTCA or CABG.

❍ **What is the concept of "hibernating myocardium"?**

Hibernating myocardium refers to a chronically hypoperfused and hypocontractile left ventricular segment that improves functionally only after coronary revascularization.

❍ **Are thrombolytic agents effective in non-Q wave MI?**

No, there is no evidence to support their use. In fact, some published data suggest that their use may be detrimental.

❍ **What is the prognosis of patients presenting with Q wave MI complicated by acute mitral regurgitation?**

Prognosis is quite compromised with an approximate one-year survival of only 50%.

❍ **A 68 year old man with a history of angina at three blocks exertion presents with onset of chest pain typical of his agnina occurring after breakfast. He says this is his usual pain except that it has never occurred at rest. Physical exam is unremarkable, and the ECG reveals only non-specific findings. His pain is relieved with IV nitroglycerine and a dose of metoprolol. Laboratory findings: Total CK 110 (upper limit of normal is 150), CK-MB is 10% (upper lilmit of normal is 6%). What is the patients prognonis?**

The patient appears to have unstable angina and does not meet the criteria for thrombolhtic therapy. However, the CK findings suggest he actually developed a non-Q wave MI. The diagnosis remains unclear in this circumstance. Whatever the diagnosis, the prognosis is worse in these patients compared to that of patients with UA without CK-MB elevation. Thus, these patients are probably better off if evaluated as if the diagnosis is non-Q wave MI.

❍ **A 77 year-old man presents complaining of chest pain. He states that he was playing racquet-ball, and slipped and hit his head on the wall. After this he noted the onset of chest pain radiating to the arm. A hot shower did not relieve his symptoms. He notes that he has continued to have dull ache in his chest. He also reports an episode of diaphoresis after the shower and mild nausea. ECG reveals acute anterior wall MI. What would you do to treat him?**

Administer aspirin immediately. The choice for additional therapy is complicated by the presence of head trauma. In the proper setting, direct PTCA is the treatment of choice, since it produces higher TIMI-3 flow rates and defines the coronary anatomy, with lower stroke risk. The benefits of direct PTCA over thrombolytic therapy, while still debated, required a high volume operator and access to a lab within 60-90 minutes. If direct PTCA was not available for this patient, the decision to give thrombolytic therapy is a difficult one.

❍ **A 58 year-old woman without past medical history presents with complaints of one day of dull ache in the center of her chest that is unrelieved with aspirin or antacids. She states that the day prior to admission she had about three hours of severe discomfort in the chest associated with sweating which resolved spontaneously and she is now left with the symptoms described. Her blood pressure is 120/80, pulse is 100 and she is mildly diaphoretic. A pan-systolic murmur is heard at the left sternal border. Her lungs are clear. ECG reveals Q-Waves in leads VI-V4. Over the next twelve hours, you note that she becomes cold and clammy to palpation with signs of decreased peripheral perfusion. Her lungs remain clear. What is the diagnosis?**

Acute ventricular septal defect. Patients with acute mitral regurgitation usually have pulmonary congestion, making this diagnosis less likely. Risk factors for development of VSD include: female gender and hypertension. Despite pathological reports that VSD most often occurs about day 4 post-myocardial infarction, clinical observations suggest that the risk is higher in the first 24 hours. Definitive treatment is surgical, but operative mortality ranges from 20 to 70%. The diagnosis should be confirmed by echocardiography. Following this, vasodilator therapy with nitroprusside and insertion of an intra-aortic balloon-pump and Swan-Ganz catheter should be performed.

❍ **What affects ventricular remodeling?**

Ventricular remodeling is the change in size, shape and thickness of both the infarcted and non-infarcted regions of myocardium. The primary factors determining remodeling are: infarct size, scar formation and left ventricular filling pressure. The contribution of the latter may be part of the explanation of the effect of ace inhibitors in preserving left ventricular function when administered in the peri-infarct setting.

❍ **What is infarct expansion?**

An increase in the size of the infarct zone unrelated to additional myocardial necrosis. Causes may include slippage of the muscle bundles, disruption of the normal cellular array and tissue loss in the infarct zone. This occurs almost exclusively in transmural MIs, is more common in anterior infarction, and the degree of expansion may be related to pre-existing wall thickness (hypertrophy may be protective). Infarct expansion has been shown to be associated with increased mortality and increased incidence of non-fatal complications.

❍ **What are the major precipitants of AMI?**

In over half of patients with AMI, no precipitantant can be indentified. However, some precipitatory factors which have been identified include emotional stress, surgical procedures, neurological disturbances and perhaps extreme physical excertion. Circadian changes in plasma catecholamines and cortisol may also play a precipitatory role.

❍ **What is the most common presenting symptoms of AMI?**

Chest pain. Unlike aortic dissectioin, this pain often waxes and wanes, and over time will become severe. It usually lasts greater than 30 minutes and is frequently described as crushing, constricting, or as pressure. The pain is typically retrosternal and frequently radiates to the jaw and the ulnar aspect of the left arm. In some patients, particularly the elderly, AMI may present as a sumptoms of acute left ventricular failure rather than chest pain.

❍ **What are the other typical symptoms of AMI?**

Diaphoresis, apprehension, sense of doom, nausea and vomiting, which occur in greater than 50% of patients with transmural infarction. These latter symptoms, and perhaps the others to some extent, occur presumably due to the Bezold-Jarisch reflex. Nausea and vomiting occur more frequently in inferior myocardial infarction.

❍ **What are the chief differential diagnoses of AMI?**

Acute pericarditis, aortic dissection and acute GI illness. Acute pulmonary embolism and costochondritis are also frequently considered in the differential.

❍ **What are the most common atypical presentations of AMI?**

Congestive heart failure, angina without a prolonged or severe episode and atypical pain location.

❍ **What is a silent AMI?**

Population studies suggest that 20 to 60% of non-fatal MIs are unrecognized by the patient and are found on subsequent routine ECG. About one-half of these MIs are truly silent with no identifiable symptoms recalled by the patient. Unrecognized or silent infarction occurs more often in patients without previous anginal syndromes and is more common in diabetics and hypertensive patients.

❍ **What are the most common physical findings in AMI?**

There really aren't any, and findings depend upon the absence or presence of actue complications such as congestive heart failure, acute mitral regurgitation or cardiogenic shock. Most patients will appear to be in some distress. Of note, a fourth heart sound is almost universally present in ptients with acute MI.

❍ **Describe the chactaresistic pattern of creatine phospkokinase (CK-MB) elevation in AMI.**

CK exceeds normal levels in 4 to 8 hours after onset of MI. The mean peak for CK is 24 hours, but can range from 8 to 58 hours. Peak levels occur earlier in patients who receive reperfusion therapy, with mean peak CK rise occurring at approximately 12 hours. In gnereal, CK levels normalize 3 to 4 days after onset of pain.

❍ **What are the main causes of false positive CK elevation?**

Muscle disease, alcohol intoxication, diabetes mellitus, skeletal muscle trauma, vigorous exercise, convulsion, PE and thoracic outlet syndrome.

❍ **Desribe the characteristics pattern of lactate dehydrogenase (LDH) elevation after onset of AMI.**

Levels exceed normal by 24 to 48 hours after AMI onset, peak 3 to 6 days after onset and normalize 8 to 14 days after onset. Total LDH, while sensitive, is not specific. Fractionation into its isoforms increases specificity, since myocardium contains primarily LDH-1, where other sources contain primarily the other LDH isoforms. Thus, an LDH-1 to LDH-2 ratio of greater than 1.0 is a commonly used cutoff for diagnosing recent MI. Use of LDH analysis should be limited to those patients with normal CK measurements.

❍ **What other serum markers are important in diagnosing AMI?**

Recently, it has been shown that the Troponins demonstrate high concordance with CK-MB, and they appear a bit earlier in the course of MI. Also, subsets of the Troponins are highly specific for myocardial damage. Lastly, recent published data suggest that the amount of Troponins released may be an independent marker of survival.

❍ **What are the most common findings on chest X-ray in AMI?**

The chest X-ray is often normal, but pulmonary vascular congestion and cardiomegaly are the most common abnormalities found.

❍ **How sensitive is the ECG for detecting AMI?**

The initial ECG is 50 to 70% sensitive for AMI. Serial ECGs increase the sensitively to about 80%. The presenting ECG is important in determining the acute treatment. All patients with suspected AMI should receive aspirin. ST-elevation AMI or new left bundle branch block are generally considered for reperfusion therapy.

❍ **What defines high risk EDG changes in AMI?**

Anterior location, previous MI and complex ectopy.

❍ **What is the differential diagnosis of "ischemia at a distance"?**

ST-depression in a territory subtended by a coronary artery other than the one presumed to be responsible for the ST elevation diagnostic of MI is termed ischemia at adistance. The differential diagnosis: true ischemia, reciprocal ECG changes without ischemia or, in the case of anterior ST depression with inferior infarction, posterior wall infarction.

Importantly, differentiation cannot be reliable made by ECG or even vectorcardiography. Surprisingly, regardless of whether the ECG changes represent ischemia in another territory or electrocardiographic changes only, they imply a worse prognosis.

❍ **Does the use of thrombolytic therapy in the pre-hospital setting reseul in better reperfusion rates?**

Probably not. Although not well studied, data from several trials suggest that a thorough pre-hospital assessment, including 12 lead ECG, which prepares the receiving Emergency Department for the patient, saves enough time that pre-hospital thrombolysis is unnecessary. There are some trials however, which did show some advantage to pre-hospital thrombolytic administration. In addition, where a hospital is greater than 60 minutes away, pre-hospital thrombolysis may be advantageous.

❍ **What factors contribute to defining patients at high risk for complications from thrombolytic therapy? (This is <u>not</u> the same as contraindications).**

Advanced age, systollic blood pressure greater than 200 and/or diastolic blood pressure greater than 110 that is not effectively lowered with medical therapy in the emergency depaprtment, history of definite stroke and recent surgery. There are many other factors which add incremental risk, such as CHF, hypotension and anterior locations, to name a few. It should be noted that high risk patients receive the greatest benefits from thrombolytic therapy.

❍ **What are key findings of the GUSTO-I trial as related to choice of thrombolytic agent?**

GUSTO-I showed that accelerated t-PA provided a 14.5% relative risk reduction in 30 day mortality compared with streptokinase. The absolute risk reduction for mortality was 1%. This was seen in patients receiving thrombolytic therapy within 4 hours of onset of chest pain. Stroke occurred slightly less frequently in streptokinase-treated patients, and the difference reached statistical significance in patients greater than 75 years of age.

❍ **Routine use of oxygen is or is not beneficial in acute MI?**

The rationale is that hypoxemia is bad for myocardial necrosis and that ventilation perfusion mismatch is common in patients with acute MI, particularly after heparin administration. However, the routine use of oxygen in non-hyproxemic patients has not been proven beneficial. Regardless, most centers recommended routine use of oxygen per 6 to 12 hours to ensure adequate oxygenation of the patient.

❍ **What are the major contraindications to beta-blocker therapy in AMI?**

All patients with AMI should be considered for beta-blocker therapy, and only patients with a major contra-indication should be excluded. These contraindications include pulmonary edema with rales greater than one-third of the lung fields, marked hypotension, PR-interval greater than 24 seconds or advanced hear block, bradycardia (heart rate less than 55-60 bpm) or known bronchospasm (active or history of severe bronchospasm). Several studies have repeatedly shown that beta-blocker therapy reduces mortality and recurrent ischemia when administered early in acute myocardial infarction.

❍ **Which agent for the treatment of AMI has the best cost-benefit ratio with regard to improved survival?**

Aspirin. When all MIs are considered, overall acute mortality is about 13 to 14%. Administration of aspirin reduces this to about 10 to 11% (a relative reduction of about 20%). The only thrombolytic agent studied without concomitant aspirin use was streptokinase, which reduced mortality to about 10.4% The combination of aspirin plus thrombolytic agent has reduced overall mortality to 7-8 %.

❍ **What are the indications for temporary transvenous pacing in AMI?**

Temporary pacing is indicated in patients at high risk with developing complete heart block, particularly new bifascicular bundle branch block or LBBB. Patients who develop a systole, Mobitz type II and complete heart block will may also benefit from temporary transvenous pacing. It should be noted, however, that the use of temporary pacing has never been statistically proven to improve prognosis.

❍ **What is the most common sustained supraventricular arrhythmia in AMI?**

Sinus tachycardia. About one-third of patients will develop sinus tachycardia in the first days after acute AMI. The most common causes are anxiety, persistent pain, and left ventricular failure.

❍ **What is the least common sustained supraventricular arrhythmia AMI?**

Atrial flutter, occurring in 1-3%.

❍ **What is the most common sustained arrhythmia in AMI?**

Probably ventricular fibrillation, occurring in up to 10% of patients, and is seen more commonly in transmural infarction. The majority (60%) of VF events in AMI patients occur within 4 to 6 hours, and 80% by 12 hours. This "primary" VF have been thought not to affect prognosis when treated rapidly, but some investigators have suggested this may indicate a worse prognosis.

❍ **What is the best treatment for accelerated idioventricular rhythm (AIVR)?**

AIVR, characterized by a wide QRS rhythm with a rate faster than the atrial rate and less than 150 bpm, should not be treated, unless associated with a very significant drop in blood pressure. This rhythm is seen frequently in the early stages of AMI and occurs more often in patients with early reperfusion. However, it is neither sensitive nor specific enough to be considered a reliable marker for reperfusion.

❍ **What is reperfusion injury?**

The acceleration of myocardial cell necrosis after reperfusion. It is characterized by rapid cellular swelling and wide spread architectural disruption. It is likely the acceleration of necrosis occurs in cells already destined to die, but it is possible that reperfusion may cause necrosis of reversably injured myocardial cells as well.

❍ **What factors predict development of pericarditis in AMI patients?**

Pericarditis usually occurs 1 day to 6 weeks after AMI. It is more common in males, Q wave infarction and patients with congestive heart failure. Some reports suggest that pericarditis occurs in 10 to 20% of patients, but pericardial effusion without evidence of pericarditis is far more common.

❍ **In AMI patients surviving their event, what is the most powerful predictor of long-term survival?**

This is still debated, but the degree of increase in end systolic volume <u>may</u> be the strongest. The extent of underlying left ventricular dysfunction (LVEF) and congestive heart failure are also strong predictors.

❍ **How common is acute myocardial infarction (AMI)?**

It is estimated that one and a half million myocardial infarctions occur every year in the U.S. Approximately one third of the patients with these events will die, with one half of deaths occurring prior to institution of medical therapy.

❍ **What is the pathophysiology of acute MI?**

In general, acute occlusion secondary to thrombosis is considered the most common cause of AMI. Most transmural MIs are associated with complete obstruction whereas non-transmural MIs may be done to thrombosis alone, spasm with associated thrombosis, or, in significantly obstructed arteries, may be done to hypoxemia or hypotension.

❍ **What is the most common cause of acute coronary thrombosis?**

Plaque disruption. Not all plaques have the same propensity to rupture. Characteristics rendering plaques "vulnerable" to disruption include: high lipid content, thin (as opposed to thick) fibrous cap, monocyte content and shear forces present.

❍ **What are the most common non-atherosclerotic causes of AMI?**

Embolization, arteritis, trauma, aortic or coronary dissection and congenital anomalies.

❍ **What is the most common cause of myocardial infarction in patients with angiographically normal coronary arteries?**

Approximately 6% of all MI patients, and as many as 25% of MI patients less than age 35 will have normal coronaries by arteriography. Possible explanations for this include oxygen demand supply mismatch, prolonged hypotension, anatomic abnormalities of the copronary arteries and hematologic disorders. It has been theorized that coronary spasm and small vessel disease may also be possible causes.

❍ **What are the most common metabolic disorders associated with increased risk of myocardial infarction?**

Hurler's disease, homocystinuria, Fabry's disease, amyloidosis and pseudoxanthoma elasticum.

❍ **What is the most common congenital anomaly associated with AMI?**

Anomalous origin of the left coronary artery from the pulmonary artery. If the left of right coronary artery originates from the contralateral aortic sinus, aberrant passage of the vessel between the aorta and the right ventricle outflow tract may result in MI, but more often results in sudden death.

❍ **Describe the difference between "supply" and "demand" ischemia.**

Supply ischemia is due to occlusion or critical narrowing of the coronary artery, and it usually occurs in acute transmural MI. Demand ischemia is esentially due to a mismatch in oxygen supply and demand when coronary narrowing does not allow sufficient delivery of oxygen associated with the increased oxygen demand of an active myocardium. This move often occurs in unstable anginal syndromes and clinically defined non-Q wave MI.

❍ **Why is the difference between supply and demand ischemia important?**

While the difference is a bit artificial, and both frequently occur together, the difference is important because different metabolic and mechanical changes occur in the myocardium depending upon the type of ischemia. The consequence of supply ischemia is the simultaneous development of cellular hypoxia and impaired washout of metabolites. As a result, the ischemia tissue becomes flacid. In demand ischemia, while hypoxia also develops, washout of metaboloties is relatively preserved, so contractility (which is related to a balance between calcium and inorganic phosphate and protons) is maintained.

❍ **List the most common causes of myocardial oxygen supply-demand mismatch?**

Severe coronary artery disease, aortic stenosis, aortic insufficiency, carbon monoxide poisoning, thyrotoxicosis and prolonged hypotension.

❍ **What are the phases of contraction abnormalities seen with acute cessation of blood flow to the myocardium?**

They occur sequentially and are generally catagorized as dysynchrony, hypokinesis, akinesia and dyskinesis.

❍ **How much of the left ventricle needs to be involved before hemodynamic signs of left ventricular failure are present?**

Clinical congestive heart failure can occur with amost any overall left ventricular dysfunction. In AMI, hemodynamic evidence of left ventricular dysfunction occurs when 20 to 25% of the LV exhibits abnormal wall.

❍ **What percentage of arteries successfully opened with thrombolytic therapy for acute myocardial infarction reocclude?**

15% of arteries successfully opened reocclude during the first few days following thrombolytic therapy.

❍ **What is the mortality benefit from aspirin alone in acute myocardial infarction with thrombolytic therapy and in subsequent reinfarction?**

Aspirin reduced mortality from acute myocardial infarction by 23% and reduced non-fatal reinfarction by 49%. When used with thrombolytic therapy, there was a 40-50% reduction in mortality from acute myocardial infarction.

❍ **A 63 year-old gentleman presents to the Emergency Department with moderate substernal chest pressure and lightheadedness for 90 minutes. His BP on admission is 80/40 and his HR is 110/min and regular. Physical exam reveals JVD to the angle of the jaw, a right parasternal S3**

gallop, an apical S4 gallop and clear lungs on auscultation. ECG reveals 2 mm ST elevation in leads II, III, and aVF with reciprocal ST depression in V1-V3. What is the most likely diagnosis and what is the most appropriate initial therapy?

Inferior myocardial infarction with right ventricular infarction. Following 160-325 mg of aspirin administration, thrombolytic therapy and a large bolus of intravenous saline followed by a moderately high infusion rate of saline are indicated. If the patient remains hypotensive despite adequate intravenous saline, as measured by the development of lung congestion on auscultation, intravenous Dobutamine is indicated.

❍ **A 47 year-old woman is admitted to you with substernal chest pressure for 1 hour. Serial ECGs and CK measurements confirm a non-Q wave anterior wall myocardial infarction. She has no arrhythmias, no evidence of heart failure and no recurrent chest pain while in the hospital. You discharge her on Diltiazem and aspirin on the fifth hospital day after she had a normal pre-discharge low-level treadmill exercise test. You schedule her for a symptom-limited treadmill test in two weeks. Three days after discharge, she reports a ten-minute episode of substernal chest pressure while walking across the room, relieved with one sublingual nitroglycerin. What should you advise her to do?**

Readmit her to the hospital, place her on intravenous heparin and nitroglycerin and perform cardiac catheterization with coronary angiography the following morning.

❍ **A 56 year-old gentleman presents to your office three weeks after suffering an inferior wall myocardial infarction, treated successfully with r-TPA. He has non-insulin-dependent diabetes mellitus. He denies any post-infarct symptoms. You supervise a symptom-limited treadmill exercise test which reveals 2 mm horizontal ST depression in the inferior and lateral leads after three minutes of exercise on Bruce protocol. On your recommendation, he undergoes a coronary angiogram and cardiac catheterization which reveals >70% stenosis of the proximal LAD, mid-RCA and first obtuse marginal branch of the circumflex. The LVEF on ventriculogram is 44%. What should you advise your patient at this time?**

Undergo 3-vessel coronary artery bypass graft surgery.

❍ **A 70 year-old man is admitted to the hospital with chest pain of 3 hours duration. ECG demonstrates anterior ST elevation for which he is given aspirin, r-TPA, heparin and intravenous nitroglycerin. His symptoms resolve. Serum chemistries reveal a peak CPK of 1800 and a CK-MB fraction of 15%. He is eventually transferred out of the CCU and his hospitalization is uneventful until day 5, when he develops sudden, severe shortness of breath. BP is 110/75 and his pulse is 125 and regular. Examination reveals a new systolic murmur. What would the most appropriate therapeutic intervention be?**

Intravenous sodium nitroprusside. This patient is most likely suffering from rupture of the left ventricular septum and subsequent defect, a not uncommon complication of MI. Afterload reduction is key to stabilization until surgical repair of the VSD can be performed, usually in about 8-12 weeks, after the infarct has healed. If nitroprusside fails to stabilize the patient, intra-aortic balloon counterpulsation and intravenous nitroglycerin should be employed.

❍ **What are the major complications of left ventricular aneurysms?**

LV thrombus formation (with the subsequent risk of thromboembolic events), CHF and ventricular arrhythmias.

❍ **What ECG changes arise in a true posterior infarction?**

Large R wave and ST depression in V1 and V2.

❍ **What conduction defects commonly occur in an anterior wall MI?**

The dangerous kind. Damage to the conducting system results in a Mobitz II second or third degree AV block.

❍ **How should PSVT be treated during an AMI?**

Vagal maneuvers, adenosine, or cardioversion. Stable patients may be able to tolerate negative inotropes, such as verapamil or even beta-blockers.

❍ **A patient presents one day after discharge for an AMI with a new, harsh systolic murmur along the left sternal border and pulmonary edema. What is the diagnosis?**

Ventricular septal rupture. Diagnosis is confirmed with Swan-Ganz catheterization or echo. The treatment regime includes nitroprusside, for afterload reduction, and possibly an intra-aortic balloon pump followed by surgical repair.

❍ **When does cardiac rupture usually occur in patients who have suffered acute MIs?**

50% ari
se within the first 5 days, and 90% occur within the first 14 days post-MI.

❍ **Which type of infarct commonly leads to papillary muscle dysfunction?**

Inferior wall MI. Signs and symptoms include a mild transient systolic murmur and pulmonary edema.

❍ **A patient presents two weeks post AMI with chest pain, fever and pleuripericarditis. A pleural effusion is detected by on CXR. What is the diagnosis?**

Dressler's (post-myocardial infarction) syndrome. This syndrome is caused by an immunologic reaction to myocardial antigens.

❍ **What percentage of patients over age 80 experience chest pain with an AMI?**

Only 50%. 20% experience diaphoresis, stroke, syncope and/or acute confusion.

❍ **Which type of thrombolytic agent is fibrin-specific?**

Tissue plasminogen activator. This agent is a human protein with no antigenic properties.

❍ **What is unstable angina (UA)?**

In the presence of ECG or enzyme evidence of AMI, the term UA is usually applied in three historical circumstances: 1) New onset angina of Canadian class III or worse; 2) Angina at rest as well as with minimal exertion; 3) More severe or prolonged angina in the context of a previous stable pain pattern. The more traditional definitions require one or more of these historical features with electrocardiographic changes, but many centers will classify patients as having unstable angina in the absence of ECG cardio findings.

❍ **What is the primary pathophysiologic disturbance in UA?**

In general, patients presenting with UA tend to have more severe and/or extensive CAD, and UA may be precipitated by a decrease in oxygen supply or an increase in demand. Typically, reduction in oxygen supply is the primary problem and is usually the result of thrombosis (often with spontaneous recanalization) and less often the result of progression of atherosclerosis or vasoconstriction.

❍ **How does one treat unstable angina?**

UA, like AMI, is usually due to plaque rupture followed by platelet aggregation and thrombosis. Thus, the use of aspirin, heparin, or both is essential. Of note, while aspirin and heparin are both effective, there has not been definitive proof that one is better than the other, or that the combination is better than either agent alone. Use of nitroglycerin, beta-blockers and calcium channel blockers are also standard therapy.

❍ **Are thrombolytic agents affective in non-Q wave MI?**

No, there is no evidence to support their use. In fact, some published data suggest that their use may be detrimental.

❍ **What is the prognosis of patients presenting witn Q-wave MI complicated by acute mitral regurgitation?**

Prognosis is quite compromised with an approximate one year survival of only 50%.

❍ **What is the best treatment of cardiogenic shock (SBP <90 and/or evidence of peripheral hypoperfusion)?**

The best treatment has not been established. Use of ionotropic agents and vasopressor agents is standard. The role of direct PTCA is still unresolved. Observational studies suggest a better outcome, but other studies have identified a selection bias in patients chones for direct PTCA. Although survival remains dismal in patients presenting with shock, meta-analyses suggest there may be some benefit with administration of thrombolytic agents (particularly streptokinase).

❍ **What is the definition of unstable angina?**

Unstable angina is an intermediate coronary syndrome between angina pectoris and acute myocardial infarction. Its presence depends on one or more of the following three historical features: 1) crescendo angina (more severe, prolonged or frequent) superimposed on a pre-existing pattern or relatively stable, exertion-related angina pectoris, 2) angina pectoris of new onset (within one month) which is brought on by minimal exertion or 3) angina pectoris at rest as well as minimal exertion. Variant angina, which is also characterized by angina at rest, has sometimes been considered to be a form of unstable angina, but it is pathogenetically different from unstable angina.

❍ **What is the classification of unstable angina?**

Class I: New onset, severe or accelerated angina occurring within two months of presentation without rest pain. Also included in this class are patients whose angina is more frequent, severe, longer in duration or precipitated by substantially less exertion than previously.

Class II Patients with angina at rest during the preceding two months but not within the last 48 hours.

Class III Patients with rest angina at least once within the preceding 48 hours.

❍ **What are some of the clinical circumstances in which unstable angina occurs?**

Secondary unstable angina refers to patients, usually with underlying obstructive CAD, in whom the imbalance between myocardial oxygen supply and demand causing the instability results from conditions that are extrinsic to the coronary vascular bed. This includes patients who have anemia or hypoxemia that cause reduced myocardial oxygen supply, as well as patients with fever, infection, aortic stenosis, uncontrolled hypertension, thyrotoxicosis, extreme emotional upset and tachyarrhythmias that cause increased myocardial oxygen demand.

Primary unstable angina, the most common form of unstable angina, occurs in the absence of an identifiable extracoronary condition and in patients who have not suffered an acute myocardial infarction within the preceding two weeks. Post-infarction unstable angina is present in patients who develop unstable angina within two weeks of a documented acute myocardial infarction; it occurs in approximately 20% of patients following infarction.

❍ **What is the etiology of primary unstable angina?**

Atherosclerotic plaque rupture followed by platelet aggregation and thrombus formation. Aggregation of platelets and thrombus formation, usually superimposed on an atherosclerotic plaque, obstructs blood flow to the affected myocardium sufficiently long enough to cause ischemia and clinical symptoms, but not long enough to result in myocardial necrosis and infarction, as recanalization of the affected coronary artery occurs, usually within 20 minutes to one hour after the onset of plaque rupture. Unstable angina is often a precursor of acute myocardial infarction, and the two conditions share a common pathophysiologic link.

❍ **Among all patients with unstable angina, what percentage of patients have three-vessel coronary artery disease?**

Approximately 40%.

❍ **Among all patients with unstable angina, what percentage of patients have left main coronary artery disease (> 50% stenosis)?**

Approximately 20%.

❍ **Among all patients with unstable angina, what percentage of patients have no critical coronary obstruction on coronary angiogram?**

Approximately 10%.

❍ **Among all patients with unstable angina, what percentage of patients have two-vessel coronary artery disease? Single-vessel CAD?**

Approximately 20% have two-vessel CAD and 10% have single-vessel disease.

❍ **What percentage of patients with unstable angina present with unstable angina as their initial manifestation of CAD?**

Approximately 50%.

❍ **Of patients who present with unstable angina as their initial manifestation of CAD, what percentage have single-vessel CAD? Three-vessel disease?**

Approximately 50% have single-vessel disease (the majority have left anterior descending involvement) and less than 20% have three-vessel disease.

❍ **What is the short-term prognosis of patients with unstable angina and no critical obstruction of a coronary artery on coronary angiogram (no intraluminal stenosis > 60%)?**

Excellent.

❍ **What is the percentage of intracoronary thrombus found on coronary angiography in patients with unstable angina?**

50-70%.

❍ **When a prior angiogram is available, the lesion responsible for an episode of unstable angina with documented ischemia is formerly greater than a 50% stenosis what percentage of the time? Formerly greater than 70% stenosis?**

Lesions responsible for acute ischemic episodes are formerly greater than 50% stenotic only 33-50% of the time and formerly greater than 70% less than 25% of the time.

❍ **What percentage of patients with acute myocardial infarction have a prodrome of unstable angina shortly before infarction?**

Approximately 50%.

❍ **What percentage of patients with unstable angina develop myocardial infarction in the short-term?**

Approximately 5%.

❍ **What is the 5-year survival of patients with unstable angina rendered asymptomatic on medical therapy prior to discharge from the hospital who have a normal resting electrocardiogram and an exercise electrocardiogram negative for ischemia?**

Greater than 95%.

❍ **Can patients with unstable angina, who have been stabilized and rendered asymptomatic on medical therapy prior to discharge from the hospital, be safely evaluated by exercise testing?**

Absolutely. However, coronary angiography is indicated for the vast majority of patients with unstable angina as the first diagnostic test, even in patients rendered asymptomatic by medical therapy.

❍ **What factors portend a worse prognosis and signify a high-risk patient in those with unstable angina?**

Older patients, patients with continued rest pain despite medical therapy, and patients with thrombi, complex coronary morphology or multivessel disease on coronary angiography. Patients who have ischemia detected on ambulatory electrocardiographic monitoring and those with significant ST-T wave abnormalities at presentation are also at higher risk and tend to have an unfavorable outcome.

❍ **What is the most useful diagnostic test in the evaluation of patients with unstable angina?**

Coronary angiography.

❍ **What is the hallmark of drug therapy for patients admitted with unstable angina?**

Intravenous low molecular-weight heparin and at least 81 mg of aspirin daily. Intravenous nitroglycerin is strongly recommended for patients with Class II or Class III unstable angina, but one must keep in mind to increase the dose of intravenous heparin during intravenous nitroglycerin administration as nitroglycerin reduces the efficacy of heparin.

❍ **What is the role of thrombolytic therapy in unstable angina?**

None. To date, no clinical trial has shown any benefit of thrombolytic therapy, presumably because thombi in unstable angina tend to be platelet-rich, not fibrin-rich, and thus resistant to thrombolytic therapy.

❍ **What are some other highly efficacious drug therapies in patients with unstable angina?**

Beta-blockers have been shown to be highly effective in reducing the frequency and duration of both symptomatic and silent myocardial ischemic episodes. Calcium channel antagonists, while not as efficacious as beta-blockers in reducing myocardial oxygen demand, are highly effective in reducing symptoms and ischemic episodes, but should not be used as monotherapy. In fact, monotherapy with nifedipine in unstable angina is associated with an increase in non-fatal myocardial infarctions within the first 48 hours after initiation of therapy.

❍ **What percentage of patients with unstable angina are refractory to maximal medical therapy?**

Approximately 9%. These patients are quite vulnerable to adverse results during PTCA and CABG and should be strongly considered for intra-aortic balloon counterpulsation prior to any further intervention.

❍ **What is the strategy for managing patients with unstable angina?**

All patients should receive immediate medical therapy with an eye to stabilization. Patients who remain unstable and those deemed candidates for invasive management should be referred for cardiac catheterization within 48 hours of presentation, provided there are no contraindications to invasive therapy. Patients who stabilize easily and who are not at high risk for complications, and those patients who prefer continued medical management, or those who are not candidates for invasive therapy because of contraindications should continue on intensive medical therapy. Patients should be strongly considered for cardiac catheterization if they have one or more of the following high-risk indicators: prior revascularization, associated congestive heart failure or depressed LVEF (< 50%) by non-invasive study, malignant ventricular arrhythmias, persistent or recurrent pain/ischemia, and/or a functional study indicating a high risk.

❍ **What percentage of patients who have sudden cardiac death have a prior history or angina, myocardial infarction or congestive heart failure?**

50%.

❍ **In patients with sudden cardiac death, what percentage of patients are found to have a coronary thrombus on autopsy?**

30-75%. It is most commonly found in patients with single-vessel CAD and those with acute myocardial infarction or recent unstable angina. It is less common in patients with previous myocardial infarction or three-vessel CAD.

❍ **What medical regimen can one use in patients with unstable angina who have a contraindication or a major complication to intravenous heparin?**

Ticlodipine, at a dose of 250 mg twice daily, or clopidogrel at 75 mg per day are very suitable alternatives to heparin. Furthermore, unlike intravenous heparin, they can be feasibly continued in the outpatient setting.

❍ **Among survivors of sudden cardiac death without myocardial infarction, which group of patients are more likely to have complex coronary atherosclerotic lesions: those with inducible ventricular tachycardia or those without inducible ventricular tachycardia on electrophysiology testing?**

Those patients without inducible ventricular tachycardia, suggesting those survivors of sudden cardiac death without inducible ventricular tachycardia on electrophysiology testing had ischemia as their precipitating event, while those who had inducible ventricular tachycardia had an arrhythmic etiology of their sudden cardiac death episode.

❍ **Which is the most common type of cardiac failure, high or low output?**

Low output failure. Reduced stroke volume, lowered pulse pressure, and peripheral vasoconstriction are all signs of low output failure.

❍ **Rales are present on exam in a 50 year-old man with recent anterior wall MI. What can you say about the pulmonary artery occlusion ("wedge") pressure?**

It is likely above 20 to 25 mmHg.

❍ **A 30 year-old woman with long-standing idiopathic cardiomyopathy has faint basilar crackles on lung exam. What would you expect her pulmonary wedge pressure to be?**

In chronic heart failure, patients may have elevated wedge pressures (a reflection of elevated left ventricular end diastolic pressure) greater than 30mmHg with only minor findings on lung exam. This is likely due to increased pulmonary lymphatic drainage.

❍ **Can the chest radiograph show signs of systolic heart failure when the physical exam is negative?**

Rales on exam develop when there is extravasated fluid within the alveoli. The first site fluid accumulates in hydrostatic pulmonary edema is the interstitial space that surrounds blood vessels and bronchi. This interstitial fluid is visible on X-rays before the exam becomes positive.

❍ **A 65 year-old man 3 days post an uncomplicated inferior wall MI is noted to have basilar crackles on lung exam that mostly clear with coughing. His creatinine is 2.1, and he weighs 75 kg. Approximately how much furosemide should you administer for adequate diuresis?**

Probably none. In the proper clinical context, rales are obviously a useful sign of heart failure, even in its incipient stage. Since most ICU patients are bed-bound and will experience atelectasis of dependent lung tissue, the patient should be reexamined after a few vigorous coughs and gentle pulmonary toilet. Very often rales and diuretics will soon disappear from the bedside.

❍ **You suspect severe LV systolic dysfunction in a new ICU admission. A pulmonary artery catheter is placed. However, your pressure transducer is malfunctioning and your cardiac output machine is broken. What laboratory test will confirm your suspicions?**

Measurement of the mixed venous saturation is an extremely useful measure of low-output state in heart failure. With reduced systolic function, peripheral tissues will extract more oxygen; this will reduce the mixed venous oxygen saturation, often dramatically.

❍ **A 65 year-old man complains of fatigue and shortness of breath. Exam: rales and edema; a displaced PMI with a systolic murmur at the left sternal border radiating to the aortic area and a holosystolic murmur at the apex radiating to the axilla. Echo: low normal LV function, aortic valve sclerosis with a peak gradient on continuous wave doppler study of 40 mmHg. Color doppler not performed. Pulmonary artery catheter findings: cardiac output 2.4: mixed venous oxygen saturation: 45% (Normal: ≈65%). How do you explain the patient's low-output state by pulmonary artery catheterization, given preserved LV function and non-critical AS on echocardiogram?**

This patient emphasizes the importance of the mixed venous oxygen saturation: this low number, suggesting increased extraction of oxygen from the periphery and a low output state, appears to contradict the echo data. However, the patient has mitral regurgitation (MR) on exam, the severity of which was not reported on echo. A repeat study demonstrated severe MR, and revealed an important contributing factor to the patient's low output state.

❍ **A 70 year-old admitted four days ago with an inferior wall MI is short of breath. A recent echocardiogram reports (but does not grade the severity of) mitral regurgitation (MR). You insert a pulmonary artery catheter and note a giant V wave on wedge tracing. Can you correlate the height of the V wave with the degree of MR?**

Beware! Giant V waves may not even indicate MR! V wave size is related to the volume of blood entering the left atrium (as it is reflected back in the wedge tracing) and also to left atrial compliance. Severe MR with a large, distended left atrium may not exhibit a giant V wave. Alternatively, a hypervolemic patient with no MR may acutely distend a normal-sized LA and demonstrate giant V waves. The present patient actually has a ventricular septal defect (VSD) as a complication of MI; increased pulmonary blood flow through the VSD produced a "hypervolemic" state, giant V waves and CHF.

❍ **What is preload?**

The wall stress that the ventricle (LV) sees at the end of diastole, which is determined by venous return. In the normal heart, when preload increases, the LV distends, the resting length of the sarcomere increases and the LV can generate greater pressures more rapidly, augmenting stroke volume.

❍ **What is afterload?**

The load against which the LV must contract as systole begins—that is, the pressure the LV must generate to open the aortic valve and then eject blood.

❍ **You are asked to evaluate hypotension in an elderly woman. On evaluation, the patient complains of chest pain. She is diaphoretic; her lips are dusky; her radial pulse is faint and slow. Jugular venous distension is present, but the lung fields are clear. Glancing at her bedside monitor, you conclude that her central venous line has migrated distally, since there is a right ventricular pressure tracing. What's going on?**

The patient is having a right ventricular infarction with hypotension secondary to right ventricular failure. The physical exam findings are classic. The central line has not migrated, but is showing a characteristic "ventricularized" tracing.

❍ **Sustained ventricular tachycardia is well controlled in a 55 year-old man post non-Q wave MI with lidocaine 2 mcg/mL. He has a known history of ischemic cardiomyopathy. Day 3 of his admission, his speech becomes slurred, he is lethargic, and, when aroused, becomes very agitated. What should you do?**

This patient has classic findings of lidocaine toxicity, and you should strongly consider stopping this drug. Elderly patients and patients with heart failure of hepatic insufficiency are especially at risk.

❍ **An elderly man with progressive symptoms of shortness of breath is intubated for respiratory failure. He has a 100 pack/year smoking history. On exam, he is agitated and "bucking the vent". Breath sounds are coarse throughout, heart sounds faint. External jugular veins are prominently distended. His liver edge is palpable; his extremities are dusky, with lower extremity pitting edema. EKG shows sinus tachycardia and poor R wave progression. The BUN/creatinine ratio is elevated. You have concluded that the patient has systolic heart failure. What is your next step?**

Reconsider your diagnosis! The ICU is fraught with physical exam pitfalls. JVD may be difficult to interpret—especially in a patient who is increasing his intrathoracic pressure by breathing out of synch with the ventilator. Patients with COPD can have dusky extremities; they may have coarse breath sounds throughout their lung fields; pulmonary hypertension and RV dysfunction may lead to peripheral edema; diaphragmatic or abdominal viscera displacement may alter the axis of the heat and affect EKG interpretation. Under such circumstances, a bedside echo may be very helpful.

❍ **A 60 year-old man with a recent syncopal episode is hospitalized with congestive heart failure and chest pain. His BP is 165/85 mm Hg, his pulse is 85/min and there is a grade III/VI harsh systolic murmur at the apex and aortic area. An echocardiogram reveals a disproportionately thickened septum and anterior systolic motion of the mitral valve. What is this patient's diagnosis and what physical findings would most likely be present?**

Obstructive hypertrophic cardiomyopathy (IHSS). The murmur typically decreases with handgrip and Valsalva, and increases with vasodilators, standing, nitroglycerin, diuretics and digoxin. Mitral regurgitation is frequent as a result of anterior systolic motion of the mitral valve. Congestive heart failure is present because of diastolic dysfunction, thus an S4 gallop is common.

❍ **A 72 year-old woman admitted to the ICU with pulmonary edema is much improved after overnight diuresis. Soon after you note that she is 4L negative in fluid balance, she develops polymorphic VT requiring cardioversion. Her regular medications include 80 mg bid of furosemide. What is a likely etiology?**

Beware of electrolyte abnormalities, especially hypokalemia, inducing torsades pointes in CHF patients after vigorous diuresis – especially in patients on chronic diuretics.

❍ **You correct the electrolyte imbalances in the above patient, and she is carefully diuresed another 2L. Vital signs are stable, with BP 120/80 HR 80. Echo reveals EF'35% and you initiate captopril 25 mg every eight hours. Two hours later, the patient complains of dizziness; BP 80/60 HR 100. What happened?**

ACE inhibitors can have a profound first dose effect and lead to symptomatic hypotension, especially in patients, like this one, who have been aggressively diuresed. The peak effect with a short acting agent such as captopril will occur 1 to 2 hours after the initial dose. Careful volume expansion usually reverses this effect. It's best to initiate ACE therapy with a low dose of short acting drug (i.e., captopril 6.25 mg) especially in acutely ill patients.

❍ **A 65 year-old man with known severe hypertension, past CHF and COPD is intubated for acute pulmonary edema and suspected pneumonia. BP is 190/110; 92 saturation is 94% on 60% O_2. You successfully lower his blood pressure to 140/80 with intravenous sodium nitroprusside. However, the patient develops chest pressure and you note that his O_2 saturation is now 86%. What happened?**

Two effects of nitroprusside are likely culprits. Non selective dilation of the pulmonary arteriolar bed can worsen ventilation-perfusion mismatch, especially in patients with COPD or pneumonia, and cause desaturation. "Coronary steal" (reduced perfusion to coronary arteries with fixed obstruction in the setting of arteriolar dilation by nitroprusside) may lead to ischemia and chest pain.

❍ **Despite appropriate medical therapy, including combination diuretics, a 75 year-old woman with reduced systolic function in acute pulmonary edema remains oliguric. What "mechanical" intervention may increase her urine output?**

Intubation or CPAP, if she can tolerate it. A large portion of her (already decreased) cardiac output is going to her overworked diaphragm. Decreasing her work of breathing will allow better perfusion of her kidneys, and can lead to dramatic diuresis.

❍ **The above patient has a 2.5L diuresis after intubation. She is placed on a CMV mode with 10 of PEEP. The next morning, her lungs are clear. You attempt a T-piece wean, but note rales throughout both lung fields within minutes. What are three possible explanations.**

1) You've increased her work of breathing prematurely (i.e., before maximizing other therapies). 2) Coronary artery disease with concomitant ischemia may be contributing. 3) You've abruptly withdrawn potent cardiopulmonary effects of positive pressure ventilation. By increasing intrathoracic pressure, CMV and PEEP decrease the pressure gradient for venous blood flow from the great vessels to the right atrium, thereby decreasing preload; positive pressure against the heart can also have afterload-reducing effects.

❍ **What are two reasons why dobutamine, in general, is a superior inotrope in heart failure to dopamine?**

Dobutamine acts as a peripheral dilator and reduces systemic vascular resistance, whereas dopamine, even at intermediate infusion rates, may cause peripheral vasoconstriction. Tachycardia and arrhythmias tend to occur more frequently with dopamine than dobutamine.

❍ **What are the most common causes of atrial fibrillation?**

Hypertension with hypertensive heart disease is very common. Ischemic heart disease, mitral or aortic valvular heart disease, cor pulmonale, dilated cardiomyopathy, hypertrophic cardiomyopathy (particularly the obstructive type), alcohol intoxication ("holiday heart syndrome"), hypo- or hyperthyroidism, pulmonary embolism, sepsis, hypoxia, pre-excitation syndrome and pericarditis are also common causes.

❍ **How is atrial fibrillation treated?**

The treatment of atrial fibrillation consists of three major considerations: 1) control of ventricular rate, 2) conversion, if possible or feasible, to sinus rhythm and 3) prevention of thromboembolic events, particularly CVA. Rate control is best managed with beta-adrenergic blockers or calcium channel blockers (diltiazem or verapamil), or less desirable, digoxin. Digoxin should be used in patients with poor LV systolic function and those with a contraindication to beta-blockers <u>and</u> calcium channel blockers. Digoxin provides good rate control at rest but often suboptimal rate control during exertion. Conversion to sinus rhythm, in the stable patient, is best managed, initially, with antiarrhythmic agents, such as 1A agents like quinidine or procainamide, 1C agents such as propafenone or Class III agents like amiodarone or sotalol. In the unstable patient or the patient with acute ischemia, hypotension or pulmonary edema, immediate synchronized electrical cardioversion, starting at 200 joules should be performed. If, in the stable patient, cardioversion with antiarrhythmic agents is unsuccessful, synchronized electrical cardioversion should be performed without interruption of antiarrhythmic therapy. Patients with atrial fibrillation of 1 year duration or longer, or those with left atrial size of >5.0 cm on echocardiography should not be cardioverted because of the extremely low success rate. Patients with recent atrial fibrillation >3 days duration should be started on Warfarin and anticoagulated to an INR between 2-3.5 for at least three weeks before any attempt to cardiovert to sinus rhythm because of the significant risk of embolic CVA. Those patients with chronic atrial fibrillation should be on lifelong Warfarin, unless an absolute contraindication to Warfarin exists or the patient cannot reliably take Warfarin.

❍ **What percentage of patients with atrial fibrillation converted to sinus rhythm will revert back into atrial fibrillation?**

50% will revert back to atrial fibrillation within one year of cardioversion, regardless of medical therapy.

❍ **What are the common causes of SVT?**

Myocardial ischemia, myocardial infarction, congestive heart failure, pericarditis, rheumatic heart disease, mitral valve prolapse, pre-excitation syndromes, COPD, ethanol intoxication, hypoxia, pneumonia, sepsis and digoxin toxicity.

❍ **What is the treatment of paroxysmal SVT?**

In a hemodynamically stable patient, intravenous adenosine. If unsuccessful, then intravenous verapamil, beta-blockers or procainamide. In the unstable patient with hypotension, angina or heart failure, immediate synchronized cardiversion should be performed.

❍ **What is the most common supraventricular arrhythmia in the perioperative setting?**

Atrial fibrillation.

❍ **You are called to the CCU to evaluate the sudden onset of hypotension in an 80 year-old woman. She received a porcine aortic valve for severe aortic stenosis less than 24 hours ago. The bedside monitor reveals atrial fibrillation at a rate of 120 bpm. What is the pathophysiology?**

A rapid ventricular response and loss of AV synchrony, as can be seen in new-onset atrial fibrillation, can have devastating hemodynamic consequences, especially in patients with impaired diastolic filling – often including the elderly, and patients with left ventricular hypertrophy, which this patient with long-standing aortic stenosis most likely has.

❍ **What pharmacotherapy is most appropriate in the above patient?**

None. Hemodynamically unstable patients with tachyarrhythmias are best treated with electrical cardioversion.

❍ **What is the key feature of Mobitz Type I 2° AV block (Wenkebach)?**

A progressive prolongation of the PR interval until the atrial impulse is no longer conducted through to the ventricle, resulting in a dropped QRS. Almost always transient, atropine and transcutaneous/transvenous pacing is required for the rare instances of symptoms or cardiac instability.

❍ **What is the feature of Mobitz II 2° AV block?**

A constant PR interval until one sinus beat fails to conduct through to the ventricule, resulting in a dropped QRS. Since this rhythm is indicative of His bundle damage, and 85% of patients with this rhythm eventually develop complete heart block, temporary followed by permanent pacing is usually required.

❍ **What is the most common cause of Mobitz Type II 2° AV block?**

Coronary artery disease with acute myocardial ischemia. In the absence of coronary artery disease, the most common cause is degenerative AV node and His bundle disease.

❍ **What is the appropriate management of the above arrhythmia in a patient on no SA or AV nodal suppressant drugs?**

Temporary transvenous pacemaker insertion followed by permanent pacemaker implantation.

❍ **A 57 year-old male is scheduled for a total colectomy for ulcerative colitis. He has stable angina for several years and has hypertension. His pre-op ECG reveals NSR, LVH and 1° AV block. What is the likelihood of high degree AV block occuring in the perioperative period?**

Patients with 1° AV block have an extremely low incidence of developing high degree AV block in the perioperative period or any other period. Thus, no temporary pacing in the perioperative period is required.

❍ **What is the agent of choice for the immediate pharmacologic conversion of atrial fibrillation to sinus rhythm of less than 48 hours duration?**

Ibutilide.

❍ **What is the treatment of Torsades de Pointes?**

Torsades de Pointes is a polymorphic form of ventricular tachycardia that occurs in the setting of long repolarization. Treatment usually requires removal of the reversible triggers that caused Q-T prolongation, such as hypokalemia and drugs, such as quinidine and other antiarrhythmic agents, pacing the atrium or ventricle to increase cardiac rate and rapidly infusing magnesium sulfate.

❍ **Name five useful ECG criteria for identifying VT.**

- AV dissociation – often best seen in lead V1 and rare in SVT with aberrancy.
- Capture of fusion beats – often noted as a "narrow" premature beat occurring during a wide complex tachycardia.
- A QRS with a RBBB morphology greater than 140 ms in duration, or a LBBB morphology greater than 160 ms in duration.
- Extreme right or left axis deviation ("northwest axis") is seldom seen outside of VT.
- Positive or negative concordance of QRS complexes in the precordial leads.

❍ **Which antiarrhythmic agents increase defibrillation threshold (i.e., increase the energy requirement for successful defibrillation)?**

Lidocaine, mexiletine, encainide, flecainide, propafenone, amiodarone and verapamil.

❍ **What are the most common initial rhythms in adults with cardiac arrest?**

VF and VT.

❍ **For VF or unstable VT, what is the most important intervention to optimize chances for successful resuscitation?**

Defibrillation.

❍ **What percentage of individuals successfully resuscitated from sudden cardiac death will succumb to a second episode within 2 years?**

60%.

❍ **What is the primary indication for atropine?**

Symptomatic bradycardia.

❍ **A 28 year-old presents with hemodynamically stable paroxysmal supraventricular tachycardia (PSVT) at a rate of 170. What is the drug of choice?**

Vagal maneuvers are tried first. If unsuccessful, adenosine is the drug of choice.

❍ **What is the treatment of choice for rapid atrial fibrillation in a patient with Wolff-Parkinson-White syndrome?**

Cardioversion if the patient is unstable, otherwise procainamide (20 to 30 mg/min up to 17 mg/kg) is the treatment of choice. The infusion should be stopped if further widening of the QRS or hypotension occurs.

❍ **What percentage of Americans experiencing cardiac arrest are resuscitated? What percentage of these suffer neurological damage?**

Up to one-third are resuscitated and survive to discharge. Of this group, 20 to 40% develop permanent brain damage ranging from subtle to severe.

❍ **Tachycardia occurs after a cardiac arrest and is treated successfully with defibrillation and epinephrine. Would you treat this post-resuscitation rhythm?**

If the patient has a pulse and is hemodynamically stable, no treatment may be necessary. If epinephrine is responsible for the tachycardia, it should resolve quickly. Sustained sinus tachycardia should not be allowed to persist, however, as it increases myocardial oxygen consumption.

❍ **T/F: An AICD (automated implantable cardioverter-defibrillator) is a contraindication to defibrillation.**

False. If functioning, the AICD should assess, charge and shock within 30 seconds. If the patient is in ventricular fibrillation (VF) and a shock is not being delivered, proceed with external defibrillation.

TRAUMA PEARLS

"The only missing clotting factor is silk."
Donald Trunkey, M.D.

❍ **Following blunt trauma to the chest, what type of injury is implied by the presence of pneumomediastinum, subcutaneous emphysema and a large air leak following tube thoracostomy?**

Tracheobronchial tear or disruption.

❍ **What is the definitive method for diagnosing a tracheobronchial injury?**

Bronchoscopy.

❍ **What is a flail chest?**

When a segment of the thoracic cage becomes anatomically and functionally separated from the rest of the cage. It is caused by double fractures of 3 or more contiguous ribs, most often due to blunt trauma. The flail segment moves inward when the rest of the chest moves outward. This results in ineffective ventilation.

❍ **What is the major cause of hypoxemia in patients with flail chest?**

Pulmonary contusion.

❍ **How is flail chest treated?**

Analgesics and ventilatory support when respiratory failure occurs. The use of stabilizing devices is controversial.

❍ **What is the eponym for a C1 burst fracture from vertical compression?**

Jefferson fracture.

❍ **A patient in a motor vehicle accident sustains a hyperextension injury to the neck. The x-rays reveal a C2 bilateral pedicle fracture. What is this fracture called?**

A Hangman's fracture.

❍ **A patient has an avulsion fracture of the spinous process of C7 with a history of a hyperflexion mechanism. What is the diagnosis?**

Clay shoveler's fracture, which is a fracture involving the spinous process of the lower cervical vertebrae. The mechanism is usually flexion or a direct blow.

❍ **A patient suffers a bilateral facetal dislocation. What is the major concern?**

Very unstable injury with disruption of the anterior longitudinal ligament and the annulus fibrosis. The mechanism is flexion.

❍ **Name some stable cervical spine fractures.**

Simple wedge, clay shoveler's, transverse process fracture, isolated fracture of articular pillar and an isolated and mild burst fracture of a vertebral body (not of C1).

❍ **A patient presents after receiving a blow to the forehead. Her neck is hyperextended and she complains of weakness in her arms and minimal weakness in her lower extremities. What is the most likely diagnosis?**

Central cord syndrome.

❍ **What is the most common cause of shock in patients with blunt chest trauma?**

Pelvic or extremity fracture.

❍ **What organ is most commonly injured in blunt trauma?**

The spleen. Generalized abdominal pain with radiation to the left shoulder subsequent to blunt trauma suggests splenic rupture. Splenic rupture can also occur following minor trauma in a patient with infectious mononucleosis.

❍ **What sign should be charted when performing a neurological exam on a patient with a suspected anterior dislocation of the shoulder?**

Sensation over the lateral deltoid, which demonstrates an intact sensory component of the axillary nerve.

❍ **T/F: Chemical burns to the eyes are not true ophthalmological emergencies.**

False. These must be irrigated immediately.

❍ **What is the most common cause of laryngeal trauma?**

Blunt trauma secondary to motor vehicle accidents.

❍ **What are the signs and symptoms of a fracture to the zygomaticomaxillary complex?**

Subcutaneous emphysema, edema, ecchymosis, facial flattening, subconjunctival hemorrhage, ecchymosis around the orbit, unilateral epistaxis, anesthesia of the maxilla, upper lip and gum from infraorbital nerve injury, step deformity, decreased mandibular movement and diplopia.

❍ **What are the two most common findings with an orbital floor fracture?**

Diplopia and enophthalmos.

❍ **Bilateral mental fractures may cause what acute complication?**

The tongue may cause acute airway obstruction because of loss of anterior support.

❍ **A child falls and knocks out his front tooth. How would treatment differ if the child were age 3 versus age 13?**

With primary teeth, no reimplantation should be attempted because of the risk of ankylosis or fusion to the bone. However, with permanent teeth reimplantation should occur as soon as possible. Remaining periodontal fibers are a key to success. Thus, the tooth should not be wiped dry as this may disrupt the periodontal ligament fibers still attached.

❍ **What is the best transport medium for an avulsed tooth?**

Hank's solution, which is a pH balanced cell culture medium, can help maintain cell viability if the tooth has been avulsed for more than 30 minutes. Milk is an alternative or the patient may place the tooth underneath his/her tongue if the patient is able to avoid aspirating.

❍ **A patient complains of a tongue irritation from a slightly chipped tooth after a fall. No dentin is exposed. What treatment can be offered to this patient?**

Tooth fractures only involving the enamel are called Ellis Class I fractures. The sharp edges can be filed with an emery board for immediate relief and the patient is referred to a dentist for cosmetic repair.

❍ **How can one differentiate Ellis class II and III fractures?**

Class II: Fractures involving the dentin and enamel. The exposed dentin will be pinkish.
Class III: Fractures involving the enamel, dentin and pulp. A drop of blood is frequently noted in the center of the pink dentin.

❍ **Why should topical analgesics not be used in Ellis class III tooth fractures?**

Severe tissue irritation or sterile abscesses may occur with their use. Treatment includes application of tinfoil, analgesics and immediate dental referral.

❍ **What is Volkmann's ischemia?**

Ischemia induced by compartment syndrome.

❍ **What is Volkmann's contracture?**

It is the result of untreated Volkmann's ischemia - a contracture deformity secondary to muscle necrosis.

❍ **What clinical features differentiate partial thickness from full thickness burns?**

Partial thickness: Pink to mottled red, blisters, bullae, moist weeping surface and painful.
Full thickness: Waxy white, charred or dark red, dry leathery and insensate.

❍ **In estimating the size of a burn, which body part varies most as a percent body surface area with age?**

The head. At birth the head accounts for 19% BSA. At age 1 it is 17%, age 5 = 13%, age 10 = 11%, age 15 = 9% and adult = 7%.

❍ **What are the five major musculoskeletal emergencies?**

1) Open fracture
2) Open joint injuries
3) Dislocation
4) Vascular injuries
5) Neurologic injuries

❍ **What injury is associated with knee dislocations?**

Injury to the popliteal artery.

❍ **What is a defect in the chest wall into which air is pulled during inspiration called?**

Sucking chest wound.

❍ **How big does a chest wall defect have to be to redirect the incoming air away from the trachea?**

If the wound is > two-thirds the diameter of the trachea it will become the path of least resistance and become a sucking chest wound, making effective spontaneous ventilation impossible.

❍ **What percentage of patients with traumatic disruption of the aorta will have an abnormal initial chest x-ray?**

90 %.

❍ **What are some of the radiographic findings seen in traumatic aortic disruption?**

Mediastinal widening, prominent aortic knob, obliteration of the aortic window, tracheal deviation, loss of the normal aortic outline, downward deviation of the left mainstem bronchus, widening of the paravertebral stripe and hemothorax.

❍ **What is the usual mechanism by which traumatic diaphragmatic hernias occur?**

Penetrating wounds to the lower chest and upper abdomen cause the majority of diaphragmatic hernias. Children are more likely to suffer this injury from blunt trauma.

❍ **What are some of the radiographic findings seen in traumatic diaphragmatic hernias?**

Visceral herniation, loss of the normal diaphragmatic contour and apparent elevation of the diaphragm.

❍ **In which portion of the diaphragm are traumatic hernias most commonly seen?**

The left posterolateral portion.

❍ **How should a DPL be performed for a trauma victim with a fractured pelvis?**

Open supraumbilical incision to avoid a rectus sheath hematoma.

❍ **When does a subdural hematoma become isodense?**

Between 1 to 3 weeks after the bleed. At that time it may not show up on CT.

❍ **What spinal level innervates the diaphragm?**

C3, C4, C5. Remember: "3–4–5 keep the diaphragm alive!"

❍ **Define increased intracranial pressure.**

ICP > 15 mmHg.

❍ **What is the most common site of a basilar skull fracture?**

Petrous aspect of the temporal bone.

❍ **What cardiovascular injury is commonly associated with sternal fractures?**

Myocardial contusions.

❍ **What valve is most commonly injured with blunt trauma?**

Aortic valve.

❍ **What is the most likely cause of a new systolic murmur and ECG infarct pattern observed in a patient with chest trauma?**

Ventricular septal defect.

❍ **A patient cannot actively abduct her shoulder. What injury does this suggest?**

Rotator cuff tear. The cuff is comprised of the supraspinatus, infraspinatus, subscapularis and the teres minor muscles and tendons.

❍ **Why is a displaced supracondylar fracture (of distal humerus) in a child considered a true emergency?**

The injury often results in injury to brachial artery or median nerve. It can also cause compartment syndrome.

❍ **What is the significance of the anterior fat pad sign with an elbow injury?**

Fat pad sign or radiolucency just anterior to the distal humerus is indicative of effusion or hemarthrosis of the elbow joint. This suggests an occult fracture of the radial head.

❍ **What is the most commonly feared complication of a scaphoid fracture?**

Avascular necrosis. The more proximal the fracture, the more common is avascular necrosis.

❍ **What type of Salter-Harris fracture has the worst prognosis?**

Type V- compression injury of the epiphyseal plate.

❍ **What fracture is frequently missed when the patient complains of an ankle injury?**

Fracture at the base of the fifth metatarsal, caused by plantar flexion and inversion. Radiographs of the ankle may not include the fifth metatarsal.

❍ **What fracture is associated with avascular necrosis of the femoral head?**

Femoral neck fractures. Avascular necrosis occurs with 15% of non-displaced femoral neck fractures and with nearly 90% of displaced femoral neck fractures.

❍ **What is a stress fracture?**

Small, repetitive forces usually involving the metatarsal shafts, the distal tibia and the femoral neck cause a stress or "fatigue" fracture. These fractures may not be visible on initial radiographs.

❍ **What are the features of anterior cord syndrome?**

Loss of anterior cord function, which involves complete motor paralysis and loss of pain and temperature sensation. Posterior column function, which includes light touch, vibration and proprioception, is preserved.

❍ **What are the features of central cord syndrome?**

There is a loss of motor function worse in the upper extremities than the lower extremities. The perianal area is often spared. Cervical hyperextension is the usual mechanism.

❍ **What are the features of the Brown-Sequard syndrome?**

Caused by penetrating injury to one side of the spinal cord, it presents with an ipsilateral motor deficit and contralateral loss of pain and temperature sensation. Light touch is usually absent on the side of the lesion.

❍ **Which pattern of partial cord injury has the worst rate of functional recovery?**

Anterior cord syndrome.

❍ **What is the most common type of incomplete spinal cord injury?**

Central cord syndrome.

❍ **What is a teardrop fracture and is it considered stable?**

It is an avulsion of the anterior-inferior portion of the vertebral body caused by flexion and is unstable.

❍ **By what mechanism are unilateral facet dislocations caused?**

Severe flexion-rotation.

❍ **Describe a Jefferson fracture.**

A burst fracture of the ring of C1, usually from a vertical compressive force. Best seen on odontoid view.

❍ **Describe a Hangman's fracture.**

C2 bilateral pedicle fracture caused by hyperextension.

❍ **When should ED thoracotomy be considered in trauma?**

In a patient with penetrating trauma who arrests en route to the hospital or in the emergency department.

❍ **A radial pulse on exam indicates a BP of at least _____.**

80 mmHg.

❍ **A femoral pulse on exam indicates a BP of at least_____.**

70 mm Hg.

❍ **A carotid pulse indicates a BP of at least_____.**

60 mm Hg.

❍ **What is the most common long bone fractured?**

The tibia.

❍ **A trauma patient presents with decreasing level of consciousness and an enlarging right pupil. What is the most likely diagnosis?**

Uncal herniation with oculomotor nerve compression.

❍ **What does the corneal reflex test?**

Ophthalmic branch (V_1) of the trigeminal (5th) nerve and the facial (7th) nerve.

❍ **Name the clinical signs of basilar skull fracture.**

Periorbital ecchymosis (raccoon's eyes), retroauricular ecchymosis (Battle's sign), otorrhea or rhinorrhea, hemotympanum, bloody ear discharge, hearing loss and anosmia.

❍ **A trauma patient presents with anisocoria, neurological deterioration or lateralizing motor findings. What is the treatment?**

Hyperventilation, mannitol IV and phenytoin.

❍ **How is posterior column function tested and why is it significant?**

Position, light touch and vibration are transmitted in the posterior columns, which are spared in the anterior cord syndrome.

❍ **At what point of airway obstruction will inspiratory stridor become evident?**

70% occlusion.

❍ **What nerve should be avoided during pericardiotomy?**

The phrenic nerve is avoided by opening the pericardium along the cranial to caudal axis.

❍ **Differential diagnosis of distended neck veins in a trauma patient?**

Tension pneumothorax, pericardial tamponade, air embolism and cardiac failure. Neck vein distention may not be present until hypovolemia has been treated.

❍ **What should be checked prior to inserting a chest tube in an intubated patient with respiratory distress and decreased breath sounds on one side?**

Position of the endotracheal tube.

❍ **Should a chest tube be placed into a bullet hole apparent in the 4th lateral interspace?**

No. The tube might follow the bullet track into the diaphragm or lung.

❍ **A trauma patient presents with subcutaneous emphysema. What is the diagnosis?**

Pneumothorax or pneumomediastinum. If subcutaneous emphysema is severe, consider major bronchial injury.

❍ **A pneumothorax is suspected but does not show up on PA and lateral CXR. What other x-rays should be considered?**

Expiratory films. A pneumothorax is usually best seen on expiratory films.

❍ **What rib fracture has the worst prognosis?**

First rib. First and second rib fractures are associated with bronchial tears, vascular injury and myocardial contusions.

❍ **How much fluid needs to collect intrapleurally before it is visible on decubitus or upright chest x-rays?**

200 to 300 ml.

❍ **Describe Beck's triad.**

Diminished heart tones, hypotension and distended neck veins. Classically described for pericardial tamponade, may also occur with myocardial contusion, AMI and tension pneumothorax.

❍ **T/F: Electrical alternans is suggestive of pericardial tamponade.**

True.

❍ **What is the most accurate plain film x-ray finding indicating traumatic rupture of the aorta?**

Deviation of the esophagus > 2 cm right of the spinous process of T4.

❍ **What is the basic disorder contributing to the pathophysiology of compartment syndrome?**

Increased pressure within closed tissue spaces compromising blood flow to muscle and nerve tissue.

❍ **What are the two basic mechanisms for elevated compartment pressure?**

1) External compression: by burn eschar, circumferential casts, dressings or pneumatic pressure garments.
2) Volume increase within the compartment: hemorrhage into the compartment, IV infiltration or edema due to post-ischemic swelling.

❍ **Which two fractures are most commonly associated with compartment syndrome?**

Tibial (anterior compartment involvement) and supracondylar humeral fractures.

❍ **What are the early general signs & symptoms of compartment syndrome?**

Early findings:
1. Tenderness and pain out of proportion to the injury
2. Pain with active and passive motion
3. Hypesthesia (paresthesia)

Late findings:

1. Compartment tense, indurated and erythematous
2. Slow capillary refill
3. Pallor and pulselessness

❍ **What are the four compartments of the leg?**

Anterior, lateral, deep posterior and superficial posterior compartments.

❍ **What signs & symptoms would be noted for a compartment syndrome involving the superficial posterior compartment of the leg?**

Pain on active and passive foot dorsi-flexion and plantar-flexion and hypesthesia of the lateral aspect of the foot (sural nerve).

❍ **What intracompartmental pressure raises concern?**

Normal pressure is less than 10 mm Hg. A level > 30 mm Hg mandates consideration of emergent fasciotomy. There probably is no numerical value that dictates fasciotomy in all patients. The development of compartment syndrome appears to depend upon the intracompartment pressure, the mean arterial pressure and the degree of tissue injury.

❍ **Is the heat of firing significant enough to sterilize a bullet and its wound?**

No. Contaminants from body surface and from a nonsterile body compartment as the viscera can be carried along the bullet's path.

❍ **What anatomic locations of bullets/pellets are associated with lead intoxication?**

Within bursa, joints or disc spaces.

❍ **Other than lead intoxication, why should intraorticular bullets be removed?**

Potential for lead synovitis leading to severe damage of articular cartilage.

❍ **What is the most common artery involved with an epidural hematoma?**

Meningeal artery, specifically the middle.

❍ **Where are epidural hematomas located?**

Between the dura and inner table of the skull.

❍ **Where are subdural hematomas located?**

Beneath the dura and over the brain and arachnoid. Caused by tears of pial arteries or of bridging veins.

❍ **For a trauma victim, which test is most helpful for evaluating retroperitoneal organs?**

CT.

❍ **What type of contrast medium should be used to evaluate the esophagus if traumatic injury is suspected?**

Gastrografin.

❍ **Describe the 3 zones of the neck and their evaluation for penetrating trauma.**

I - Below the cricoid cartilage: Arteriogram and consideration of bronchoscopy and esophagoscopy.

II - Between the cricoid and the mandible: Surgery is the classical method of evaluation.

III - Recently, some have utilized arteriography and others have utilized an observatory approach in select patients.

❍ **A stress fracture is suspected of the 2nd or 3rd metatarsal, but none is found on initial x-rays. How long before a 2nd set of x-rays will likely be positive?**

14 to 21 days.

❍ **What are the three steps of bone healing after a fracture?**

Union, consolidation, remodeling.

❍ **What is the purpose for arthrocentesis of a knee with an acute hemarthrosis?**

Relieve pressure and pain and see if fat globules are present indicating a fracture.

❍ **Where is the most common site of compartment syndrome?**

Anterior compartment of the leg, which contains the tibialis anteriorsus, extensor digitorum longus, extensor hallucis longus and peroneus muscles, as well as the anterior tibial artery and deep peroneal nerve.

❍ **How are sprains classified?**

1st° - stretching of ligament, normal x-ray.
2nd° - severe stretching with partial tear, marked tenderness, swelling, pain and normal x-ray.
3rd° - complete ligament rupture, marked tenderness, swelling and deformed joint. X-ray may show an abnormal joint.

❍ **Name the function of and spinal level innervating the biceps, triceps, flexor digitorum, interossei, quadriceps, extensor hallucis, biceps femoris, soleus and gastrocnemius and rectal sphincter.**

Muscle	Action	Spinal Level
Biceps	Forearm flexion	C 5,6
Triceps	Forearm extension	C7
Flexor digitorum	Finger flexion	C8
Interossei	Finger Add/Abd	T1
Quadriceps	Knee extension	L3,4
Extensor hallucis	Great toe dorsiflexion	L5
Biceps femoris	Knee flexion	S1
Soleus and gastrocnemius	Foot plantar flexion	S1,2
Rectal sphincter	Sphincter tone	S2-4

❍ **What is the dose of methylprednisolone used to treat acute spinal cord injury?**

30 mg/kg load over 15 min in the first hour followed by 5.4 mg/kg per hour over the next 23 hour.

❍ **What is the sensory innervation to the nipple, umbilicus and perianal region?**

Nipple - T5.
Umbilicus - T10.
Perianal - S2-4.

❍ **What percentage of cervical spine fractures are seen on lateral, odontoid and AP films of the cervical spine?**

Lateral 80%
Odontoid < 10%.
AP < 10%.
Some are only seen on CT.

❍ **On lateral cervical spine x-ray, how much soft tissue prevertebral swelling is normal at C2?**

Greater than 7 mm is suggestive of a vertebral fracture.

❍ **What is suggested by anterior subluxation of a vertebral body more than one half its width?**

Bilateral facet dislocation.

❍ **How much angulation is normal in an adult lateral cervical spine x-ray measured across a single interspace?**

Up to 10°.

❍ **On lateral cervical spine x-ray, what does "fanning" of the spinous processes suggest?**

Posterior ligamentous disruption.

❍ **What are the three most unstable cervical spine injuries?**

Transverse atlantal ligament rupture, dens fracture and burst fracture with posterior ligament disruption.

❍ **What is the most common thoracolumbar wedge fracture in the elderly?**

L1. Wedge > 50% usually requires admission for pain control and observation for ileus.

❍ **Describe the key features of spinal shock.**

Hypotension with bradycardia.

❍ **A trauma patient has blood at the urinary meatus. What test should be ordered?**

Retrograde urethrogram.

❍ **In blunt trauma, what is the most common renal pedicle injury?**

Renal artery thrombosis.

❍ **Describe the leg position in a patient with a femoral neck fracture.**

Shortened, abducted and slightly externally rotated.

❍ **Describe the leg position in a patient with an anterior hip dislocation.**

Hip is abducted and externally rotated. 10% of hip dislocations. Mechanism is forced abduction. If anterior superior, hip is extended. If anterior inferior, hip is flexed.

❍ **Describe the leg position in a patient with a posterior hip dislocation.**

Shortened, adducted and internally rotated. 90% of hip dislocations. Force applied to a flexed knee directed posteriorly. Associated with sciatic nerve injury (10%) and avascular necrosis of the femoral head.

❍ **A pneumatic tourniquet can be inflated on an extremity to more than a patient's systolic blood pressure for how long?**

2 hours without damage to underlying vessels or nerves.

❍ **What mechanisms of injury create wounds that are most susceptible to infection?**

Compression or tension injuries.

❍ **Bacterial endocarditis secondary to soft tissue infections may be caused by which two organisms?**

Staphylococcus aureus and Staphylococcus epidermidis.

❍ **What factors increase the likelihood of wound infection?**

Dirty or contaminated wounds, stellate or crushing wounds, wounds longer than 5 cm, wounds older than 6 hours and infection prone anatomic sites.

❍ **A tennis player presents to your "fast-track" after stepping on a nail that went right through her favorite, oldest pair of tennis shoes. What organism might infect her puncture wound?**

Pseudomonas aeruginosa.

❍ **What is the most common bacteria seen in cat bite wounds which can also occur with dog bites?**

Pasteurella multocida.

❍ **What types of wounds result in the majority of tetanus cases?**

Lacerations, punctures and crush injuries.

❍ **What is the risk associated with not treating a septal hematoma of the nose?**

Absorption of the septal cartilage resulting in septal perforation.

❍ **What is the resultant deformity if an auricular hematoma is not properly treated?**

Cauliflower ear.

❍ **What should be the first maneuver in treating a long bone fracture in which distal pulses are absent?**

Gentle reduction of the fracture in an attempt to restore distal circulation.

❍ **What steps are involved in evaluating an extremity after a traumatic insult?**

Assessment of the circulation, neurologic function, bony deformities and soft tissue defects.

❍ **Pain with motion in an extremity without an apparent fracture is best studied with what modality?**

Motion or stress X-rays, which help identify ligamentous injuries.

❍ **What is the proper exam for testing motor function of the radial nerve?**

Thumb extension and abduction.

❍ **Which nerve supplies sensation to the dorsal aspect of the web space between the first to second toes?**

Deep peroneal nerve.

❍ **T/F: Fractures associated with open wounds should be explored surgically.**

True. These are classified as open fractures and require adequate debridement and irrigation. They are assumed to be contaminated. Antibiotics alone cannot replace adequate debridement of necrotic and contaminated tissues.

❍ **In general, what is the maximum time limit for salvaging an ischemic limb?**

Six hours. Less if all the arterial collaterals are injured as well.

❍ **T/F: When a posterior dislocation of the knee is reduced and a normal vascular exam is obtained, one may be assured that no vascular injury is present.**

False. These injuries are often associated with intimal disruption within the popliteal artery which can lead to thrombosis. Further investigation using arteriography or duplex sonography should be employed to rule out such injuries.

❍ **What are the treatment modalities used to minimize the risk of infection in an open fracture?**

Antibiotic therapy, aggressive surgical debridement, fracture stabilization and meticulous wound care.

❍ **In the multiply injured trauma patient who has sustained a femur fracture, what is the preferred timing of intramedullary fixation: early (<24 hours) or late (> 48 hours)?**

Early intramedullary nailing has been associated with decreased pulmonary complications, decreased blood loss and shorter ICU stays.

❍ **What is the incidence of developing a compartment syndrome with an open tibial fracture?**

10%. It is more common with the more severe injuries, such as open fractures.

❍ **What associated injuries must be considered in the presence of calcaneal fractures?**

Vertebral compression or burst fractures.

❍ **What are typical clinical findings of a compartment syndrome?**

Tenseness of the involved compartment to palpation, pain with passive motion, paresis and intact distal pulses. Loss of distal pulses is a late sign.

❍ **T/F: There is an absolute value for a compartment pressure which is diagnostic of a compartment syndrome.**

False. There is no specific value. In general an abnormal compartment pressures is > 30 mm Hg, but this does not take into account systemic pressures. Some have suggested that when the difference between the mean arterial pressure and the compartment pressure is less than 40 mm Hg a compartment syndrome should be expected.

❍ **How should amputated parts be transported to the hospital?**

The part should be stored on saline moistened gauze in a plastic bag and placed on ice. It should not come into contact with the ice. "Dry ice" should never be used.

❍ **T/F: Human bite wounds to the hands are relatively benign.**

False. These injuries need to be treated with antibiotics and, if necessary, surgery.

❍ **T/F: Nerve injury associated with low velocity missile wounding is generally permanent.**

False. Nerve injury associated with low velocity is most often a neuropraxia and typically recovers.

❍ **What clinical findings are suggestive of arterial injury after penetrating trauma?**

Physical findings such as a cold limb, absent or diminished pulse, difference in extremity systolic pressures or the presence of a bruit or thrill may indicate an arterial injury. Some arterial injuries are best treated in the operating room without the delay of an arteriogram, especially when there is threatened viability of the limb.

❍ **What percentage of gunshot related arterial injury is associated with concomitant nerve injury?**

Arterial injury secondary to a gunshot wound is associated with nerve injury in 70% of cases.

❍ **Irreversible changes to muscle occur at what point after traumatic ischemia?**

Muscle ischemia is most often associated with arterial injury or compartment syndrome. Irreversible changes occur after six hours of ischemia, potentially earlier if the collaterals are also injured.

❍ **T/F: Pulse deficit is a reliable sign of axillary artery injury.**

False. Studies found pulse deficits present in only 54% of axillary artery injuries, compared to 75% or greater in other extremity arterial injuries.

❍ **What are absolute indications for exploration of extremity stab wounds?**

Absolute indications for exploration of extremity stab wounds include: 1) arterial bleeding 2) limb ischemia 3) nerve deficit.

❍ **The majority of neurologic deficits associated with penetrating trauma to the brachial artery involve which nerve?**

The median nerve.

❍ **Which joint dislocation is associated with the highest rate of arterial injury?**

Knee dislocation has the highest incidence of arterial injury. As many as 30% of high energy knee dislocations injure the popliteal artery.

❍ **Among venous injuries the most commonly injured vein is in which anatomic location?**

The superficial femoral vein.

❍ **Humeral shaft fractures are associated with injury to which upper extremity nerve?**

Radial nerve.

❍ **T/F: Neural injury associated with fractures have a good chance of spontaneous recovery.**

True. Recovery is much less common with injuries associated with dislocations.

❍ **T/F: Every attempt should be made to salvage a mangled extremity. A delay in amputation does not affect outcome.**

False. Delay in amputation can result in increased risk of sepsis, death, disability and number of surgical procedures.

❍ **What is fat embolism syndrome?**

A clinical syndrome characterized by respiratory insufficiency, mental status changes and thrombocytopenia with petechiae. Fat emboli arise primarily from the marrow of fractured long bones. The pulmonary findings are essentially indistinguishable from that of adult respiratory distress syndrome (ARDS).

❍ **What landmarks define the abdominal cavity?**

The space marked by the nipple to inguinal crease anteriorly and tip of scapula to buttock crease posteriorly.

❍ **T/F: The physical exam is a reliable diagnostic tool for abdominal injury.**

False. The physical exam can miss up to 40% of abdominal injuries.

❍ **T/F: Any penetrating trauma from the nipple line to the inguinal ligament can produce an intra-abdominal injury.**

True. Due to the upward movement of the diaphragm during normal respiration to the level of the fifth intercostal space, any penetrating injury below this can cause an abdominal injury.

❍ **What are the appropriate tests to evaluate the abdomen for hemoperitoneum in hemodynamically unstable patients?**

Diagnostic peritoneal lavage or ultrasound.

❍ **What constitutes a positive diagnostic peritoneal lavage (DPL) following blunt trauma?**

> 10 ml gross blood on aspiration, >100,000 red blood cells (RBC/mm^3), bacteria, bile or food particles.

❍ **What are the RBC criteria for DPL in penetrating trauma?**

100,000 RBCs or more for stab wounds to the anterior abdomen, flank and back. 5,000 RBCs or more for chest stab wounds and gunshot wounds.

❍ **T/F: The false negative rate for DPL in stab wounds using a 100,000 RBC cutoff is 20%.**

False. The false negative rate for DPL is less than 10%.

❍ **T/F: The false positive rate for DPL in stab wounds is 5 to 10%.**

True.

❍ **What is the one absolute contraindication to diagnostic peritoneal lavage?**

Obvious need for laparotomy.

❍ **What injuries are most commonly missed by CT scan?**

Hollow viscus, pancreas and diaphragm.

❍ **T/F: Recent experience has shown CT scanning to be specific for solid organ and hollow viscus injuries.**

False. Even with the advent of high-resolution helical CT scans the test still lacks sensitivity for hollow viscus injury.

❍ **What is the likelihood that a stab to the abdomen will inflict an injury requiring operative repair?**

50% of stab wounds to the abdomen actually penetrate the peritoneal cavity. However, only 25% of stab wounds to the abdomen result in injury necessitating operative repair.

❍ **What is the most commonly injured organ following penetrating trauma to the abdomen?**

The liver followed by the small bowel.

❍ **What is the incidence of colon injury following penetrating trauma to the abdomen?**

The colon is injured in 25% of gunshot wounds and 5% of stab wounds to the abdomen.

❍ **What is the significance of rectal examination following penetrating injury to the abdomen?**

Gross blood on digital rectal exam is indicative of a colorectal injury.

❍ **When is primary repair of a colon injury not warranted?**

This is controversial. If gross fecal contamination, shock, massive blood loss, other associated abdominal injuries or delay in diagnosis greater than eight hours is present, primary repair may not be indicated.

❍ **What percentage of pancreatic injuries have associated intra-abdominal injuries?**

Greater than 90% of pancreatic injuries have associated vascular or solid organ injury.

❍ **T/F: Serum amylase is a useful marker for ruling out pancreatic injury.**

False. Amylasemia is neither sensitive nor specific for pancreatic injury.

❍ **What is the critical issue in operative management of pancreatic trauma?**

Identification of injury to the major duct.

❍ **What type of injury is suggested by retroperitoneal gas on plane abdominal radiograph along the right psoas margin or over the right pole of the kidney?**

Duodenal injury.

❍ **What are the indications for pancreatoduodenectomy in abdominal trauma?**

1) Massive hemorrhage from head of pancreas or adjacent vascular structures.
2) Unreconstructable ductal injury in head of pancreas.
3) Combined injuries of duodenum and head of pancreas.

❍ **What is the "coiled spring" sign?**

The radiological appearance of a duodenal hematoma on upper GI series.

❍ **What does the initial treatment of a duodenal hematoma found on upper GI series consists of?**

Observation with nasogastric suction.

❍ **When is primary closure of the duodenum contraindicated?**

Gunshot injuries of greater than 50% of the duodenal circumference or when associated bile duct injury is present.

❍ **With all types of abdominal injury, what is the organ most often injured?**

Liver.

❍ **How sensitive is a physical exam in identifying injuries to the liver?**

As many as 45% of liver injuries can be missed with clinical exam alone.

❍ **What is the overall mortality rate for liver injuries?**

10%. Low for grades 1 & 2, higher for grades 3, 4, & 5.
Grade 3 = 25%.
Grade 4 = 46%.
Grade 5 = 80%.

❍ **What types of liver injuries should be drained post-operatively?**

Closed suction drainage is only required for grade III or greater liver injuries.

❍ **What is the Pringle maneuver?**

Occlusion of the portal triad which includes the hepatic artery and portal vein.

❍ **What is the diagnostic purpose of the Pringle maneuver?**

To demonstrate that hepatic hemorrhage is coming from the hepatic artery or portal vein as opposed to the hepatic veins or inferior vena cava.

❍ **How is the common bile duct evaluated intraoperatively with respect to hepatic trauma?**

Cholangiography.

❍ **What is the most frequent extrahepatic biliary structure injured in abdominal trauma?**

The gallbladder, treated by cholecystectomy.

❍ **What is the treatment of choice for complex bile duct injury (greater than 50% circumference)?**

Roux-en-Y choledochojejunostomy or hepaticojejunostomy.

❍ **What is the most appropriate maneuver in an unstable patient found to have a liver injury during exploratory laparotomy?**

Perihepatic packing should be performed in unstable patients, i.e., those with hemorrhage, hypothermia and coagulopathy.

❍ **What is the most common indication for exploratory laparotomy following blunt trauma?**

Splenic injury.

❍ **What percentage of splenic injuries in children can be managed expectantly?**

Nonoperative management of splenic injury in children is successful in greater than 90% of cases.

❍ **Splenectomy carries a lifelong risk of overwhelming postsplenectomy sepsis. What are the main organisms associated with postsplenectomy sepsis?**

Pneumococcus, meningococcus and Haemophilus influenza. All three are encapsulated organisms.

❍ **What is the mortality rate for overwhelming postsplenectomy sepsis?**

50%.

❍ **Do the current pneumococcal polyvalent vaccines protect against all known serotypes of S. pneumoniae?**

No. It covers serotypes responsible for approximately 90% of bacteremias.

❍ **What is the likelihood that an abdominal gunshot wound will require operative therapy?**

80 to 95%.

❍ **What are contraindications for the use of laparoscopy in the evaluation of the abdomen in the trauma patient?**

Multiple previous operations, shock or head injury with elevated ICP.

❍ **What is the most common injury missed by the use of laparoscopy in the trauma patient?**

Hollow viscus injury.

❍ **What is considered optimal treatment for an impalement injury to the abdomen?**

Secure the object until it can be removed in the operating room under direct vision with the abdomen open.

❍ **Which retroperitoneal hematomas require mandatory exploration after blunt abdominal trauma?**

Those centrally located.

❍ **What determines surgical management of retroperitoneal hematomas?**

Zonal distribution and mechanism of injury. All zone 1 (central) hematomas should be explored regardless of mechanism. Zone 2 (flank) and zone 3 (pelvic) hematomas resulting from penetrating injury should be explored. Expanding hematomas in zone 2 in blunt trauma should be explored as well. However, stable hematomas in zones 2 and 3 in blunt injury should not be explored.

❍ **What are the clinical manifestations of abdominal compartment syndrome?**

Respiratory: decreased compliance, increased airway pressures, increased pulmonary vascular resistance, hypercarbia and hypoxemia.
Cardiovascular: decreased cardiac output.
Abdomen: decreased splanchnic flow.
Renal: oliguria.

❍ **What formula should be used to calculate fluid requirements for resuscitation of a burn victim?**

4 ml/kg / %TBSA / day.
One-half of this is given in the first 8 hours.

❍ **What number of points is the best verbal response worth in the Glasgow coma scale?**

5.

❍ **What number of points is the best motor response worth in the Glasgow coma scale?**

6.

❍ **A patient opens his eyes to voice, makes incomprehensible sounds and withdraws to painful stimulus. What is his GCS?**

9.
Glasgow coma scale:

Eye opening	Best verbal response	Best motor response
4 spontaneously	5 oriented x 3	6 obeys command
3 on request	4 confused conversation	5 localizes pain stimulus
2 to pain	3 inappropriate words	4 flexes either arm appropriately
1 no opening	2 incomprehensible sounds	3 flexion withdrawal
	1 no response	2 extension withdrawal
		1 no response

❍ **What electrolyte is depleted in a victim of a hydrofluoric acid burn?**

Hydrofluoric acid results in hypocalcemia.

❍ **A patient has sustained blunt trauma to the chest that results in pneumothorax. Multiple chest tubes have not controlled the air leak. What complication should you suspect?**

A Bronchial tear. Bronchoscopy is necessary for diagnosis, followed by emergency thoracotomy.

❍ **Can tetanus occur after surgical procedures?**

Yes. While most cases of tetanus in the US occur after minor trauma, there have been numerous reports of tetanus following general surgical procedures, especially those involving the GI tract.

❍ **What are the risk factors for the development of tetanus in a wound?**

Age of wound:	> 6 hours
Configuration:	Stellate wound
Depth:	> 1 cm
Mechanism of injury:	Missile, crush, burn, frostbite
Signs of infection:	Present
Devitalized tissue:	Present
Contaminants:	Present
Denervated or ischemic tissue:	Present

❍ **A 15 year old fire victim is burned over both legs, his entire back and his right arm. What percentage of his body is burned?**

63%. Follow the adult rule of 9s. Head = 9%. Arms = 9% each. Front = 18%. Back = 18%. Legs = 18% each.

❍ **A 14 year old patient who has been burned over the entire top of his body (arms and torso, front and back) develops severe difficulty breathing and appears to be going into respiratory arrest. What should you do?**

Perform an escharotomy. The patient is most likely suffering ventilatory restriction due to the circumferential eschar about his chest that is constricting the chest cavity. Escharotomies need not be performed with anesthesia, not even local anesthesia, because third degree burns involve the nervous tissue and are thus insensitive to pain.

❍ **What is the required dose of Ringer's solution in a 16 year old with 20% body surface burn?**

4 liters in the first 8 hours (500 ml per hour). The patient should receive 250 ml/hour over the next 16 hours. The Parkland formula = (4 ml)(kg body weight)(% burned). Give 1/2 the volume in the first 8

hours and the other half in the next 16 hours. Management after this should be judged clinically. Urine output should be maintained at 50 ml/hr in adults and 0.5 to 1 ml/kg/hour in children.

❍ **You stabilize a multiple trauma victim whose injuries include mild head injury, scalp lacerations and a femur fracture. The next morning you note a new right hemiparesis and confusion. Furthermore his oxygen saturation has dropped to the low 90s and his urine output is declining. The patient is noted to have petechiae on his chest and in his conjunctivae. What is the most likely diagnosis?**

Fat embolism.

Angiotensin-converting enzyme inhibitor. Although angioneurotic edema may occur anytime during therapy, it is most likely to occur within in first month when using and ACE inhibitor.

❍ **A patient presents with sudden onset of vision loss in one eye that quickly returns. What is the most likely diagnosis?**

Amaurosis fugax. Usually caused by central retinal artery emboli from extracranial atherosclerosis.

❍ **What conditions have been associated with central retinal vein occlusion?**

Hyperviscosity syndromes, diabetes and hypertension. Funduscopic examination shows a chaotically streaked retina with congested dilated veins. There are superficial and deep retinal hemorrhages, cotton wool spots and macular edema.

❍ **A patient presents with traumatic pain behind the left eye, a left pupil afferent defect, central visual loss and a left swollen disc. What is the diagnosis and potential causes?**

Optic neuritis. This may be idiopathic or may be associated with multiple sclerosis, Lyme disease, neurosyphilis, lupus, sarcoid, alcoholism, toxins or drug abuse.

❍ **After entering a dark bar, a patient developed eye pain, nausea, vomiting, blurred vision and he sees halos around lights. Why would this patient be given mannitol, pilocarpine and acetazolamide?**

This patient has acute narrow angle glaucoma. The goal of treatment is to decrease intraocular pressure. To accomplish this, one should:

1) Decrease the production of aqueous humor with a carbonic anhydrase inhibitor.
2) Decrease intraocular volume by making the plasma hypertonic to the aqueous humor with mannitol.
3) Constrict the pupil with pilocarpine, allowing increased flow of the aqueous humor out through the previously blocked canals of Schlemm.

❍ **A patient presents with ptosis and ipsilateral miosis of the pupil and has pain in the ipsilateral arm. Where is the lesion?**

The clinical diagnosis is Horner's syndrome. This can be confirmed with topical pharmacologic testing with cocaine drops. If the involved pupil does not dilate, the patient has an ipsilateral Horner's syndrome. The presence of arm pain suggests that the lesion involves the sympathetic chain at the level of the brachial plexus. An apical lung tumor (Pancoast tumor) should be suspected in this setting.

❍ **A 45 year-old patient presents with painless variable diplopia and ptosis. There is moderate weakness of eyelid closure bilaterally. The pupils and the remainder of the exam are normal. What is the next most appropriate evaluation?**

Myasthenia gravis may mimic any pupil-spared, non-proptotic, painless ophthalmoplegia. It may occur with or without ptosis. An edrophonium (Tensilon) test reverses the ptosis and ophthalmoplegia.

❍ **A 55 year-old diabetic patient develops acute onset of proptosis, chemosis and ophthalmoplegia. A black eschar is seen on the palate. What is the most likely diagnosis?**

An acute ophthalmoplegia with orbital signs in a diabetic patient is mucormycosis until proven otherwise. Early recognition is crucial as the disease may be life threatening.

❍ **A 40 year-old horse-racing jockey, weighing 105 lbs., was brought to the emergency room because of slowly progressive confusion and imbalance of several days duration. He is disoriented**

and confused and frequently repeated himself and has an unsteady gait. He has a full range of eye motion and has no ocular misalignment. However, he had a primary position upbeat nystagmus, which became downbeating with convergence and mild horizontal end gaze nystagmus. What is the likely etiology for his confusion and eye findings?

The patient probably has Wernicke's encephalopathy caused by thiamine deficiency. Although most often seen with nutritional deprivation associated with chronic alcoholism, the disorder may also be seen with eating disorders, bulimia, hyperemesis gravidarum and maintaining low weight (e.g., jockeys). Characteristic findings include the classic triad of ophthalmoplegia (bilateral lateral rectus weakness), ataxia and mental changes. The ocular motor signs are quite varied in Wernicke's disease and include bilateral abducens palsies, gaze-evoked or primary position vertical nystagmus, various combinations of horizontal and vertical gaze palsies and internuclear ophthalmoplegia, convergence disorders and ocular bobbing. Thiamine therapy must be urgently instituted.

❍ **What are the ocular manifestations of Lyme disease?**

Uveitis, keratitis and optic neuritis.

❍ **What is the most common cause of endogenous fungal endophthalmitis?**

Candida species.

❍ **What are the two major risk factors for ocular candidiasis?**

Indwelling venous catheters and intravenous drug abuse.

❍ **What systemic bacterial infection is associated with granulomatous uveitis and yellow-white choroidal nodules?**

Tuberculosis.

❍ **What is the most frequent condition associated with orbital cellulitis?**

Sinusitis.

❍ **Why must the anesthesiologist be informed, prior to general anesthesia, that a patient is taking echothiophate?**

Phospholine iodide inhibits plasma pseudocholinesterase (as well as acetylcholinesterase), the enzyme responsible for metabolism of succinylcholine. Intraoperative administration of succinylcholine might lead to cardiovascular collapse and respiratory arrest.

❍ **What are the findings in a pseudotumor cerebri patient?**

An obese, young, female patient complaining of chronic headaches, transient visual obscurations, who on examination has papilledema, an enlarged blind spot on visual field testing and has a normal brain CT scan, except for smaller ventricles. Pseudotumor cerebri is a classic example of the idiopathic intracranial hypertension. A high opening pressure during lumbar puncture is both diagnostic as well as therapeutic. Treatment consists of acetazolamide and repeat lumbar puncture.

❍ **Sudden loss of vision in one eye - what to do?**

In an elderly patient with polymyalgia rheumatica, jaw claudication, decreased appetite, weight loss and tender temporal arteries, the diagnosis of giant cell arteritis must be considered as an emergency and an ESR must be obtained. A vascular event, consisting of central retinal artery occlusion, manifests as a cherry red spot in the funduscopic exam. Urgent massage of the globe and paracentesis by an ophthalmologist may be immediately required. Amaurosis fugax is a transient loss of vision in one eye, usually due to embolic event from the carotid or heart. Several ophthalmic conditions that may cause unilateral loss of vision include vitreous hemorrhage, nonarteritic anterior ischemic optic neuropathy, branch retinal artery occlusion, posterior ischemic optic neuropathy, papilledema, migraine and age related macular degeneration.

❍ **Sudden loss of vision in both eyes - what to do?**

A hypotensive event, due to cardiac arrest, blood loss or intraoperative hypotension, may produce bilateral occipital infarction, leading to bilateral loss of vision. Rare conditions include Leber's optic atrophy and thrombotic thrombocytopenic purpura. Transient bilateral visual loss can also be due to vertebral-basilar insufficiency.

❍ **How do you differentiate metabolic coma from herniation?**

Pupillary pathways are relatively resistant to metabolic insults, so the presence or absence of light reflex is the single most important physical sign to distinguish structural from metabolic coma. Uncal herniation will produce unilateral dilated fixed pupil with localizing neurologic signs.

❍ **Define Ellis Class I, II and III.**

I - Enamel exposed.
II - Enamel plus dentin exposed (pink). Patients complain of sensitivity to heat and cold.
III - Enamel, dentin and pulp exposed (drop of blood). Patients complain of pain or no pain depending on nerve involvement. Treat by application of tinfoil, analgesics and immediate referral. Avoid topical analgesics which may cause sterile abscesses.

❍ **What five lid lacerations should be referred to an ophthalmologist?**

1. Near the lacrimal canaliculi (between the medial canthus and the punctum).
2. Near the levator (transverse lacerations of the upper lid).
3. Near the orbital septum (upper lid deep wounds, between the tarsus and the superior orbital rim).
4. Canthal tendons (wounds penetrating the lateral and medial canthi).
5. Lid margins (wounds through the tarsal plate and lid margins).

❍ **A patient presents with a history of trauma to the orbit with a dull ocular pain, decreased visual acuity and photophobia. Exam reveals a constricted pupil and ciliary flush. What will be found on slit-lamp exam?**

Flare and cells in the anterior chamber are present with traumatic iritis.

❍ **A patient presents with ear pain. On exam, the tympanic membrane has blisters which appear to contain fluid. What is the most likely diagnosis?**

Bullous myringitis, commonly caused by Mycoplasma or viruses. Treat with erythromycin.

❍ **A 16 year old former "Golden Gloves" champ presents with right ear pain and swelling after receiving a blow to the ear. Treatment?**

If the ear is not treated appropriately, cauliflower deformity may result. As such, the ear should be aseptically drained by incision or aspiration and a mastoid conforming dressing should be applied. ENT follow-up is mandatory.

❍ **A patient presents with a swollen, tender, red left auricle. What is the most likely diagnosis?**

Perichondritis caused by Pseudomonas.

❍ **What potential complication of a nasal fracture should always be considered on physical exam?**

Septal hematoma. If not drained, aseptic necrosis of the septal cartilage or septal abscess may develop.

❍ **In what age group is retropharyngeal abscess most common?**

Children less than six years old. Symptoms may include difficulty breathing, fever, enlarged cervical nodes, difficulty swallowing and a stiff neck. Exam may reveal a mass or fullness in the posterior pharyngeal area.

❍ **In what age group are peritonsillar abscesses most common?**

Adolescents and young adults. Symptoms may include ear pain, odynophagia, dysphagia, trismus, drooling and hot potato voice.

❍ **A 5 year old child presents with a history of sinus infection. On exam, the child's eyelid is red and swollen, the globe is displaced laterally and inferiorly and proptosis is present. What is the most likely diagnosis?**

The child may have orbital cellulitis and an abscess associated with ethmoid sinusitis.

❍ **A patient presents with gingival pain and foul odor and taste in the mouth. On exam, fever and lymphadenopathy are present. The gingiva is bright red and the papillae are ulcerated and covered with a gray membrane. What is the most likely diagnosis?**

Acute necrotizing ulcerative gingivitis.

❍ **What are the signs and symptoms of a mandibular fracture?**

Malocclusion, pain, decreased range of motion, bony deformity, swelling, ecchymosis and mental nerve anesthesia.

❍ **Describe a Le Fort I fracture.**

Fracture line starting at the nasal apertures to the wall of the maxillary sinuses bilaterally, across the pterygomaxillary tissue and involving the lateral pterygoid plates. X-rays often miss this fracture.

❍ **Describe the physical findings of a Le Fort II fracture.**

Swelling of the nose, lips, eyes and midface. Sub-conjunctival hemorrhage may be present with blood in the nares. Suspect cerebrospinal involvement and check for rhinorrhea. Water's view and CT should be ordered. Fracture involves facial aspects of the maxillae extending to the nasal and ethmoid bones. Fracture also involves the maxillary sinuses and infraorbital rims bilaterally across the bridge of the nose.

❍ **Describe the fracture line in a Le Fort III fracture.**

Runs through the frontozygomatic suture lines bilaterally, through the orbits and through the base of the nose and ethmoid region. Also called a "dishface" fracture. Movement of the zygoma and midface is suggestive. Water's view and CT confirm the diagnosis.

❍ **Cerebrospinal rhinorrhea is most common with which type of Le Fort fracture?**

III.

❍ **What is the commonest cause of acute epiglottitis in children and adults?**

Hemophilus influenzae type b.

❍ **What form of prophylaxis should be given to household contacts of patients with acute epiglottitis?**

Rifampin.

❍ **What class of drugs is contraindicated in Ludwig's angina?**

Neuromuscular blocking agents. Because they may cause relaxation of pharyngeal muscles and thereby narrow the airway.

❍ **What is the most important risk factor for malignant external otitis?**

Diabetes mellitus.

❍ **What is the most common bacterial cause of malignant external otitis?**

Pseudomonas aeruginosa.

❍ **What physical finding is highly suggestive of endophthalmitis?**

Anterior chamber hypopyon.

❍ **What are the most common presenting symptoms of endophthalmitis?**

Loss of vision, eye pain, redness and eyelid swelling.

❍ **What are the two most important risk factors for rhinocerebral mucormycosis?**

Neutropenia and diabetic ketoacidosis.

❍ **What local findings are most characteristic of rhinocerebral mucormycosis?**

Black nasal discharge and cranial nerve palsies.

❍ **Which antifungal agent is considered the drug of choice for rhinocerebral mucormycosis?**

Amphotericin B.

❍ **Is surgical debridement required for effective management of rhinocerebral mucormycosis?**

Yes.

❍ **What local signs are strongly suggestive of orbital cellulitis?**

Proptosis and pain.

❍ **What are the most common local signs of cavernous sinus thrombosis?**

Bilateral proptosis and ophthalmoplegia.

❍ **What two diagnostic studies are most helpful in establishing the diagnosis of cavernous sinus thrombosis?**

Computed tomography or magnetic resonance imaging.

❍ **What is the most common local complaint in adults with acute epiglottitis?**

Dysphagia.

❍ **What local signs are most associated with peritonsillar abscess?**

Unilateral swelling of the soft palate.

❍ **What is the preferred method of treatment of peritonsillar abscess?**

Incision and drainage.

❍ **What infection is associated with the "lumpy jaw" syndrome?**

Actinomycosis.

PULMONARY PEARLS

"We rarely gain a higher or larger view except when it is forced upon us through struggles which we would avoid if we could."
Charles Cooney

❍ **What is the American-European Consensus Conference definition for the diagnosis of ARDS?**

PaO_2/FIO_2 ratio < 200, bilateral infiltrates and wedge pressure < 18.

❍ **What is the cause of hypoxemia in ARDS?**

An increase in alveolar fluid that causes a reduction in the diffusion of oxygen into the capillaries, increasing the shunt.

❍ **What is the mortality of ARDS?**

40 to 60%.

❍ **What are the major risk factors for ARDS?**

Sepsis, trauma, aspiration, multiple transfusions, shock and pulmonary contusions. Many other systemic and local insults may trigger ARDS.

❍ **Why is the pulmonary artery wedge pressure an important feature in the diagnosis of ARDS?**

The presence of a significantly elevated wedge pressure implies that the pulmonary edema is due to left ventricular dysfunction rather than alveolar dysfunction.

❍ **Does PEEP improve ARDS?**

PEEP commonly improves oxygenation. However, it does not reduce the amount of total lung water.

❍ **What is the distribution of pulmonary edema in ARDS?**

Routine chest x-ray appears to show a diffuse distribution. However, CT scan studies reveal an increased involvement in the dependent portions of the lung fields.

❍ **What are the x-ray findings in ARDS?**

Commonly, patchy bilateral peripheral infiltrates. Cardiogenic pulmonary edema typically demonstrates an enlarged heart, pleural effusions and peribronchial cuffing with septal lines.

❍ **What complications are associated with ARDS?**

Pneumothorax, pulmonary infection, pulmonary hypertension and multisystem organ failure.

❍ **What is the advantage of pressure controlled ventilation in ARDS?**

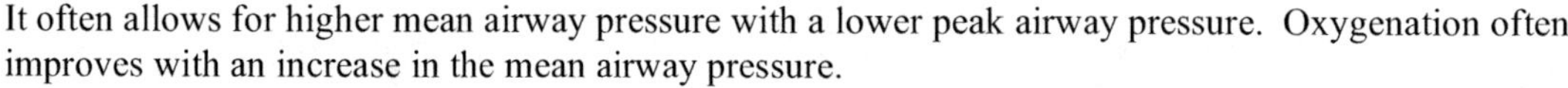

It often allows for higher mean airway pressure with a lower peak airway pressure. Oxygenation often improves with an increase in the mean airway pressure.

❍ **Has the strategy of minimizing plateau pressures been demonstrated to improve outcome in ARDS?**

This strategy is commonly employed. It is controversial as to whether such a strategy improves the clinical outcome.

❍ **What is the theory behind the strategy to minimize plateau pressures for ARDS?**

Decreasing plateau pressures decreases the propensity for alveolar overdistention. Animal studies have demonstrated that alveolar overdistention will result in the same pathological changes as ARDS. The most practical way to currently estimate alveolar overdistention is by measuring plateau pressure.

❍ **Is surfactant therapy helpful in ARDS?**

While there is some evidence that exogenous surfactant is helpful in some pediatric cases, the studies in adults have failed to show a benefit.

❍ **What are the three phases of ARDS?**

Acute or exudative, proliferative and fibrotic phase.

❍ **What is the role of PEEP in ARDS?**

To maintain alveolar inflation and functional residual capacity. This optimizes V/Q matching and improves oxygenation.

❍ **What is compliance and how is it calculated?**

Compliance measures of the elasticity of the lungs. It is calculated by measuring the change in volume for a given change in pressure.

❍ **What are the changes in compliance in ARDS?**

The compliance is decreased due to increased fluid and debris in the alveoli.

❍ **What are the negative effects of PEEP on cardiac output?**

PEEP may reduce cardiac output by reducing venous return, by increasing pulmonary vascular resistance and by shifting the interventricular septum to the left, thus reducing the left ventricular end diastolic volume.

❍ **What are the ways that the optimal level of PEEP can be determined?**

Compliance, oxygenation, calculation of oxygen delivery and elucidation of the lower inflection point on the volume-pressure curve.

❍ **What is the role of corticosteroids in ARDS?**

Steroids have not been shown effective in the early phase of ARDS. In the later stages of ARDS, steroids may have a role by reducing lung fibrosis.

❍ **What interventions have been shown to reduce the mortality of ARDS?**

There never has been a clinically useful interventional study completed in adults that has clearly demonstrated an improved mortality in ARDS.

❍ **Which drugs can cause ARDS?**

Opiates, salicylates, cocaine, protamine and certain chemotherapeutic agents.

❍ **How long after an initial insult does ARDS usually occur?**

12 to 72 hours.

❍ **What does ARDS stand for?**

Acute Respiratory Distress Syndrome is a better term than Adult Respiratory Distress Syndrome as this syndrome occurs in children.

❍ **What is the characteristic histologic change in ARDS?**

Pathologists call this diffuse alveolar damage. It is characterized by a process of diffuse lung inflammation that progresses to fibrosis. Interestingly, the number of inflammatory cells observed is not large. There is heterogeneity both in time and space as to which alveoli are in the inflammatory phase and which are in the fibrotic phase. Another name for ARDS is hyaline membrane disease, which refers to the hyaline membranes seen histopathologically. These are collections of sloughed type 1 pneumocytes and other cellular debris.

❍ **In patients diagnosed with ARDS, what are the most common causes of death?**

Multisystem organ failure or sepsis syndrome, not respiratory failure.

❍ **T/F: Any cause of shock can cause ARDS.**

True.

❍ **T/F: Too much oxygen can cause ARDS.**

True.

❍ **What is a safe level of oxygen for prolonged use?**

An FiO_2 of 0.50 is safe and 0.60 is probably safe.

❍ **If a patient with ARDS has all the ventilator settings optimized, including the PEEP, but the FIO_2 is 0.90 with an oxygen saturation of 90%, should the FIO_2 be lowered to avoid the potential of lung injury?**

No. Hypoxemia is a real threat that must be avoided even to the extent of accepting the risk of oxygen toxicity.

❍ **T/F: A patient with ARDS can have a fever without having a source of infection.**

True.

❍ **What is in the differential diagnosis of ARDS?**

Broadly three categories - cardiogenic pulmonary edema, pneumonia (PCP, fungi, bacteria, legionella, miliary TB) and inflammatory lung conditions (drug reaction, collagen vascular disease, BOOP, acute eosinophilic pneumonia).

❍ **What is the optimal fluid management strategy in ARDS?**

No such strategy has been clearly demonstrated as the preferred strategy. Current thinking is to avoid hypervolemia while maintaining an adequate intravascular volume to optimize oxygen transport to peripheral organs.

❍ **How does the pressure-volume curve appear in a patient with ARDS?**

Generally, with pressure on the horizontal axis and volume on the vertical axis, the curve has three components. Initially, the curve is relative flat, until shifting to a steeper rising curve. The changeover is called the lower inflection point and is thought to reflect the opening of atelectatic alveoli in the dependent portions of the lungs. The curve continues to rise until it flatens again. This second change is called the upper inflection point and is thought to reflect the overdistention of alveoli.

❍ **What is the current ventilator strategy in ARDS utilizing the lower and upper inflection points?**

To give enough PEEP to exceed the lower inflection point, thereby minimizing sheer forces on alveoli that results from the atelectatic alveoli being excessively opened and closed. This has an additional benefit of optimizing oxygenation by keeping the atelectatic alveoli open. The second component is to minimize the lung volume by keep the peak pressure below the upper inflection point, thereby avoiding overdistention of the alveoli.

This strategy makes pathophysiological sense but has not been clinically demonstrated to be clearly advantageous. Clinical trials are underway.

❍ **Does nitric oxide improve oxygenation in ARDS?**

Yes, but outcome studies have not been completed.

❍ **T/F: ECMO improves the mortality in ARDS.**

False.

❍ **What is permissive hypercapnia?**

The ventilator strategy of protecting the lungs from alveolar overdistention by reducing lung volumes and accepting, as a cost, the rise in pCO_2 and fall in pH. This is a controversial strategy, although two consensus conferences suggested that this strategy be utilized when plateau pressures are elevated. Studies are underway which will hopefully resolve the controversy.

❍ **What is the plateau pressure? What is the peak airway pressure?**

The plateau pressure is the static pressure that exists when, at end inspiration, the airway is occluded. Occlusion of the airway creates a static column of air from the endotracheal tube to the alveoli. Because a static column of air is in pressure equilibrium, the pressure measured at the endotracheal tube is the same as that in the alveoli. The plateau pressure is a method to measure the alveolar distending pressure. An excessive elevation of this pressure is thought to reflect alveolar overdistention.

Peak airway pressure is the maximal excursion of the airway pressure gauge during the inspiratory and expiratory cycle.

❍ **Does inverse ratio ventilation improve oxygenation in ARDS? Does it improve mortality?**

Inverse ratio ventilation is the strategy to reverse the normal 1:2 inspiration to expiration ratio in spontaneous breathing. This has been shown to improve oxygenation by increasing mean airway pressure at a lower peak pressure. The controversy is whether it has any beneficial effect over simply increasing PEEP. It is unknown if this strategy improves mortality.

❍ **What is the effect of PEEP on right ventricular preload and afterload? How about on left ventricular preload and afterload?**

PEEP decreases preload to both ventricles, increases RV afterload and decreases LV afterload.

❍ **What is the long term lung function in ARDS survivors?**

Mild reduction of DLCO and mild restrictive ventilatory defect. Some have normal lung function.

❍ **T/F: Patients with ARDS do not develop auto-PEEP.**

False.

❍ **Why does PEEP improve oxygen exchange in ARDS?**

PEEP reverses atelectasis and redistributes lung water from the alveoli to the interstitium.

❍ **How does prone positioning improve oxygenation in ARDS?**

Prone positioning recruits dorsal lung units and improves V/Q matching.

❍ **Are there any side effects noted with prone positioning?**

Yes. Although unusual, hypotension, desaturation and arrhythmias have occurred after prone positioning.

❍ **What level is suggested as the maximal transalveolar pressure (as estimated by the plateau pressure) that will avoid barotrauma in a patient with ARDS?**

35 cm H_2O is commonly suggested in the literature. A recent editorial suggested that higher levels may be acceptable. Randomized trials addressing this are ongoing.

❍ **What is the equation for the A-a gradient?**

A-a $= ((713 \text{ mmHg} \times FIO_2) - pCO_2/.8 - pO_2)$

The normal A-a gradient is 5 to 15 mmHg. The A-a gradient increases with pulmonary embolism.

❍ **Most pulmonary emboli arise from what veins?**

The iliac and femoral veins.

❍ **What does normal ventilation with mismatched decreased lung perfusion suggest?**

Pulmonary embolus.

❍ **Can a patient with a PE have a pO_2 greater than 90 mmHg?**

Yes, but rarely (5%).

❍ **What are two relatively specific CXR findings in PE?**

Hampton's hump: a wedge shaped infiltrate abutting the pleura.
Westermark's sign: decreased lung vasculature markings on the side with a PE.

❍ **How long should chronic warfarin therapy for DVT be given?**

Warfarin should be administered for at least 3 to 6 months after a DVT.

❍ **What is the risk of PE in a patient with an axillary or subclavian vein thrombus?**

About 15%.

❍ **What is Virchow's triad?**

1) Injury to the endothelium of the vessels.
2) Hypercoagulable state.
3) Stasis.

❍ **What is the classical ECG finding in pulmonary embolism?**

$S_1Q_3T_3$ pattern.

❍ **A 48 year old woman is transferred from another hospital a week and a half after sustaining a left upper extremity fracture, a complex pelvic fracture, bilateral lower extremity femur fractures and a left tibial fracture. While sitting in bed, she experiences severe dyspnea, tachypnea and tachycardia. Pulse oximetry reveals an oxygen saturation of 88% on room air. She is given supplemental oxygen and transferred to the ICU. What is your diagnosis?**

Pulmonary embolism secondary to deep vein thrombosis.

❍ **What risk factors for deep vein thrombosis did she have?**

Trauma or surgery of pelvis or lower extremities, indwelling vascular catheters and prolonged immobility.

❍ **What preventative measures can be taken in patients at risk for developing DVTs?**

Early ambulation, elastic stockings that provide graded compression from ankle to thigh, low-dose heparin, intermittent pneumatic compression and prophylactic inferior vena cava filters.

❍ **What tests can be used to diagnosis pulmonary embolism?**

Pulmonary angiogram is the gold standard. V/Q (ventilation/perfusion) scans are the best non-invasive tests to establish or exclude the diagnosis of PE. A high probability scan in a clinical scenario of high likelihood for PE is an indication to treat. An intermediate or low probability scan necessitates further studies. Duplex ultrasound is used to detect DVT not to diagnose PE. However, if the duplex ultrasound is positive, then therapy for DVT will also treat PE.

❍ **What are the indications for pulmonary angiography?**

Non-diagnostic non-invasive lower extremity venous study with a non-diagnostic ventilation-perfusion scan or anticipated embolectomy.

❍ **What are the indications for vena cava filter placement?**

Contraindication to anticoagulation, hemorrhage after anticoagulation, failure of anticoagulation to prevent recurrent pulmonary embolism and prophylaxis for extremely high-risk patients.

❍ **What is the diagnostic test of choice for documenting DVT?**

Duplex ultrasound. The accuracy of physical examination for DVT is generally quoted to be 50%.

❍ **What are the risk factors for DVT?**

Surgery (knee and hip greater than abdominal and urological)
Pregnancy
Cardiac disease, especially post-MI
Age greater than 50 years
Prior DVT
Immobilizaton
Acute paraplegia (but not chronic paraplegia)
Oral contraceptives (but not hormonal replacement therapy)
Major trauma
Malignancy, especially adenocarcinoma
Factor deficiency state
Antiphospholipid antibodies
Nephrotic syndrome
Paroxysmal nocturnal hemoglobinuria
Protein losing enteropathy

❍ **Which factor deficiency states predispose to DVT?**

Activated protein C resistance
Protein C deficiency
Protein S deficiency
Plasminogen deficiency
Antithrombin III deficiency

❍ **What is activated protein C deficiency?**

A point mutation in factor V results in resistance of factor V to the natural anticoagulant effects of protein C. This is the most common deficiency state known to predispose to DVT.

❍ **T/F: The more risk factors a patient has, the greater the chances of developing a DVT.**

True.

❍ **T/F: Only patients with known risk factors develop DVTs.**

False.

❍ **What are the symptoms of a PE?**

Dyspnea, pleurisy, cough, hemoptysis and syncope.

❍ **Which symptom is more common in massive PE than submassive PE?**

Syncope.

❍ **What are the signs of PE?**

Crackles, increased P2, thrombophlebitis, heart gallop, peripheral edema, cardiac murmur and cyanosis.

❍ **What is the most common CXR finding in PE?**

Atelectasis or pulmonary parenchymal defect.

❍ **What are other CXR findings in PE?**

Pleural effusion, pleural based opacity, elevated diaphragm, Westermark's sign and normal.

❍ **Is a normal CXR the most common finding in a PE?**

No. It occurred 16% of the time in the PIOPED database.

❍ **What are the two most common ECG finding in PE?**

Sinus tachycardia and nonspecific ST-T wave changes.

❍ **What are other ECG findings in PE?**

Normal, left axis deviation, RBBB, atrial fibrillation, pseudo-infarction pattern and S1Q3T3.

❍ **T/F: A patient can have a pO_2 greater than 100 or an A-a gradient less than 10 and still have a PE.**

True.

❍ **T/F: The pO_2 or A-a gradient differentiates between a patient with a PE and a patient without a PE.**

False.

❍ **T/F: A blood gas is indicated in every patient suspected of having a PE.**

False.

❍ **What is the primary utility in getting an ECG and CXR in a patient suspected of have a PE?**

To rule out other causes for their respiratory symptoms.

❍ **In a patient with a high probability V/Q scan and a high clinical risk for PE, are any other studies needed?**

No.

❍ **In a patient with a normal V/Q scan and a low clinical risk for PE, are any other studies needed?**

No.

❍ **What is the probability of a PE in all patients with a low probability V/Q scan?**

14%. This varies from 4% to 40%, depending on the clinical likelihood of a PE.

❍ **In a patient with high clinical and V/Q scan probabilities for pulmonary embolism and being considered for thrombolysis, is an angiogram necessary prior to thrombolysis?**

No. The prevalence of PE in patients with high clinical and V/Q scan probabilities for PE is 96%.

❍ **What can be performed in a patient whose post V/Q test probability is still uncertain?**

A lower extremity ultrasound can be performed. If positive, the patient will be treated the same as for a PE. If negative, a pulmonary angiogram can be performed. Some support the use of serial lower extremity ultrasounds in patients with adequate cardiopulmonary reserve. For those with limited reserve, an angiogram is recommended. The use of serial lower extremity ultrasound in such a setting has not been commonly practiced in the United States. The role of D-dimers in the setting of suspected PE has yet to be clarified.

❍ **What is the difference between D-dimer ELISA and latex assays?**

The ELISA is thought to be more accurate.

❍ **What are the accepted indications for the use of thrombolytics in PE?**

Definitely accepted: hemodynamic instability.
Controversial: 40% or more of pulmonary vasculature involved with PE, obstruction of blood flow to one lobe or multiple pulmonary segments, severe hypoxia and right heart failure seen echocardiographically.

❍ **What is the advantage of using thrombolytic agents for PE?**

The only proven benefits have been short-term hemodynamic parameters. No randomized study has been performed with a large enough sample size to assess the impact on mortality.

❍ **Which drugs prolong the effect of coumadin?**

Alcohol (with liver disease), amiodarone, cimetidine, erythromycin, fluconazole, INH, metronidazole, omeprazole, phenylbutazone, propafenone and propranolol.

❍ **Which drugs shorten the effect of coumadin?**

Barbiturates, carbamazepine, griseofulvin, nafcillin, rifampin, sucralfate and vitamin K.

❍ **What are the modified PIOPED criteria for a high probability V/Q scan?**

2 large V/Q mismatches
1 large and 2 or more moderate mismatches
4 or more moderate mismatches
(Large = >75% of a segment)

❍ **What are the modified PIOPED criteria for an intermediate probability V/Q scan?**

1 large V/Q mismatch, with or without 1 moderate mismatch
1-3 moderate mismatches
1 matched defect with a normal CXR
(Moderate = 25% to 75% of a segment)

❍ **What are the modified PIOPED criteria for a low probability V/Q scan?**

1 or more perfusion defect that is smaller than the CXR defect
2 or more matches with a normal CXR and some areas of normal perfusion in lung
1 or more small perfusion defect with a normal CXR
Perfusion defects thought to be caused by effusions, cardiomegaly, aortic dilatation, hila, mediastinum and elevated hemidiaphragms
(Small = <25% of a segment)

❍ **Has one type of IVC filter been proven to be superior to the other types?**

No.

❍ **What is the goal for heparin therapy?**

To maintain the PTT between 1.5 and 2.5 times control.

❍ **What is the goal for coumadin therapy?**

To maintain the INR between 2 and 3.

❍ **What is the treatment for chronic thromboembolic pulmonary hypertension?**

Pulmonary thromboendarterectomy.

❍ **What is the pathophysiology of chronic thromboembolic pulmonary hypertension?**

A pulmonary embolism that results in symptoms secondary to obstruction or stenosis of the pulmonary arteries due to unresolved clot. Typically pulmonary emboli are naturally lysed by the fibrinolytic system resulting in no or minimal residual clot.

❍ **Do calf vein thrombi embolize to the lung?**

Generally no, but they may propagate to the popliteal vein. Popliteal vein thrombi can embolize to the lung.

❍ **How is a subclavian vein thrombosis usually diagnosed?**

With ultrasonography.

❍ **What are the ultrasonographic findings in acute DVT?**

Presence of echogenic material in vein lumen, noncompressibility of vein, venous distention, free-floating thrombus and absence of Doppler tracing.

❍ **What is the rate of PE in patients who have had IVC filters placed?**

2 to 3%.

❍ **What is the best initial method for localizing hemoptysis in a patient who is actively bleeding?**

Bronchoscopy.

❍ **What is the location for aspiration pneumonias?**

In the supine patient, it is in the posterior segment of the upper lobe and in the superior segment of the lower lobe. In the upright patient, it is in the basilar segments of the lower lobes. The right lung is favored over the left because of the straighter takeoff of the right mainstem bronchus.

❍ **What are the common directly toxic (non-infected) respiratory tract aspirates?**

Gastric contents, alcohol, hydrocarbons, mineral oil, animal and vegetable fats. All of these produce an inflammatory response and pneumonia. Gastric contents are the most common offender.

❍ **What are the consequences of aspirating acid?**

The response is rapid, with near immediate bronchitis, bronchiolitis, atelectasis, shunting and hypoxemia. Pulmonary edema may occur within 4 hours. The clinical manifestations are dyspnea, wheezing, cough, cyanosis, fever and shock.

❍ **What is the antibiotic of choice for gastric acid aspiration?**

None.

❍ **What is the role of corticosteroids in gastric acid aspiration?**

None.

❍ **What is the main priority in treating gastric acid aspiration?**

Maintenance of oxygenation. Intubation, ventilation and PEEP (positive end expiratory pressure) may be required.

❍ **What are the radiographic manifestations of acid aspiration?**

Varied. There may be bilateral diffuse infiltrates, irregular "patchy" infiltrates or lobar infiltrates.

❍ **What outcomes occur in patients who do not rapidly resolve gastric acid aspiration pneumonitis?**

ARDS (adult respiratory distress syndrome), progressive respiratory failure and bacterial superinfection.

❍ **What is the predominant oropharyngeal flora in outpatients?**

Anaerobes. Community acquired aspiration is usually anaerobic. The most common aerobes involved are streptococcal species.

❍ **What is the antibiotic of choice for outpatient acquired infectious aspiration pneumonia?**

Clindamycin.

❍ **What is the bacteriology of inpatient acquired infectious aspiration pneumonia?**

Mixed aerobic and anaerobic organisms. Unlike outpatients, Staphylococcus aureus, Escherichia coli, Pseudomonas aeruginosa and Proteus species are common.

❍ **What are the major causes of massive hemoptysis?**

Tuberculosis, bronchiectasis and lung cancer.

❍ **What causes hemoptysis in patients with tuberculosis (either active or healed)?**

Pulmonary artery (Rasmussen's) aneurysm, bronchiolar ulceration and necrosis, bronchiectasis, broncholithiasis and mycetoma (fungus ball).

❍ **What is the purpose of bronchoscopy in hemoptysis?**

Localization and diagnosis.

❍ **What are the invasive therapies for massive hemoptysis?**

Thoracotomy, embolization, balloon tamponade (via bronchoscopy), double-lumen tube for lung separation and independent ventilation and laser bronchoscopy.

❍ **What is the most feared complication of bronchial artery embolization?**

Anterior spinal artery embolization.

❍ **When is surgery indicated for massive hemoptysis?**

Localized massive hemoptysis unresponsive to other therapy or electively, after stabilization, for long term control of localized bleeding.

❍ **What tumor other than squamous cell, adeno-, large cell or small cell carcinoma is likely to cause hemoptysis?**

Bronchial carcinoid.

❍ **What is the most common cause of hemoptysis in patients with leukemia?**

Fungal infections, often aspergillus.

❍ **T/F: Bacterial pneumonia never causes hemoptysis.**

False.

❍ **What are the major cardiovascular causes of hemoptysis?**

Mitral stenosis, pulmonary hypertension and Eisenmenger's complex.

❍ **How does pulmonary artery catheterization produce hemoptysis?**

By pulmonary artery rupture, aneurysm formation and leakage and pulmonary infarction.

❍ **What is the frequency of hemoptysis in pulmonary embolism?**

20%.

❍ **What is a common definition for massive hemoptysis?**

Coughing of more than 600 ml of blood in 24 hours.

❍ **What are the most common causes of hemoptysis in non-hospitalized patients?**

Bronchitis, bronchogenic carcinoma and idiopathic.

❍ **What systemic illnesses cause hemoptysis?**

Amyloidosis, CHF, mitral stenosis, sarcoidosis, SLE, vasculitis, coagulation disorders and pulmonary-renal syndromes.

❍ **How can aspiration be prevented when intubating?**

By avoiding unnecessary increase in intragastric pressure from overzealous bag-valve-mask ventilation and by applying cricoid pressure during intubation.

❍ **When is aspiration most likely to occur during surgery?**

During the induction of anesthesia.

❍ **What is the clinical significance of fixed, dilated pupils in a near-drowning victim?**

Don't give up the ship! Ten to twenty percent of patients presenting with coma and fixed, dilated pupils recover completely.

❍ **What are the expected blood gas findings of a near-drowning victim?**

Metabolic acidosis from poor perfusion and hypoxia.

❍ **Are abdominal thrusts, such as the Heimlich maneuver, indicated in a near-drowning victim?**

No. Near-drowning victims usually aspirate small quantities of water and no drainage procedure is helpful.

❍ **Liquids pass from stomach to duodenum in 2 hours. Solids pass from stomach to duodenum in ________.**

4 to 6 hours

❍ **What may delay gastric emptying?**

Anxiety, pain, drugs, diabetes mellitus, gastric outlet obstruction and pregnancy.

❍ **Under what circumstances is aspiration of vomitus, oral secretions or foreign material likely?**

Anything resulting in an altered level of consciousness (e.g., alcohol, overdose, general anesthesia and stroke), impaired swallowing, abnormal gastrointestinal motility or disruption of esophageal sphincter function.

❍ **T/F: Nasogastric tubes increase the risk of aspiration.**

True.

❍ **T/F: Healthy people may aspirate small amounts of oral contents without developing clinical complications.**

True.

❍ **What are the signs of a large obstructing foreign body in the larynx or trachea?**

Respiratory distress, stridor, inability to speak, cyanosis and loss of consciousness.

❍ **What are the symptoms of a smaller (distally lodged) foreign body?**

Cough, dyspnea, wheezing, chest pain and fever.

❍ **What is the procedure of choice for foreign body removal?**

Rigid bronchoscopy. Fiberoptic bronchoscopy is an alternate procedure in adults, not in children.

❍ **What are the common radiographic findings in foreign body aspiration?**

Normal film, atelectasis, pneumonia, contralateral mediastinal shift (more marked during expiration) and visualization of the foreign body

❍ **T/F: Aspiration of fluids with a pH less than 5 produces chemical pneumonitis.**

False. Aspirate pH less than 2.5 produces chemical injury.

❍ **The chemical pneumonitis produced by aspirated gastric acid is called ____________ ____________.**

Mendelson's syndrome.

❍ **T/F: Aspiration of liquid gastric contents with a pH greater than 2.5 produces no clinical consequences.**

False. Hypoxemia, bronchospasm and atelectasis may develop.

❍ **What are the consequences of aspirating small (non-obstructing) food particles?**

Inflammation and hypoxemia that may result in chronic bronchiolitis or granulomatosis.

❍ **Name the commonly aspirated hydrocarbons.**

Gasoline, kerosene, furniture polish and lighter fluid

❍ **What are the effects of hydrocarbon aspiration?**

Hypoxemia, intrapulmonary shunting, pulmonary edema, hemoptysis and respiratory failure.

❍ **What is the role of emesis induction or gastric lavage in hydrocarbon ingestion?**

These maneuvers are not recommended as the patient may aspirate during regurgitation.

❍ **Can drowning occur without aspiration of water?**

Yes. 10% of victims die from intense laryngospasm.

❍ **Why is rigid bronchoscopy preferred in massive hemoptysis?**

Better suctioning ability, vision, airway control and larger port.

❍ **What are the advantages of fiberoptic bronchoscopy?**

Less invasive, better access to upper lobes and ability to visualize to fifth or sixth generation bronchi.

❍ **What non-invasive bedside maneuver may assist management of massive hemoptysis?**

Positioning the bleeding lung in a dependent position

❍ **How does hemoptysis differ from hematemesis?**

Blood in hemoptysis is often frothy and bright red. Alveolar macrophages may be seen on microscopy. Hematemesis is often acidic with a pH less than 2.5

❍ **What is the major complication of a double lumen tube for independent lung ventilation?**

The tube may slip distally, such that no ventilation is provided to one lung or proximally, so that separation of the 2 sides is lost.

❍ **An asthmatic patient suddenly develops a supraventricular tachycardia. Blood pressure is normal and the QRS complex is also narrow. What therapy is most appropriate?**

Verapamil. Avoid the use of adenosine as it is relatively contraindicated and may exacerbate bronchospasm in asthmatic patients. Also avoid ß-blockers.

❍ **How is decompression sickness treated?**

Primarily by re-exposing the victim to a pressure similar to or greater to that experienced prior to the onset of symptoms. Usually this is done in a hyperbaric chamber and usually it involves breathing 100% oxygen. Treatment duration and pressure are a matter of clinical judgment and protocol and depend greatly on the pressure to which the victim was exposed prior to onset of symptoms.

❍ **Can the hematocrit "overcompensate" or go dangerously high in patients chronically exposed to high altitudes?**

Hematocrits in excess of 60 to 65% do occur with chronic exposure to altitude. This is associated with "sludging" in the cerebral circulation.

❍ **What illness may occur as a result of exposure to altitude?**

Acute mountain sickness is an illness attributed directly to hypobaric hypoxemia.

❍ **What are the symptoms of acute mountain sickness?**

The syndrome covers a spectrum from mild headache and fatigue to life threatening cerebral and pulmonary edema. Headache is throbbing, worse at night and early after awakening. Loss of appetite and nausea are frequent.

❍ **What causes pulmonary and cerebral edema in acute mountain sickness?**

The mechanism is not certain but is generally accepted to be a cytotoxic injury as a direct result of the hypoxemia.

❍ **How does one treat acute mountain sickness?**

Avoid further ascent. The presence of neurologic problems or symptoms or signs of pulmonary edema dictate immediate descent. Stable mild and generalized symptoms without suggestion of pulmonary or cerebral edema can be observed without ascent for 24 hours. Acclimatization will take place within 12 hours to 3 days.

❍ **Is any drug therapy indicated?**

Acetazolamide produces a central stimulation of respiration. When available, oxygen usually provides prompt improvement in symptoms but may not be available where the problem exists (on the side of a mountain). Dexamethasone is associated with improvement.

❍ **Name some processes that cause the work of breathing to increase markedly in patients with COPD.**

Increased dead space ventilation requiring a higher minute ventilation, decreased respiratory muscle efficiency due to hyperinflation and increased airway resistance.

❍ **A patient has severe status asthmatics associated with 20 mmHg of pulsus paradoxus. After another half-hour the degree of pulsus paradoxus decreases to 5 mmHg and the degree of wheezing heard over the chest diminishes. What two exactly opposite ventilatory conditions can produce this identical picture?**

The bronchospasm may be resolving, such that the swings in intrathoracic pressure that caused the pulsus paradoxus decrease along with the intensity of wheezing. The swings in intrathoracic pressure could also decrease if the patient were tiring, such that the respiratory efforts decrease as the patient slipped into a hypercarbic acidosis.

❍ **What conditions or commonly used medications result in an increase in serum theophylline concentration?**

Cimetidine, macrolides, quinolones, verapamil, congestive heart failure and liver failure.

❍ **What conditions or commonly used medications result in a decrease in serum theophylline concentration?**

Barbiturates, phenytoin, carbamazepine, rifampin, smoking and barbecued or smoked food consumption.

❍ **How is chronic bronchitis defined?**

Daily expectoration of sputum for a minimum of three months in a year for at least two years in a patient without other underlying pulmonary disease.

❍ **If a patient with chronic bronchitis suffers an acute exacerbation of his illness, such as dyspnea, cough or purulent sputum, what type of O_2 therapy should be initiated?**

Patients with COPD are have decreased sensitivity to the hypercarbic stimulus to breathe. They are more dependent upon the hypoxic stimulus. In the case of an acute exacerbation of COPD, oxygen therapy should be guided by pO_2 levels. Adequate oxygen must be maintained such that the pO_2 is above 60 mmHg. This should be accomplished with a minimal amount of oxygen.

❍ **What spirometric test best discriminates COPD from restrictive lung disease?**

FEV_1/FVC.

❍ **Which pulmonary function tests increase in COPD?**

Residual volume and total lung capacity. All other tests (FEV_1, FEV_1/FVC, $FEV_{25-75\%}$ and DLCO) decrease.

❍ **What is the risk of placing a patient with COPD on a high FIO_2?**

Suppression of the hypoxic ventilatory drive.

❍ **If mechanical ventilation is required for a patient with status asthmaticus, what is an appropriate setting for the initial tidal volume?**

10 ml/kg.

❍ **What test is most useful to demonstrate airway caliber constriction in asthma?**

FEV_1/FVC. This test determines the amount of air exhaled in 1 second compared to the total amount of air in the lung that can be expressed. A ratio under 0.70 is consistent airway constriction seen in asthma.

❍ **What is a normal peak expiratory flow rate in adults?**

Males: 550 to 600 L/minute. Females: 450 to 500 L/minute. However, this varies somewhat with body size and age.

❍ **What should be suspected if a very young, non-smoking patient has symptoms similar to those associated with emphysema?**

Alpha-1 antitrypsin deficiency. Without alpha-1 antitrypsin, excess elastase accumulates, resulting in lung damage. Treatment for this condition is the same as that for emphysema. An alpha-1 protease inhibitor may also be useful.

❍ **Can theophylline be dialyzed?**

Yes.

❍ **What two diseases are usually seen in patients with COPD?**

Chronic bronchitis and emphysema.

❍ **What is the only known genetic abnormality that leads to COPD?**

Alpha-1 antitrypsin deficiency

❍ **What are the risks of positive pressure mechanical ventilation?**

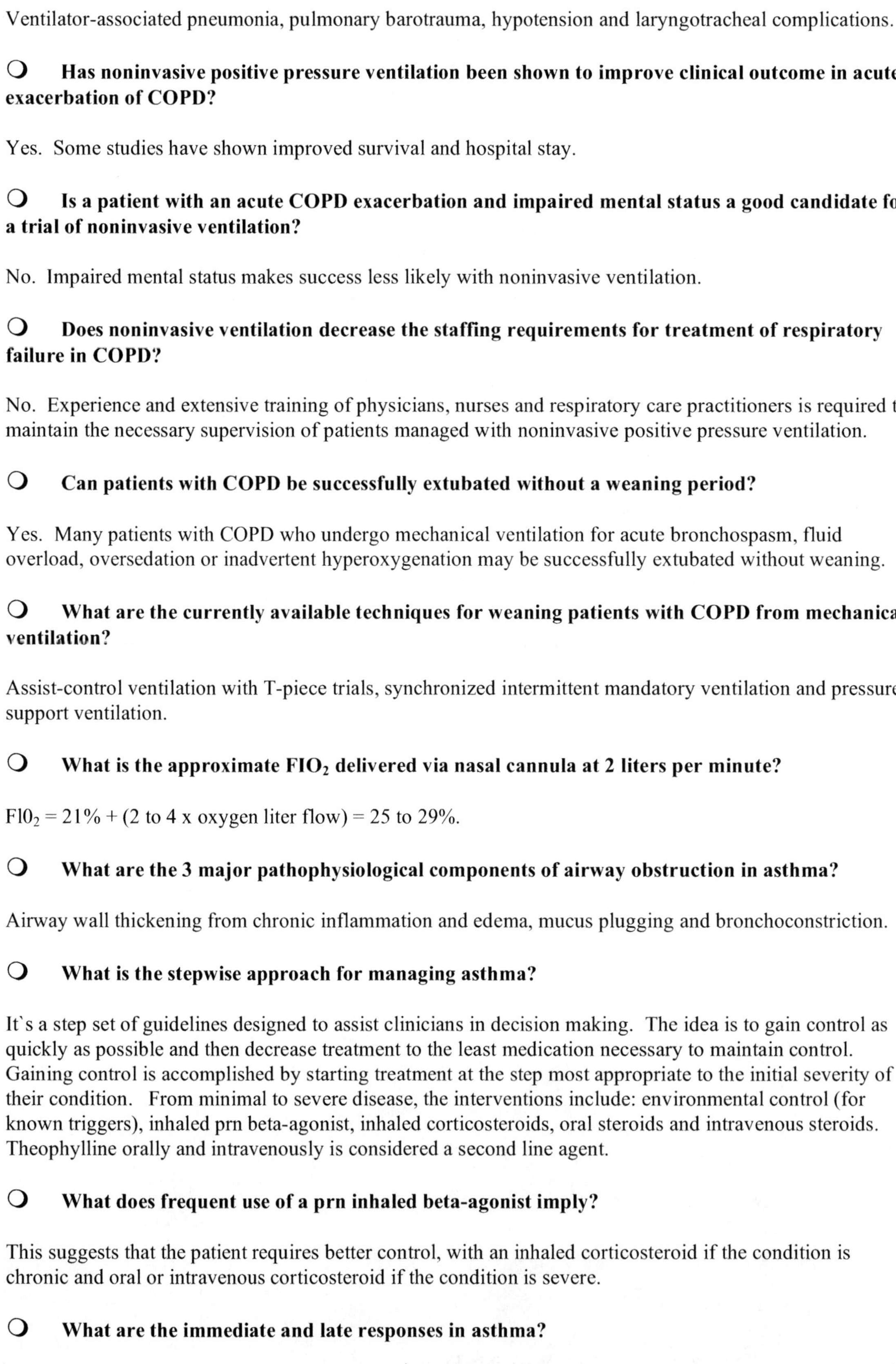

Ventilator-associated pneumonia, pulmonary barotrauma, hypotension and laryngotracheal complications.

❍ **Has noninvasive positive pressure ventilation been shown to improve clinical outcome in acute exacerbation of COPD?**

Yes. Some studies have shown improved survival and hospital stay.

❍ **Is a patient with an acute COPD exacerbation and impaired mental status a good candidate for a trial of noninvasive ventilation?**

No. Impaired mental status makes success less likely with noninvasive ventilation.

❍ **Does noninvasive ventilation decrease the staffing requirements for treatment of respiratory failure in COPD?**

No. Experience and extensive training of physicians, nurses and respiratory care practitioners is required to maintain the necessary supervision of patients managed with noninvasive positive pressure ventilation.

❍ **Can patients with COPD be successfully extubated without a weaning period?**

Yes. Many patients with COPD who undergo mechanical ventilation for acute bronchospasm, fluid overload, oversedation or inadvertent hyperoxygenation may be successfully extubated without weaning.

❍ **What are the currently available techniques for weaning patients with COPD from mechanical ventilation?**

Assist-control ventilation with T-piece trials, synchronized intermittent mandatory ventilation and pressure support ventilation.

❍ **What is the approximate FIO_2 delivered via nasal cannula at 2 liters per minute?**

$FI0_2$ = 21% + (2 to 4 x oxygen liter flow) = 25 to 29%.

❍ **What are the 3 major pathophysiological components of airway obstruction in asthma?**

Airway wall thickening from chronic inflammation and edema, mucus plugging and bronchoconstriction.

❍ **What is the stepwise approach for managing asthma?**

It`s a step set of guidelines designed to assist clinicians in decision making. The idea is to gain control as quickly as possible and then decrease treatment to the least medication necessary to maintain control. Gaining control is accomplished by starting treatment at the step most appropriate to the initial severity of their condition. From minimal to severe disease, the interventions include: environmental control (for known triggers), inhaled prn beta-agonist, inhaled corticosteroids, oral steroids and intravenous steroids. Theophylline orally and intravenously is considered a second line agent.

❍ **What does frequent use of a prn inhaled beta-agonist imply?**

This suggests that the patient requires better control, with an inhaled corticosteroid if the condition is chronic and oral or intravenous corticosteroid if the condition is severe.

❍ **What are the immediate and late responses in asthma?**

An "immediate response" occurs within minutes of exposure, is maximal within 10 to 15 minutes, will reverse with bronchodilator, will abate without treatment in one hour, may be prevented by pre-treatment with a beta-agonist and is not followed by an increase in non-specific bronchial responsiveness.

A "late response" develops within several hours of exposure, is maximal within 4 to 8 hours, may be more severe, will resolve within 12 to 36 hours, may prove more difficult to treat, may be prevented by corticosteroids and is followed by an increase in non-specific bronchial responsiveness.

Patients may demonstrate an immediate, a late or dual responses. Atypical patterns, however, may occur in up to 22% of patients.

❍ **What is extrinsic asthma?**

Asthmatic exacerbation following environmental exposure to allergens such as dust, pollen and dander.

❍ **What is intrinsic asthma?**

Asthmatic exacerbation not associated with an increase in IgE or a positive skin reaction.

❍ **What are the historical risk factors for status asthmaticus?**

Chronic steroid-dependent asthma
Prior ICU admission
Prior intubation
Recurrent ER visits in past 48 hours
Sudden onset of severe respiratory distress
Poor therapy compliance
Poor clinical recognition of attack severity
Hypoxic seizures

❍ **What should be reserved for refractory status asthmaticus after the patient has been intubated?**

Halothane anesthesia produces prompt bronchodilation, but is difficult to administer and is reserved for the most severe cases.

❍ **A 20 year-old asthmatic has had a poor response to treatment in the ER despite nebulizers and steroids. His PEFR is still 40% of predicted, his oxygen saturation is 91% and he now exhibits pulsus paradoxus on physical exam. What is your next step in management?**

Hospitalize, continue frequent inhaled beta-agonist bronchodilators and intravenous steroids.

❍ **What are the criteria for ICU admission in a severe asthma case?**

PEFR < 30% baseline
PCO_2 > 40 mmHg
O_2 saturation < 90%
Severe obstruction with evidence of decreased air movement
Pulsus paradoxus >15 mmHg.

❍ **T/F: Dynamic hyperinflation in obstructive airway disease can cause hypotension.**

True.

❍ **T/F: Briefly disconnecting the endotracheal tube from the ventilator tubing is a way to correct the hypotension associated with dynamic hyperinflation.**

True. Be careful to avoid oxygen desaturation or excessive hypercarbia.

❍ **T/F: Complications in patients with obstructive airway disease and who are mechanically ventilated have been shown to correlate with the degree of hyperinflation, as measured by the volume of gas exhaled after disconnecting the patient from the ventilator for 40 to 60 seconds.**

True.

❍ **T/F: The complications mentioned above include barotrauma (as pneumothorax) and hypotension.**

True.

❍ **What are the mainstays of therapy in asthma or COPD that has progressed to severe obstruction resulting in mechanical ventilation?**

Intravenous corticosteroids and beta-2 adrenergic agents through the endotracheal tube. Theophylline is considered a second line agent.

❍ **What method of ventilation has been recently touted as a safe way to ventilate asthmatic patients with severe obstuction?**

Permissive hypercapnia. The acceptance of mild respiratory acidosis (to 7.20) to avoid high airway pressures is thought to reduce the incidence of hypotension and pneumothorax. With this strategy, lung volumes and the respiratory rate are reduced. A reduced respiratory rate permits more time for exhalation and prevents auto-PEEP. A reduction in lung volume also prevents auto-PEEP while reducing the peak airway pressure.

❍ **A chest x-ray shows honeycombing, atelectasis and increased bronchial markings. What is the most likely diagnosis?**

Bronchiectasis, an irreversible dilation of the bronchi that is generally associated with infection. Bronchography shows dilatation of the bronchial tree but this method of diagnosis is not recommended for routine use.

❍ **What is bronchiectasis?**

An abnormal dilatation of the proximal medium sized bronchi greater than 2 mm in diameter. It is due to the destruction of the muscular and elastic components of their walls, usually associated with chronic bacterial infection

❍ **Bronchiectasis occurs most frequently in patients with what conditions?**

Cystic fibrosis, immunodeficiencies, consequent to lung infections or foreign body aspirations.

❍ **What is the sensitivity of CT scan in detecting bronchiectasis?**

At least 85%.

❍ **What are the major pulmonary function abnormalities in bronchiectasis?**

Most patients have some amount of airflow obstruction. Restriction may be noted in patients with bronchiectasis associated with restrictive lung diseases.

❍ **What is middle lobe syndrome?**

Bronchiectasis and chronic recurrent pneumonia of the right middle lobe.

❍ **What are the causes of middle lobe syndrome?**

Angulation at the origin of the right middle lobe bronchus. Extrinsic compression of the right middle lobe bronchus by enlarged lymph nodes combined with an absence of collateral ventilation.

❍ **What is cystic fibrosis (CF)?**

CF is a multisystem disorder affecting children and young adults, characterized by abnomal mucus production resulting in chronic obstruction and infection of the airways and exocrine pancreatic insufficiency.

❍ **What is the incidence of CF?**

1 in 2500 live births among whites and 1 in 17,000 live births among blacks.

❍ **What is the inheritance pattern of CF?**

Autosomal recessive.

❍ **T/F: The recovery of P. aeruginosa, particularly the mucoid form, from the lower respiratory tract of a child or young adult with chronic lung symptoms is virtually diagnostic of CF.**

True.

❍ **What other organisms have been found to colonize the respiratory tract of patients with CF?**

Pseudomonas cepacia, Escherichia coli, Xanthomonas maltophilia, klebsiella, proteus and anaerobes.

❍ **What are the initial lung function abnormalities in CF?**

Small airway obstruction as evidenced by decreased maximum mid expiratory flow.
Reduced flow at low lung volumes.
Elevation of RV/TLC ratio.
Decreased diffusion capacity.

❍ **What are the diagnostic criteria for CF?**

Primary:
Characteristic pulmonary manifestations and/or,
Characteristic gastrointestinal manifestations and/or,
A family history of CF
plus
Sweat Cl concentration > 60 mEq/L [repeat measurement if sweat Cl is 50 - 60 mEq/L].

Secondary Criteria:
Documentation of dual CFTR mutations and evidence of one or more characteristic manifestations.

❍ **What are the main treatments for cystic fibrosis?**

(1) Respiratory: bronchodilators, antibiotics (inhaled, oral or IV), inhaled DNase and chest physiotherapy.
(2) Gastrointestinal: pancreatic enzymes and vitamin (ADEK) supplementation, high calorie - high protein diet and H_2 receptor antagonists.

❍ **What is the most commonly performed transplant procedure to treat CF?**

Double lung transplant.

❍ **A 22-year-old with cerebral palsy and in a vegetative state was intubated for 10 days because of aspiration pneumonia. She was weaned from mechanical ventilation, extubated and one hour later, developed stridor and severe retractions. She is appropriately suctioned and given three aerosol treatments of racemic epinephrine. She has a pH of 7.20, PCO_2 of 80 and PO_2 of 80 on 100% oxygen. What should be done next?**

Intubation.

❍ **A 24 year-old female presents with a high fever, sore throat, hoarseness and increased stridor of 3 hours duration. Examination reveals an ill appearing woman with a temperature of 40° C, inspiratory stridor, drooling and mild intercostal retractions. She prefers to sit up. What is the most likely diagnosis?**

Epiglottitis or supraglottitis.

❍ **What is the predominant auscultatory finding in a patient with a foreign body lodged in the right mainstem bronchus?**

Expiratory wheezing.

❍ **When a radiolucent foreign body is lodged in the right mainstem bronchus with resultant incomplete obstruction, inspiratory and expiratory films show air-trapping and increased lucency of the lung on the involved side. What is the cause of this phenomenon?**

Ball-valve air trapping. Air enters around the foreign body during inspiration and is trapped as the airway closes around the foreign body during expiration, preventing emptying of that side.

❍ **What are the flow-volume characteristics of obstruction of the upper airways?**

Variable extrathoracic: decreased flow during inspiration, as with vocal cord paralysis.
Variable intrathoracic: decreased flow during expiration, as with tracheomalacia.
Fixed intra- or extrathoracic: decreased flow during both inspiration and expiration, as with scar tissue.

❍ **What causes hereditary angioedema?**

Deficiency in the production or function of C1 esterase inhibitor.

❍ **What is type 1 and type 2 hereditary angioedema?**

Type 1 patients have low serum C1 esterase inhibitor levels. Type 2 patients have abnormal C1 esterase inhibitor function.

❍ **What is the treatment for hereditary angioedema?**

C1 esterase inhibitor. Epinephrine, antihistamines and steroids are often used, although they have not been proven effective.

❍ **What is functional asthma?**

A conversion disorder in which patients present with dyspnea and voluntary adduction of the vocal cords during expiration. Patients often have a psychiatric history. Fiberoptic laryngoscopy demonstrates paradoxical adduction of the vocal cords during inspiration.

❍ **What is the treatment for angioneurotic edema due to ACE inhibitors?**

Epinephrine, antihistamines and corticosteroids.

❍ **How does inhalation of noxious fumes result in injury to the trachea?**

The initial insult results in severe tracheobronchitis that when severe enough can result in sloughing of the mucosa, granulation tissue formation and ultimately, scar and stenosis.

❍ **Where do foreign bodies most frequently lodge?**

In the right mainstem bronchus.

❍ **What is amyloidosis?**

The extracellular deposition of amyloid, a substance that has green birefringence when viewed with a polarized light after staining with Congo red. Lesions in the airway include polyp-type, submucosal masses and diffuse tracheobronchial involvement. Profuse bleeding after biopsy has been reported.

❍ **What are the characteristics of bronchiolitis obliterans (obliterative bronchiolitis)?**

Stenosis of the bronchiolar lumen that results from chronic inflammation, scarring and smooth muscle hypertrophy.

❍ **What are the most common causes of bronchiolitis obliterans?**

Toxic fume inhalation, viral, mycoplasma and legionella infection, bone marrow transplantation, lung transplantation (form of chronic rejection), rheumatoid arthritis, penicillamine, lupus, dermatomyositis and polymyositis.

❍ **How does bronchiolitis obliterans (BO) differ from bronchiolitis obliterans with organizing pneumonia (BOOP)?**

BO is characterized by an obstructive ventilatory defect, while BOOP causes a restrictive ventilatory defect. In BOOP, the exudate and granulation tissue extend into the alveoli, whereas they do not in BO. The CXR is often patchy in BOOP whereas it can show miliary, diffuse nodular or reticulonodular infiltrates or be normal in BO. BOOP is generally more responsive to corticosteroids than BO.

❍ **What is the major side effect associated with the inhalation of N-acetylcysteine?**

Cough and bronchospasm, most likely due to irritation by the low pH (2.2) of the aerosol solution.

❍ **Grunting is usually more prominent in what type of respiratory pathology?**

Typically in small airway disease such as bronchiolitis or in diseases with loss of functional residual capacity, such as pneumonia or pulmonary edema, because grunting is an effort to maintain positive airway pressure during expiration.

❍ **What is the physiologic limiting factor in a normal adult, exercising at his maximal capacity?**

The cardiac output. At that point, the lungs, if normal, should not be functioning at more than 60% of their maximal capacity.

❍ **What pre-operative arterial blood gas value implies an increased risk of respiratory insufficiency following pulmonary resection?**

$PCO_2 > 45$ torr.

❍ **T/F: A pre-operative maximal voluntary ventilation (MVV) of < 50% predicted has no impact on the decision to proceed with a pulmonary resection.**

False. It implies an increased risk of post-operative respiratory insufficiency.

❍ **T/F: A 60 year old patient with a pre-operative FEV_1 of 1.6 liters and a pulmonary ventilation-perfusion scan showing 60% function from the left lung is at increased risk of post-operative respiratory insufficiency following left pneumonectomy.**

True. The calculated post-operative FEV_1 is < 0.8 liter implying an increased risk of respiratory insufficiency.

❍ **T/F: A patient with a pre-operative maximal voluntary ventilation of 75% predicted, a normal arterial blood gas and an FEV_1 of 1.7 liters requires no further evaluation prior to pulmonary resection.**

False. Patients with a pre-operative FEV_1 < 2.0 liters should undergo a pre-operative ventilation - perfusion lung scan to ensure that the intended pulmonary resection will not result in a post-operative FEV_1 < 0.8 liter.

❍ **Does incentive spirometry prevent post-operative pulmonary function abnormalities?**

No. However, complications are reduced.

❍ **What are the common pulmonary complications after upper abdominal surgery?**

Atelectasis, bronchitis, cough, pneumonia, pleural effusion and respiratory failure.

❍ **Are pulmonary complications reduced after laparoscopic cholecystectomy compared to standard cholecystectomy?**

Yes, pulmonary function abnormalities are also reduced.

❍ **What studies best predict the risk of post-operative pulmonary complications?**

Arterial blood gases and spirometry. CO_2 retention, FEV1 less than 70% of predicted, FVC less than 70% of predicted and MVV less than 50% of predicted indicate high risk.

❍ **How is lung function assessed prior to lung resection?**

Spirometry and blood gas. If FEV1is greater than 2 liters or 80% predicted of normal and pCO_2 less than 45 mmHg, then no further testing is required.

❍ **What is the further assessment of patients with operable lung cancer who fail to meet the blood gas and spirometric criteria for resection?**

Quantitative lung scanning, to assess the relative contribution of each lung to overall function.

❍ **What is the minimum post-operative FEV1 following resection?**

800 cc or 40% of predicted normal FEV1

❍ **What is the point where exercising muscle begins anaerobic metabolism?**

Anaerobic threshold (AT).

❍ **Why do we care about post-operative atelectasis?**

If it persists for more than 72 hours, pneumonia may develop. Perioperative mortality rates are then 20%. Incentive spirometry is an important therapy for the prevention of atelectasis.

❍ **What is the post-operative FEV_1 (predicted) from quantitative lung scanning?**

Post-op FEV_1 (predicted) = Pre-op FEV_1 x % of function in lung (or segments) remaining after resection.

❍ **What is the Vital Capacity (VC)?**

It is the maximal volume of air expired from a maximal inspiratory level. It can be measured during a forced expiratory effort (FVC) or a more relaxed expiration (usually denoted as VC or SVC). The VC and FVC should be equal in a normal, non-obstructed patient. In patients with obstructive diseases the FVC is generally lower than the VC/SVC.

❍ **What is the FEV_1?**

The FEV_1 is perhaps the single most important spirometric value. It is the volume of air expired in the first second of an FVC maneuver. It can be expressed as an absolute value or as a percentage of the FVC (FEV_1/FVC ratio).

❍ **What is a normal FEV_1?**

It is usually interpreted in the context of established predicted normal mean values. A normal FEV_1 is a value greater than 80% of predicted normal.

❍ **What is maximal voluntary ventilation (MVV)?**

This is a maneuver where the patient is asked to breathe as rapidly and deeply as possible over a 12 second period. Exhaled volume is measured and extrapolated over a minute and is expressed in liters per minute. This test provides an overall assessment of pulmonary function, including respiratory muscle strength.

❍ **What is the relationship between FEV_1 and MVV?**

The MVV is usually 35 to 40 times the FEV_1.

❍ **Which spirometric value distinguishes between obstructive and non-obstructive patterns?**

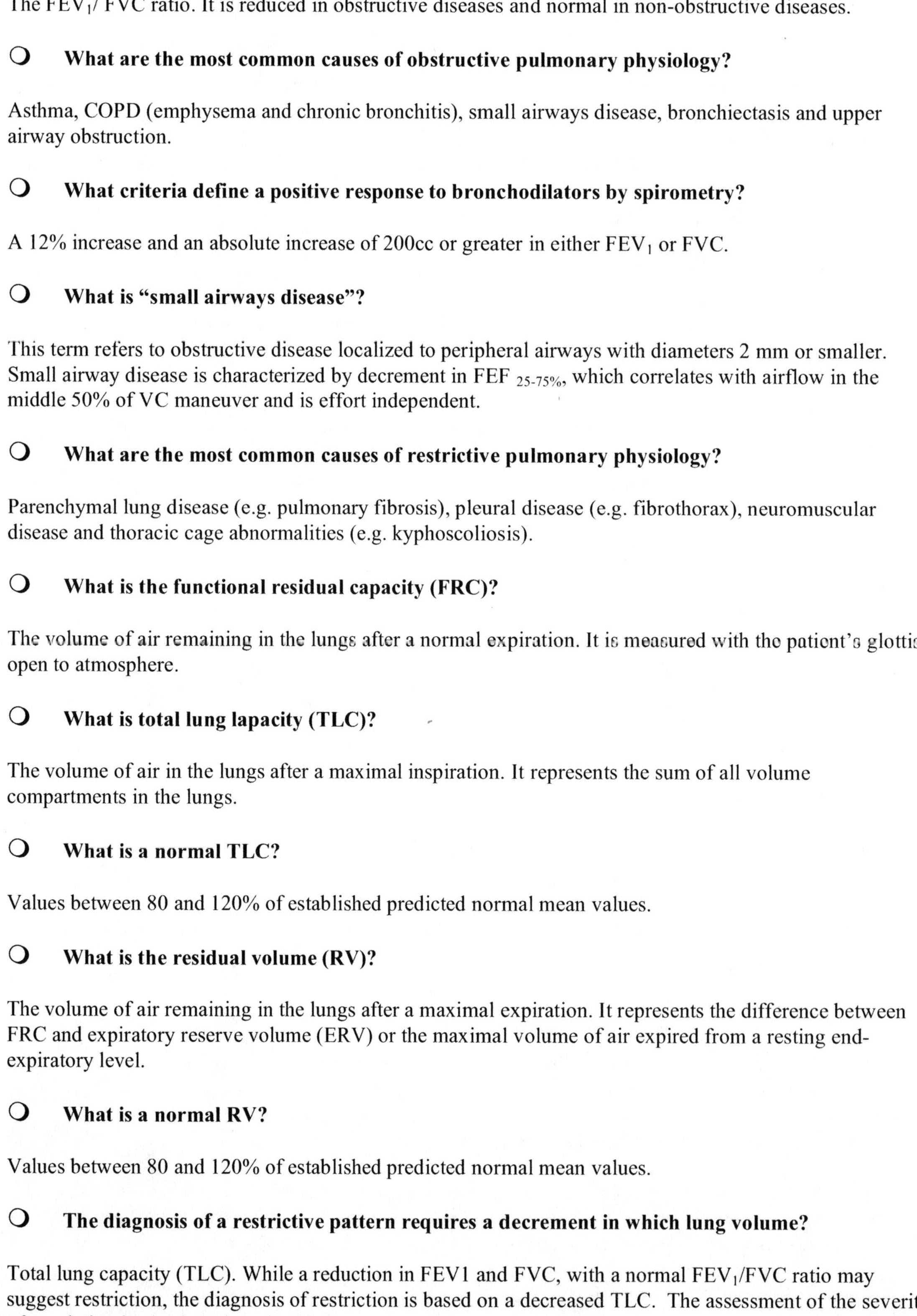

The FEV_1/ FVC ratio. It is reduced in obstructive diseases and normal in non-obstructive diseases.

❍ **What are the most common causes of obstructive pulmonary physiology?**

Asthma, COPD (emphysema and chronic bronchitis), small airways disease, bronchiectasis and upper airway obstruction.

❍ **What criteria define a positive response to bronchodilators by spirometry?**

A 12% increase and an absolute increase of 200cc or greater in either FEV_1 or FVC.

❍ **What is "small airways disease"?**

This term refers to obstructive disease localized to peripheral airways with diameters 2 mm or smaller. Small airway disease is characterized by decrement in $FEF_{25\text{-}75\%}$, which correlates with airflow in the middle 50% of VC maneuver and is effort independent.

❍ **What are the most common causes of restrictive pulmonary physiology?**

Parenchymal lung disease (e.g. pulmonary fibrosis), pleural disease (e.g. fibrothorax), neuromuscular disease and thoracic cage abnormalities (e.g. kyphoscoliosis).

❍ **What is the functional residual capacity (FRC)?**

The volume of air remaining in the lungs after a normal expiration. It is measured with the patient's glottis open to atmosphere.

❍ **What is total lung lapacity (TLC)?**

The volume of air in the lungs after a maximal inspiration. It represents the sum of all volume compartments in the lungs.

❍ **What is a normal TLC?**

Values between 80 and 120% of established predicted normal mean values.

❍ **What is the residual volume (RV)?**

The volume of air remaining in the lungs after a maximal expiration. It represents the difference between FRC and expiratory reserve volume (ERV) or the maximal volume of air expired from a resting end-expiratory level.

❍ **What is a normal RV?**

Values between 80 and 120% of established predicted normal mean values.

❍ **The diagnosis of a restrictive pattern requires a decrement in which lung volume?**

Total lung capacity (TLC). While a reduction in FEV1 and FVC, with a normal FEV_1/FVC ratio may suggest restriction, the diagnosis of restriction is based on a decreased TLC. The assessment of the severity of restriction is also based on the TLC.

❍ **What is the difference between hyperinflation and air-trapping?**

Hyperinflation refers to a significant increase in TLC or RV, while air-trapping refers to a significant increase in slow VC compared to FVC.

❍ **Which PFT data is useful for the clinical assessment of upper airway obstruction?**

The flow-volume loop.

❍ **What are the three types of upper airway obstruction (UAO)?**

Fixed: flattening of both inspiratory and expiratory limbs of the flow-volume loop.
Variable intrathoracic: flattening of the expiratory limb of the flow-volume loop.
Variable extrathoracic: flattening of the inspiratory limb of the flow-volume loop.

❍ **What may cause a fixed UAO?**

Tracheal stenosis after prolonged endotracheal intubation, goiter and tumor.

❍ **What may cause a variable extrathoracic UAO.**

Vocal cord paralysis and tumor.

❍ **What is the diffusing capacity?**

It provides a measure of volume of gas transferred across the alveolar-capillary membrane. Diffusing capacity is defined as the rate of gas flow across the lung divided by the pressure gradient for flow. Carbon monoxide (CO) is a useful gas for determining diffusing capacity as its uptake is diffusion limited. The diffusing capacity is designated as D_{LCO}.

❍ **What are three factors, other than a true diffusion defect, that can reduce the diffusing capacity?**

Anemia, elevated carboxyhemoglobin level and reduced lung volume

❍ **What are three causes of an abnormally elevated diffusing capacity?**

Polycythemia, alveolar hemorrhage and left to right shunt.

❍ **What are two common causes of an isolated reduction in diffusing capacity?**

Interstitial lung disease and occlusive pulmonary vascular disorders.

❍ **Which pulmonary function test may be useful in distinguishing emphysema from chronic bronchitis in a smoker with airflow obstruction?**

The diffusing capacity. It is reduced in emphysema due to the loss of alveolar surface area for gas exchange, but should be normal in chronic bronchitis. It should also be normal in asthma.

❍ **Which pulmonary function value best predicts prognosis/mortality in COPD?**

The FEV_1.

❍ **What is a methacholine challenge test?**

A bronchoprovocation test. It is generally used to document the presence of airways hyperreactivity in patients with clinical history suggesting bronchospasm but otherwise normal pulmonary function tests. Methacholine itself is a parasympathomimetic agent. Spirometry is first performed at baseline and after a challenge with an aerosolized diluent and then after increasing concentrations of methacholine. A test is considered positive if there is a 20% or greater drop in FEV_1 from baseline.

❍ **What is a contraindication to methacholine challenge testing?**

Abnormal baseline spirometry

❍ **What are maximal inspiratory and expiratory pressures (MIP, MEP)?**

Specific tests of respiratory muscle function. Pressures generated by maximal inspiratory and expiratory efforts are measured by a pressure gauge.

❍ **What are three causes of decrements in maximal inspiratory and expiratory pressures (MIP, MEP)?**

Poor patient effort, respiratory muscle fatigue and respiratory muscle weakness.

❍ **Interpret the following PFT data:**

FEV_1	**1.2L (42% pred)**
FVC	**2.1L (51% pred)**
FEV_1/FVC	**57%**
TLC	**115% pred**
RV	**240% pred**
D_{LCO}	**48% pred**

Severe obstruction with hyperinflation and a gas transfer abnormality. This is consistent with emphysema.

❍ **Interpret the following PFT data:**

FEV_1	**1.1L (38% pred)**
FVC	**2.6L (66% pred)**
FEV_1/FVC	**42%**
TLC	**60% pred**
RV	**66% pred**
D_{LCO}	**40% pred**

Severe obstruction with accompanying restriction and a gas transfer abnormality. There are a number of scenarios where this pattern could be seen: emphysema with concomitant pulmonary fibrosis, emphysema s/p lung resection and sarcoidosis.

❍ **Interpret the following PFT data:**

FEV_1	**2.4L (74% pred)**
FVC	**2.9L (62% pred)**
FEV_1/FVC	**83%**
MVV	**84L**

Restriction is suggested by the reduced FEV1 and FVC. There is no evidence of obstruction as the FEV1/FVC ratio is normal. The MVV is normal. Lung volume measurements are necessary to establish restriction.

❍ **Interpret the following PFT data:**

FEV_1 (pre-BD)	**2.6L (80% pred)**
FEV_1(post-BD)	**3.1L (95% pred)**
% change in FEV_1	**19%**
FVC (pre-BD)	**4.2 (105% pred)**
FVC (post-BD)	**4.4 (108% pred)**
% change in FVC	**4%**
FEV_1/FVC (pre-BD)	**62%**
FEV_1/FVC (post-BD)	**70%**

BD = bronchodilator

Obstruction with positive response to bronchodilator, indicating a significant reversible component to the obstruction. This is compatible with asthma.

❍ **Interpret the following PFT data:**

FEV_1	**1.7L (70% pred)**
FVC	**2.1L (64% pred)**
FEV_1/FVC	**81%**
MVV	**50L**
MIP	**45% pred**
MEP	**40% pred**

Restriction is suggested by reduction in FEV_1 and FVC with an otherwise normal FEV_1/FVC ratio. The MIP, MEP and MVV are all reduced, suggesting respiratory muscle weakness or fatigue.

❍ **What is the definition of normal pulmonary function?**

Normal pH, PCO_2 and PO_2, without excessive pulmonary or cardiac work.

❍ **What is the definition of restrictive lung disease?**

Decreased total lung capacity.

❍ **How are the lung volumes altered in patients with severe obstructive disease?**

The RV and TLC are increased, indicating hyperinflation.

❍ **What are the main functions of the respiratory muscles?**

Inspiratory:
Principal - external intercostals (elevate ribs) and diaphragm (descend and increase chest longitudinal dimension).
Accessory - sternocleidomastoid and scalenii (elevate and fix ribs).
Expiratory:
Passive - results from passive recoil of lungs.
Active - internal intercostals (depress ribs) and abdominal muscles (compress abdominal contents).

❍ **What are the four lung volumes and the four lung capacities?**

Lung volumes:

Tidal volume (TV)
Inspiratory reserve volume (IRV)
Expiratory reserve volume (ERV)
Residual volume (RV)

Lung capacities:
Functional residual capacity (FRC = ERV + RV)
Inspiratory capacity (IC = IRV + TV)
Vital capacity (VC = IC + ERV)
Total lung capacity (TLC = VC + RV)

❍ **T/F: Lung volumes are increased in COPD, emphysema and asthma.**

Truc.

❍ **T/F: Restrictive ventilatory defects can be broadly categorized into intraparenchymal and extraparenchymal.**

True. Any process which significantly floods the alveoli, as with blood, serum or pus, causes a restrictive ventilatory defect. Any process which restricts the expansion of the chest wall, either by increased load or decreased neuromuscular strength, causes an extraparenchymal restrictive ventilatory defect.

❍ **What happens to the airflow and the lung volumes in restrictive ventilatory defects?**

The airflow, as measured by the FEV1/FVC ratio, is unchanged or increased. The lung volumes are decreased.

❍ **What is the change in shape of the flow-volume loop in a patient with obstructive lung disease?**

The expiratory flow is reduced, the vital capacity is reduced, the shape of the expiratory flow curve is scooped out giving the appearance of a ski slope.

❍ **What percentage of predicted values for VC, FEV1, TLC and DLCO must a subject have to be considered as normal lung physiology?**

80%.

❍ **What is the value of FEV1/FVC above which subjects are considered to have normal lung physiology?**

0.70.

❍ **What will happen to the DLCO and DLCO/VA (KCO) in a patient with a pneumonectomy?**

The DLCO will be reduced. When corrected for lung volume (KCO), the value will be normal provided there is no underlying lung disease.

❍ **A patient presents with a history of CHF and COPD, related to cigarette smoking. His lung exam reveals rhonchi and crackles with a prolonged expiratory phase. CXR shows pulmonary edema. What is this patients pulmonary physiology?**

A mixed obstructive and restrictive ventilatory defect. This patient will require diuretics as well as bronchodilators.

❍ **What is a normal tidal volume?**

500 cc.

❍ **What is a normal amount of anatomic dead space?**

150 cc.

❍ **What is a normal minute ventilation?**

7,500 cc/min.

❍ **In which zone is the Pa > Pv > P alveolar?**

Zone 3.

❍ **What is Laplace's law?**

P = 4 x wall tension / radius.

❍ **What is Poiseuille's law?**

Flow rate = (P x Pi x r^4)/(8 x n x L) where P is the difference in pressure, r is the radius, n is the viscosity and L is the length.

❍ **How are airway conductance and resistance related?**

They are the inverse of one another: Conductance = 1/resistance.

❍ **What is the Fick equation for cardiac output?**

Cardiac output = VO_2 / (CaO_2 – CvO_2).
VO_2 is the oxygen consumption, CaO_2 is the arterial content of oxygen and CvO_2 is the venous content of oxygen.

❍ **What is the normal pressure around the lung (intrapleural pressure)?**

It is just subatmospheric. This is necessary to keep the lung and chest wall in close proximity.

❍ **What is the intrapleural pressure in the case of a pneumothorax?**

It is zero in a non-tension pneumothorax at end expiration. The lung collapses because of the intrinsic elastic properties of the lung. The intrapleural pressure is positive in the case of a tension pneumothorax.

❍ **Differentiate between transudate and exudate.**

Transudate: effusion to serum protein ratio is < 0.5 and for LDH the ratio is < 0.60. Also, the effusion LDH is < 2/3 of the upper limit of normal for LDH. Most commonly occurs with CHF, renal disease and liver disease.

Exudate: effusion to serum protein ratio is > 0.5 and for LDH the ratio is > 0.6. The effusion LDH is > 2/3 of the upper limit of normal for LDH. Most commonly occurs with infections, malignancy and trauma.

❍ **Why is supplemental oxygen recommended in the conservative treatment of pneumothorax?**

Absorption of a loculated pneumothorax is hastened by oxygen inhalation, which increases the pressure gradient of gases between the pleura and the capillaries.

❍ **What is the most common cause of a large pleural effusion?**

Malignancy.

❍ **What is the most common cause of a malignant pleural effusion?**

Carcinoma of the lung.

❍ **What is the volume of pleural fluid needed to obliterate the costophrenic angle on chest radiograph?**

Approximately 250 to 500 cc.

❍ **What is the most common etiology of a spontaneous pneumothorax?**

Rupture of a pulmonary bleb.

❍ **Which diseases are associated with pneumothorax?**

COPD, asthma, IPF, eosinophilic granuloma and lymphangioleiomyomatosis.

❍ **Which types of pneumonia are commonly associated with pneumothorax?**

Staphylococcus, TB, klebsiella and PCP

❍ **What is the indication for a tube thoracostomy in patients with a pneumothorax?**

Over 20 % pneumothorax or a clinical indication such as respiratory distress or enlarging pneumothorax.

❍ **What special chest x-ray may be useful for diagnosing pneumothorax?**

An expiratory film.

❍ **What is a chylothorax?**

It is a fluid collection in the pleural space due to disruption of the thoracic duct. Common causes include trauma related to cardiovascular surgery, lymphoma, Kaposi's sarcoma and other tumors. The fluid is milky and remains cloudy after centrifugation. The presence of chylomicrons verifies the diagnosis. If the fluid triglyceride level exceeds 110, then it is highly likely that a chylothorax is present. Treatment consists of spontaneous repair, pleuroperitoneal shunt, pleurodesis and duct ligation.

❍ **What is a pseudochylothorax?**

It is a long standing pleural fluid collection in which the fluid has become chyliform. The presence of cholesterol crystals verifies the diagnosis. A fluid cholesterol level above 250 suggests the diagnosis. The most common causes of this effusion are TB and RA.

❍ **What is a hemothorax?**

It is when the pleural fluid hematocrit is at least 50 % of that in the blood. All traumatic hemothoraces should have chest tube drainage. Thoracotomy is necessary for ongoing bleeding. Nontraumatic hemothorax is usually due to metastatic disease or as a complication to anticoagulation.

❍ **What is a fibrothorax?**

It is a layer of fibrous connective tissue in the pleural space. Usual causes include empyema, hemothorax, TB and collagen vascular diseases. Calcification may occur. Decortication is the only treatment.

❍ **What are some clinical disorders associated with increased capillary permeability causing exudative pleural effusion?**

Pleuripulmonary infections, systemic lupus erythematosus, rheumatoid arthritis, sarcoidosis, tumor, pulmonary infarction and viral hepatitis.

❍ **How does the presence or absence of a complicated parapneumonic effusion affect the treatment strategies?**

An uncomplicated parapneumonic effusion responds to the antibiotics directed at the pneumonia. A complicated effusion must be treated with antibiotics and a drainage procedure with or without a fibrinolytic agent.

❍ **What are the indications for the chest tube placement in parapneumonic effusion?**

Presence of a complicated parapneumonic effusion indicates the need for a chest tube. This is demonstrable by the gross appearance of purulent fluid (pus), bacterial on gram stain, positive culture of pleural fluid, low glucose (usually < 40 mg/dl), low pH (less than 7.0) and elevated LDH (>1000 IU/L; the LDH criterion alone is controversial)

❍ **What are the common features of pleural effusion associated with congestive heart failure?**

Bilateral effusions, more commonly right-sided, are associated with cardiomegaly. The fluid is transudative and serous with <1000 mononuclear cells, the pH greater than or equal to 7.4 and pleural fluid glucose levels equal to serum.

❍ **What are the characteristics of an effusion associated with pulmonary embolism?**

These may be transudative, exudative or hemorrhagic. The predominate cell type may be polymorphonuclear or mononuclear.

❍ **What are the respiratory manifestations of inhaled toxins?**

Upper airway mucosal injury, bronchitis, reactive airways disease, pneumonitis, ARDS, obliterative bronchiolitis, COPD and BOOP.

❍ **Which clinical syndromes may result from inhalation of sulfur dioxide, ammonia or nitrogen oxides?**

All of the above.

❍ **Why is acute smoke inhalation difficult to study?**

Because there are many components, including particulates, carbon monoxide, hydrogen cyanide, aldehydes and others.

❍ **What is the most common cause of death in smoke inhalation victims?**

Carbon monoxide exposure.

❍ **How does carbon monoxide exposure present?**

With a spectrum of CNS symptoms, as severe as coma and seizures. Respiratory arrest and myocardial dysfunction may occur as well.

❍ **How does cyanide toxicity present?**

With a history of an odor of bitter almonds, pink skin, tachycardia, bright red venous blood, altered mental status, hypotension and anion gap acidosis (due to lactic acid accumulation).

❍ **How is cyanide toxicity treated?**

With a combination of nitrites and sodium thiosulfate.

❍ **What are the respiratory complications of acute smoke inhalation?**

Edema of the upper airways, bronchospasm, bronchitis and ARDS.

❍ **What factors increase the bleeding complications after transbronchial lung biopsy?**

Renal failure, hemorrhagic diathesis, amyloidosis, bronchiectasis and pulmonary hypertension.

❍ **What drugs can induce a lupus reaction?**

Procainamide, hydralazine, isoniazid and phenytoin.

❍ **What rheumatologic ailments produce pulmonary hemorrhage?**

Goodpasture's disease, systemic lupus erythematosus, Wegener's granulomatosis and non-specific vasculitides.

❍ **What rheumatologic ailments more commonly produce pulmonary fibrosis?**

Ankylosing spondylitis, scleroderma and rheumatoid arthritis.

❍ **What rheumatologic ailments more commonly produce respiratory muscle failure?**

Dermatomyositis and polymyositis.

❍ **What are the pulmonary manifestations of SLE?**

Acute pneumonitis, diffuse alveolar hemorrhage, pleuritis, interstitial lung disease, pulmonary hypertension, bronchiolitis and weakness of the diaphragm.

❍ **What is the underlying histopathology of acute lupus pneumonitis?**

Diffuse alveolar damage, BOOP, cellular interstitial pneumonitis or a combination of these.

❍ **What is the treatment for acute pneumonitis or diffuse alveolar hemorrhage seen in patients with lupus?**

There are no controlled trials. Steroids, azathioprine, cyclophosphamide and plasmapheresis have all been used.

❍ **Describe the effusions seen in lupus.**

Exudative, pleural fluid positive for dsDNA and pleural fluid ANA titer greater than 1:160.

❍ **What is the shrinking lung syndrome in lupus?**

Weakness of the diaphragm that results in reduction of static lung volumes but with a normal DLCO when volumes are taken into account.

❍ **What are the pulmonary manifestations of RA?**

Pleurisy, pleural effusions, pulmonary hypertension, rheumatoid nodule, obliterative bronchiolits, interstitial lung disease, BOOP and lymphocytic interstitial pneumonia.

❍ **Characterize the pleural fluid seen in RA.**

Exudative, low pH (less than 7.2), low glucose, (often under 50), low complement levels, cytology of necrotic debris, spindle shaped macrophages, multinucleated histiocytes and the presence of rheumatoid factor (RF) in the fluid.

❍ **Arthritis of what joint may impose difficulty in dealing with airways?**

The cricoarytenoid and atlanto-axial joints.

❍ **Describe obliterative bronchiolitis seen in RA.**

Insidious onset, obstructive ventilatory defect, normal or hyperinflated CXR and a minority of patients respond to steroids and cyclophosphamide.

❍ **Can the interstitial lung disease of RA present before the articular manifestations occur?**

Yes.

❍ **Which drugs, used to treat RA, may cause interstitial lung disease?**

Gold, penicillamine and methotrexate.

❍ **What are the pulmonary manifestations of scleroderma?**

Pleural disease, interstitial lung diseases, pulmonary hypertension and aspiration pneumonitis.

❍ **Is the usual interstitial pneumonitis of scleroderma more likely to occur in the CREST syndrome or the diffuse cutaneous form?**

The diffuse cutaneous form.

❍ **Which scleroderma syndrome is more associated with pulmonary hypertension?**

CREST.

❍ **Why is aspiration a concern in scleroderma?**

The associated esophageal disorder of decreased peristalsis and dilatation, more commonly seen in the CREST variant, predisposes patients to aspiration.

❍ **What are the pulmonary manifestations of the polymyositis-dermatomyositis syndrome?**

Aspiration pneumonia, diaphragmatic weakness and interstitial lung disease.

❍ **What is the mechanism for aspiration seen in polymyositis-dermatomyositis?**

Inflammatory myositis involving the striated muscle of the hypopharynx and upper esophagus.

❍ **What are four distinct presentations of bleomycin lung toxicity?**

Chronic pulmonary fibrosis, hypersensitivity lung reaction, acute pneumonitis and acute chest pain syndrome.

❍ **What is the typical time period during which acute radiation pneumonitis develops?**

Within the first eight weeks after radiation.

❍ **What is the nature of the lung toxicity associated with the cytokine, interleukin-2?**

Fluid retention and pulmonary edema.

❍ **What are four syndromes of penicillamine induced lung toxicity?**

Chronic pneumonitis, hypersensitivity lung disease, bronchiolitis obliterans and pulmonary-renal syndrome.

❍ **What drugs are known to have caused bronchiolitis obliterans organizing pneumonia?**

Bleomycin, penicillamine, amiodarone, cocaine, cyclophosphamide, mitomycin C, methotrexate, sulfasalazine and gold.

❍ **What acute pulmonary reaction might one encounter at the time of a persantine-thallium study for cardiac ischemia?**

Bronchospasm due to dipyridamole.

❍ **After removal from cardiopulmonary bypass during coronary revascularization surgery, a patient develops severe wheezing. What drug might be responsible?**

Protamine.

❍ **What risk factors predispose to a higher incidence of pulmonary injury with amiodarone?**

A maintenance dose of amiodarone in excess of 400 mg/day, use of angiography, cardiac or lung surgery and concomitant lung disease.

❍ **The presence of foamy appearing macrophages and infiltration of inflammatory cells including lymphocytes, plasma cells, histiocytes and neutrophils suggests lung injury from what drug?**

Amiodarone.

❍ **What laboratory and radiological findings help distinguish amiodarone lung toxicity from CHF?**

Elevated ESR, reduced DLCO that dose not improve with diuretics, abnormal gallium-67 uptake and high attenuation of infiltrates on CT scan of lungs.

❍ **What is the incidence of aspirin-induced bronchospasm in patients with nasal polyps?**

Up to 75%.

❍ **T/F: In aspirin-induced bronchospasm there can be cross-reactivity with non-steroidal anti-inflammatory drugs.**

True.

❍ **T/F: Cardioselective beta-blockers avoid precipitation of bronchospasm in asthmatic individuals.**

False.

❍ **What drugs are associated with bronchospasm?**

Salicylates, NSAIDs, beta-blockers, protamine, contrast media, neuromuscular blocking agents and interleukin-2.

❍ **Which cervical nerves innervate the diaphragm?**

C3 to C5.

❍ **What are the causes of phrenic nerve injury?**

Cardiac surgery, trauma, cervical osteoarthritis, tumors, herpes zoster, vasculitis and diabetes.

❍ **What is the most common presentation of unilateral diaphragmatic paralysis?**

It is often asymptomatic or with mild dyspnea. In patients with lung disease, the symptoms are more severe.

❍ **How does bilateral diaphragmatic paralysis present?**

With significant dyspnea that is worse in the supine position.

❍ **How is unilateral diaphragmatic paralysis diagnosed?**

Usually with a sniff test under ultrasonic or fluoroscopic observation.

❍ **How is bilateral diaphragmatic paralysis diagnosed?**

The sniff test is difficult, as there is no good side to compare to. PFTs in sitting and supine position show a large difference in the two positions.

❍ **How is diaphragmatic paralysis treated?**

Usually unilateral involvement requires no treatment. Bilateral paralysis can be treated with mechanical ventilatory support (e.g., BiPAP, rocking bed or negative pressure ventilation).

❍ **In low cervical and upper thoracic spinal injuries, the diaphragm is intact. What occurs to the cough mechanism?**

It is decreased because the expiratory muscles are innervated below C8.

❍ **What diffuse neuromuscular diseases can cause respiratory muscle weakness and are acute in onset?**

Myasthenia gravis, Eaton-Lambert syndrome, organophosphate poisoning, botulism and aminoglycosides toxicity.

❍ **What diffuse neuromuscular diseases can cause respiratory muscle weakness and are gradual in onset?**

ALS, muscular dystrophies and myopathies (e.g., alcohol and diabetes).

❍ **What measurements should be assessed in these patients?**

Vital capacity and inspiratory and expiratory maximal pressures.

❍ **How many hours after an acute exposure to an antigen may a patient develop the signs and symptoms of hypersensitivity pneumonitis?**

Four to six hours.

❍ **What is the most common misdiagnosis given to patients with hypersensitivity pneumonitis?**

Bacterial or viral pneumonia.

❍ **The chronic form of hypersensitivity pneumonitis usually presents with gradual onset of symptoms including?**

Cough, dyspnea, malaise, weakness and weight loss.

❍ **Most of the etiological agents associated with hypersensitivity pneumonitis are secondary to occupational exposure. Farmer's lung disease is secondary to what organism?**

Thermophilic actinomyces such as Micropolyspora faeni or Thermoactinomyces vulgaris.

❍ **The non-caseating granuloma seen in hypersensitivity pneumonitis may mimic those seen in what disease?**

Sarcoidosis.

❍ **What are the classic chest x-ray findings in a patient with sarcoidosis?**

Stage The upper zones of the lung field.
Acute, subacute and chronic.
Fever, pulmonary crackles and possibly cyanosis.
Usually bilaterally and equally distributed (involving the upper lobes).
The establishment of a relationship between exposure to an antigen and the development of symptoms.
Bilateral hilar and paratracheal adenopathy with diffuse nodular appearing infiltrates. Sarcoidosis can be staged by the chest x-ray:
Stage 0: Normal
Stage 1: Hilar adenopathy
Stage 2: Hilar adenopathy and parenchymal infiltrates
Stage 3: Parenchymal infiltrates only
Stage 4: Pulmonary fibrosis

❍ **What other systems can be affected by sarcoidosis?**

The cardiovascular, gastrointestinal, immunological, integumental, lymphatics and ocular systems.

❍ **What are the most common symptoms of idiopathic pulmonary fibrosis (IPF)?**

Cough and dyspnea.

❍ **Where are opacities usually observed on chest radiographs of patients with IPF?**

In the lower lung zones and peripherally.

❍ **What percentage of patients with IPF improve with oral corticosteroids?**

Only about 30%.

❍ **What is the most important benefit a patient can be offered through lung biopsy for suspected IPF?**

Other more easily treatable interstitial lung diseases may be diagnosed.

❍ **What is the mean survival of patients diagnosed with IPF?**

Four to six years.

❍ **What histopathological finding in IPF correlates with better treatment response?**

Active inflammation with a cellular infiltrate suggests a better prognosis than acellular fibrosis.

❍ **A 54 year old patient with IPF has been on oral prednisone (1 mg per kg) for 12 weeks and PFTs continue to deteriorate. What is the appropriate treatment?**

Azathioprine or cyclophosphamide.

❍ **How is symptomatic sarcoidosis involving the lungs initially treated?**

Corticosteroids.

❍ **How may sarcoidosis affect the heart?**

Sarcoidosis can cause a cardiomyopathy, pericarditis, tachyarrythmias, (including sudden death) and bradyarrythmias (including complete heart block).

❍ **Which patients with sarcoidosis require more intensive corticosteroid therapy?**

Sarcoidosis patients with neurologic, opthalmologic, cardiac, renal and hematologic involvement require higher dose prednisone induction and longer courses, with appropriate clinical monitoring to gauge response and guide the decision to reduce dose.

❍ **Where are abnormalities commonly noted on chest CT of patients with sarcoidosis?**

Lung abnormalities are generally noted along the distribution of the lymphatics, mostly peribronchovascular and subpleural in location. The abnormalities can vary from small nodules to coarse reticular markings.

❍ **What is the typical pathologic finding on a biopsy specimen in a patient with sarcoid?**

Noncaseating granulomas.

❍ **What is the pattern of immunoglobulin deposition in the basement membranes of the kidneys and lungs in Goodpasture's disease?**

Linear.

❍ **Diffuse alveolar hemorrhage occurs most commonly in which connective tissue disorder?**

SLE (may also complicate scleroderma, rheumatoid arthritis and mixed connective tissue disorders).

❍ **Which interstitial lung disease occurs in premenopausal women and has an associated airflow obstruction and hyperinflation?**

Lymphangiomyomatosis (LAM).

❍ **What chest complications of LAM may occur at the time of presentation or during the patient's course?**

Chylous pleural effusion, pneumothorax and hemoptysis.

❍ **An interstitial lung disease which is pathologically identical to LAM may occur in patients who survive to adulthood and is characterized by mental retardation, adenoma sebaceum and epilepsy. What is this condition?**

Tuberous sclerosis.

❍ **Bronchiolitis obliterans may occur as a complication in which type of transplants?**

Bone marrow, heart-lung and lung transplantation.

❍ **Which connective tissue disorder is most associated with bronchiolitis obliterans?**

Rheumatoid arthritis.

❍ **What are the typical pulmonary function study abnormalities in patients with BOOP?**

A restrictive pattern with a decreased DLCO.

❍ **Infection with what organism is associated with pulmonary alveolar proteinosis (PAP)?**

Nocardia asteroides.

❍ **The amorphous material found in the alveolar space in PAP resembles what normally occurring substance?**

Surfactant.

❍ **What is the only definitively beneficial treatment for PAP?**

Whole lung lavage.

❍ **What interstitial lung disease is characterized by relatively preserved lung volumes radiographically, is complicated by pneumothorax and occurs more commonly in cigarette smokers?**

Eosinophilic granuloma.

❍ **What percentage of patients with eosinophilic granuloma are current or former cigarette smokers?**

90%.

❍ **What cell is the histopathologic hallmark of eosinophilic granuloma?**

Langerhan's histiocyte.

❍ **What interstitial lung diseases may be inherited as an autosomal dominant trait?**

Familial IPF, tuberous sclerosis and neurofibromatosis

❍ **Which interstitial lung diseases may have increased lung volumes?**

LAM, eosinophilic granuloma, neurofibromatosis, tuberous sclerosis, chronic hypersensitivity pneumonitis and chronic sarcoidosis.

❍ **What is the only CXR finding in IPF which is predictive of lung histopathology and prognosis?**

Honeycombing.

❍ **What is the major mechanism for resting hypoxemia in IPF?**

Ventilation-perfusion mismatch.

❍ **An increase in which two cell populations in BAL fluid in patients with IPF is predictive of a poor response to corticosteroids?**

Polymorphonuclear leukocytes and eosinophils.

❍ **A patient presents with cough, lethargy, dyspnea, conjunctivitis, glomerulonephritis, fever and purulent sinusitis. What is the probable diagnosis?**

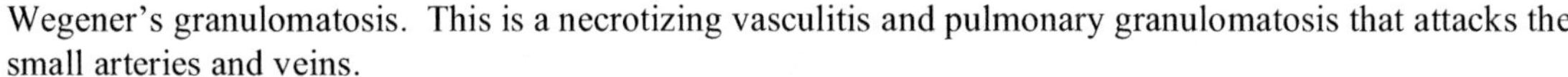

Wegener's granulomatosis. This is a necrotizing vasculitis and pulmonary granulomatosis that attacks the small arteries and veins.

❍ **What serological test is diagnostic for Wegener's granulomatosis?**

c-ANCA in association with appropriate clinical evidence. A renal, lung or sinus biopsy may also be helpful in making the diagnosis.

❍ **What are the most common causes of interstitial lung disease?**

In order: interstitial pulmonary fibrosis, collagen-vascular disease related, hypersensitivity pneumonitis, sarcoidosis, BOOP, eosinophilic granuloma and asbestosis.

❍ **What interstitial lung diseases have a predilection for the upper lobes?**

Sarcoidosis, chronic hypersensitivity pneumonitis, eosinophilic granuloma, silicosis, berylliosis, ankylosing spondylitis and chronic eosinophilic pneumonia.

❍ **How is primary pulmonary hypertension (PPH) diagnosed?**

It is diagnosed after ruling out cardiac, pulmonary and other causes of pulmonary hypertension. A right heart catherization confirms the presence of pulmonary hypertension. Echocardiography is useful to noninvasivelly follow the disease progression. A V/Q scan is useful to rule out pulmonary embolism as a cause for the elevated pulmonary arterial pressures.

❍ **What is the treatment for PPH?**

Oxygen, calcium channel blockers, prostacyclin (which can only be given intravenously) and anticoagulation. Inhaled nitric oxide is being studied.

❍ **What are the causes of secondary pulmonary hypertension?**

Cardiac disease, interstitial lung disease, COPD, hypoventilation syndromes, collagen-vascular diseases, pulmonary emboli that went undetected, HIV infection and drugs as fenfluramine and aminorex.

❍ **What is pulmonary veno-occlusive disease?**

It is characterized by pulmonary hypertension resulting from inflammation and thrombosis of the pulmonary veins and venules. The wedge pressure is often normal. The CXR may show signs of pulmonary edema without the pulmonary artery pruning seen in PPH. The diagnosis is made by catheterization and lung biopsy.

❍ **What is Wegener's granulomatosis?**

It is a multisystemic disease characterized by necrotizing granulomas of the upper or lower respiratory tract, necrotizing vasculitis of the lung and other organs and glomerulonephritis. Limited Wegener's granulomatosis excludes renal involvement and a systemic vasculitis.

❍ **What are the clinical findings in Wegener's granulomatosis?**

ENT findings include nasal obstruction, saddle nose deformity, rhinorrhea, purulent or bloody nasal discharge, nasal septal perforation and ulceration of the vomer. Lung involvement includes cough,

hemoptysis, diffuse alveolar hemorrhage, inflammation or scarring in the bronchi, ulceration of the larynx and trachea and subglottic stenosis. The CXR shows infiltrates, cavitation and nodules.
Renal involvement includes proteinuria, hematuria, RBC casts and glomerulonephritis on biopsy. The peripheral nervous system is involved with mononeuritis multiplex, occasionally involving the cranial nerves. Skin involvement includes palpable purpura, ulcerations, papules and nodules and pyoderma gangrenosum. Eye involvement includes scleritis, conjunctivis and episcleritis. Arthritis is mono- or polyarticular and symmetric or asymmetric.

❍ **What is the treatment of Wegener's granulomatosis?**

Corticosteroids and cyclophosphamide are the mainstay. In the early granulomatous phase, trimethoprim/sulfamethoxazole is beneficial. Gamma globulin is under investigation.

❍ **What are the characteristics of Churg-Strauss (allergic granulomatosis and angiitis) syndrome?**

Asthma, hypereosinophilia, necrotizing vasculitis and extravascular granulomas.

❍ **What are the clinical features of Churg-Strauss syndrome?**

Allergic manifestations including asthma occur initially. The CXR may show transient and patchy infiltrates due to eosinophil infiltration. Nodules and diffuse alveolar hemorrhage are also seen. Nasal obstruction, polyps, rhinorrhea and perforation occur. Neurologic involvement includes mononeuritis multiplex, symmetric polyneuropathy, cerebral infarction and ischemic optic neuropathy. CHF, renal failure and GI bleeding may also occur.

❍ **What is the treatment for Churg-Strauss syndrome?**

Steroids. In sicker patients the steroids are given intravenously.

❍ **What is the major etiology of pulmonary hypertension?**

Chronic hypoxia.

❍ **What is Goodpasture's syndrome?**

A multisystemic disease in which patients present with alveolar hemorrhage and rapidly progressive glomerulonephritis. A circulating antibody, anti-GBM is present. The urinalysis contains RBC, casts and proteinuria. The CXR demonstrates bilateral alveolar infiltrates. Renal biopsy shows a proliferative or necrotizing glomerulonephritis.

❍ **What is the pattern of IgG deposition in the kidneys?**

Linear.

❍ **What is the treatment for Goodpasture's syndrome?**

Plasmapheresis, steroids and cyclophosphamide.

❍ **What conditions cause diffuse alveolar hemorrhage due to capillaritis?**

Wegener's granulomatosis, Goodpasture's syndrome, microscopic polyarteritis, connective tissue diseases, Behcet's syndrome, Henoch-Schonlein purpura and lupus.

❍ **What diseases cause diffuse alveolar hemorrhage without capillaritis?**

Idiopathic pulmonary hemosiderosis, lupus, Goodpasture's, coagulopathies and pulmonary veno-occlusive disease.

❍ **What are the clinical features of fat embolism syndrome?**

It is characterized by hypoxemia, diffuse infiltrates, neurological abnormalities (confusion, seizures, coma, focal defects) and petechiae that appear on the head, neck and axillae. The syndrome usually occurs 24 to 72 hours after the inciting event.

❍ **How is the fat embolism syndrome diagnosed?**

Clinically. There are no specific tests available. The presence of fat globules in the serum is neither sensitive nor specific.

❍ **How is fat embolism syndrome treated?**

Supportively. There is no specific treatment. Some have suggested that corticosteroids are effective in preventing the occurance of the syndrome.

❍ **What are the clinical findings of Löffler's syndrome (simple pulmonary eosinophilia)?**

Pulmonary infiltrates, peripheral eosinophilia and symptoms that may include cough, wheezing, myalgia and low grade fever.

❍ **What are the known causes of Löffler's syndrome (simple pulmonary eosinophilia)?**

Nitrofurantoin, sulfonamides and para-aminosalicylic acid. Forty drugs have been found to cause it. Parasites including ascaris and strongyloides can also cause it. However, no cause is found in up to 30% of cases.

❍ **What are the classical chest x-ray findings in patients with Löffler's syndrome?**

Transient, migratory, pleural based infiltrates.

❍ **What disease has chest x-ray findings described as the "photographic negative of pulmonary edema" with central lung sparing?**

Chronic eosinophilic pneumonia.

❍ **What are the diagnostic criteria for allergic bronchopulmonary aspergillosis?**

Asthma, peripheral blood eosinophilia, increased serum IgE levels, serum precipitating antibodies against aspergillus antigen, immediate skin prick test for aspergillus antigen and chest x-ray infiltrates.

❍ **What is the presentation of a patient with acute eosinophilic pneumonia?**

It presents with fever, myalgias, cough, pleurisy, hypoxemia often requiring mechanical ventilation and a leukocystosis without an eosinophilia.

❍ **What is the prognosis of a patient with acute eosinophilic pneumonia?**

Generally good, although fatalities have occurred.

❍ **What is the treatment for a patient with acute eosinophilic pneumonia?**

Corticosteroids.

❍ **Define apnea, hypopnea and apnea/hypopnea index.**

Apnea: cessation of airflow for at least 10 sec.
Hypopnea: decrement of 50% or more in airflow with consequent 4% or more fall in O_2 saturation or electroencephalographic arousal.
Apnea/hypopnea index: number of apneas and hypopneas per hour.

❍ **When is obstructive sleep apnea present?**

When the apnea/hypopnea index exceeds 15, the patient has both daytime and nighttime symptoms that are due to obstruction of the airways.

❍ **What are the causes of central sleep apnea?**

Idiopathic, CNS disease, movement to high altitude and respiratory neuromuscular disease (as myasthenia gravis).

❍ **How is central sleep apnea diagnosed on polysomnography?**

A lack of airflow coinciding with a lack of chest and abdominal movements.

❍ **How is central sleep apnea treated?**

BiPAP ventilation and ventilatory stimulants.

❍ **T/F: Small cell lung cancer is often widely disseminated at the time of diagnosis and is infrequently treated by surgical resection.**

True.

❍ **What are the common sites for metastases of lung cancer?**

Brain, adrenal glands, bone, liver, contralateral lung and mediastinal and supraclavicular lymph nodes.

❍ **T/F: An ipsilateral pleural effusion is a contraindication to curative resection of a non-small cell lung cancer.**

False. Malignant pleural effusions (cytologically positive) confer T4 (stage IIIB) disease and preclude curative resection while non-malignant effusions do not change the tumor stage or resectability.

❍ **What is the most likely cause of severe head, neck and arm swelling in a patient with a centrally located mass on chest radiograph?**

Superior vena cava syndrome, the partial or complete mechanical obstruction of the superior vena cava by an intrathoracic tumor or nodal metastases.

❍ **Hypercalcemia in the absence of bony metastases is associated with which lung cancer?**

Squamous cell carcinoma (a paraneoplastic syndrome associated with tumor elaboration of a PTH-like substance).

❍ **The syndrome of inappropriate secretion of antidiuretic hormone is associated with which cell type of lung cancer?**

Small cell carcinoma

GASTROINTESTINAL PEARLS

Death is nature's way of saying, "Your table is ready."
Robin Williams

❍ **What is the nature of pleural fluid in pancreatitis?**

Exudate with high amylase levels.

❍ **What are the pulmonary manifestations of pancreatitis?**

Hypoxemia with normal CXR, ARDS and pleural effusions.

❍ **Contrast acute versus chronic effusions associated with pancreatitis.**

Acute: occurs when abdominal symptoms are dominant and the effusion is small to moderate.
Chronic: occurs when abdominal symptoms have resolved, chest symptoms predominate and the effusion is large. It may be due to a fistula from the pancreas to the pleural space.

❍ **What are the pulmonary manifestations of cirrhosis?**

Hypoxemia (due to V/Q mismatching and microvascular shunting), pleural effusions (transudative, usually right sided, usually associated with ascites), reduction in static lung volumes due to ascites and pulmonary hypertension.

❍ **Prophylaxis for stress ulcers includes what agents?**

Sucralfate, antacids and histamine receptor antagonists.

❍ **Diverticular disease is most common in which part of the colon?**

The sigmoid colon.

❍ **If blood is recovered from the stomach after an NG tube is inserted, where is the most likely location of the bleed?**

Above the ligament of Treitz.

❍ **Where is angiodysplasia most frequently found?**

In the cecum and proximal ascending colon. Lesions are generally singular. Bleeding is intermittent and seldom massive.

❍ **How much blood must be lost in the GI tract to cause melena?**

50 ml. Healthy patients normally lose 2.5 ml/day.

❍ **What are the most common causes of upper GI bleeding?**

Ulcer disease (45%), esophageal varices (20%), gastritis (20%) and Mallory-Weiss syndrome (10%).

❍ **What percentage of patients with upper GI bleeds will stop bleeding within hours of hospitalization?**

85%. About 25% of these patients will rebleed within the first 2 days of hospitalization. If no rebleeding occurs in five days, the chance of rebleeding is only 2%.

❍ **Where are bleeding duodenal ulcers most commonly located?**

On the posterior surface of the duodenal bulb.

❍ **Which type of ulcer is more likely to rebleed?**

Gastric ulcers are three times more likely to rebleed compared to duodenal ulcers.

❍ **What is the most common site for duodenal ulcers?**

The duodenal bulb (95%). Surgery is indicated only if perforation, gastric outlet obstruction, intractable disease or uncontrollable hemorrhage occur.

❍ **What is the most common site for gastric ulcers?**

The lesser curvature of the stomach. Surgery is considered earlier in gastric ulcers because of the higher recurrence rate after medical treatment and because of the higher potential for malignancy.

❍ **What is the most common cause of portal hypertension?**

Intrahepatic obstruction (90%), which is most often due to cirrhosis.

❍ **What organism causes amebic liver abscesses?**

Entamoeba histolytica. Amebic liver abscesses are primarily found in middle aged men living in or who have traveled to, tropical areas. Ninety percent occur in the right lobe of the liver. Treatment is with oral metronidazole.

❍ **What are the most commonly isolated organisms in pyogenic hepatic abscesses?**

E. coli and other gram-negative bacteria. The source of such bacteria is most likely an infection in the biliary system.

❍ **What clinical sign can assist in the diagnosis of cholecystitis?**

Murphy's sign, which is pain on inspiration with palpation of the RUQ. As the patient breaths in, the gallbladder is lowered in the abdomen and comes in contact with the peritoneum just below the examiner's hand. This will aggravate an inflamed gallbladder, causing the patient to discontinue breathing deeply.

❍ **What is the difference between cholelithiasis, cholangitis, cholecystitis and choledocholithiasis?**

Cholelithiasis: Gallstones in the gallbladder.
Cholangitis: Inflammation of the common bile duct, often secondary to bacterial infection or choledocholithiasis.
Cholecystitis: Inflammation of the gallbladder secondary to gallstones.

Choledocholithiasis: Gallstones, which have migrated from the gallbladder to the common bile duct.

❍ **What percentage of gallstones can be visualized on ultrasound?**

95%. Ultrasound is the diagnostic procedure of choice in patients with suspected cholecystitis.

❍ **What is Charcot's triad?**

1) Fever
2) Jaundice
3) Abdominal pain
This is the hallmark of acute cholangitis.

❍ **What is Reynolds' pentad?**

Charcot's triad plus shock and mental status changes. This is the hallmark of acute toxic ascending cholangitis.

❍ **What are the majority of gallstones composed of?**

Cholesterol (75 to 95%). The rest are made of pigment.

❍ **What are the majority of kidney stones made of?**

Calcium oxalate (60%). The other types of kidney stones are made of uric acid, calcium oxalate/calcium phosphate, struvite and cysteine.

❍ **What percentage of gallstones will be visualized by an x-ray?**

20%.

❍ **What are some abdominal x-ray findings associated with pancreatitis?**

- Sentinel loop (either of the jejunum, transverse colon or duodenum).
- Colon cutoff sign, which is an abrupt cessation of gas in the mid or left transverse colon due to inflammation of the adjacent pancreas.
- Calcification of the pancreas.

About two-thirds of patients with acute pancreatitis will have x-ray abnormalities.

❍ **What are Ranson's criteria?**

A means of estimating prognosis for patients with pancreatitis.

At initial presentation	Developing within 24 hours
Age > 55	Hematocrit falling > 10%
WBC > 16,000/mm^3	Increase in BUN > 5 mg/dl
AST > 250 IU/L	Serum Ca^+ < 8 mg/dl
Serum glucose > 200 mg/dl	Arterial PO_2 < 60 mm Hg
LDH > 350	Base deficit > 4 mEq/L
	Fluid sequestration > 6000 ml

0 to 2 criteria = 2% mortality
3 to 4 criteria = 15% mortality

5 to 6 criteria = 40% mortality
7 to 8 criteria = 100% mortality

❍ **What is Hamman's sign?**

Air in the mediastinum following an esophageal perforation. This condition produces a crunching sound over the heart during systole.

❍ **What is the most common site of rupture in Boerhaave's syndrome?**

The posterior distal esophagus. Boerhaave's syndrome is rupture of the esophagus that occurs after binge drinking and vomiting. Patients experience sudden, sharp pain in the lower chest and epigastric area. The abdomen becomes rigid and then shock may follow.

❍ **What type of contrast medium should be used to evaluate the esophagus if a traumatic injury is suspected?**

Gastrografin.

❍ **Name some common conditions that mimic acute appendicitis.**

Mesenteric lymphadenitis, pelvic inflammatory disease, Mittlesmertz, gastroenteritis and Crohn's disease.

❍ **What are the most frequent symptoms of acute appendicitis?**

Anorexia and pain. The classical presentations of anorexia and periumbilical pain with progression to constant RLQ pain are present in only 60% of the cases.

❍ **What percentage of patients with acute appendicitis cases have an elevated WBC count?**

An elevated leukocyte count is present in 85% of cases.

❍ **Until discounted, what intra-abdominal pathology should be assumed for a pregnant woman with right upper quadrant pain?**

Acute appendicitis.

❍ **Rovsing's, psoas and obturator signs can all indicate an inflamed appendix. What are these signs?**

<u>Rovsing's sign</u>: RLQ pain with palpation over the LLQ
<u>Psoas sign</u>: RLQ pain with right thigh extension
<u>Obturator sign</u>: RLQ pain with internal rotation of the flexed right thigh

❍ **What does an ultrasound show in acute appendicitis?**

Fixed, tender, non-compressible mass, but only in 60% of cases.

❍ **What does abdominal helical CT scanning with rectal contrast only show in appendicitis?**

Non-filling of the appendix with contrast, inflammatory changes, focal cecal apical thickening and the arrowhead sign.

❍ **What does abdominal CT scanning (oral and IV contrast) show in acute appendicitis?**

Not much in early appendicitis. However, the study is useful to determine the cause of a right lower quadrant mass, as is found with late appendicitis, perforation/abscess, carcinoma and pseudomyxoma. A new scanning technique (rectal contrast only combined with helical CT scanning) has been shown to have high accuracy in the diagnosis of appendicitis.

❍ **Which method is more sensitive for locating the source of GI bleeding, a radioactive Tc-labeled red cell scan or angiography?**

A bleeding scan can detect a site bleeding at a rate as low as 0.1 ml/min., while angiography requires more rapid bleeding, at least 0.5 ml/min.

❍ **Repeated violent bouts of vomiting can result in both Mallory-Weiss tears and Boerhaave's syndrome. What is the difference between the two?**

Mallory-Weiss tears: Involve the submucosa and mucosa, typically in the right posterolateral wall of the gastroesophageal junction.
Boerhaave's syndrome: A full-thickness tear, usually in the unsupported left posterolateral wall of the abdominal esophagus.

❍ **What is the most frequent complication of choledocholithiasis?**

Cholangitis (60%). Other complications are bile duct obstruction, pancreatitis, biliary enteric fistula and hemobilia.

❍ **Acalculous cholecystitis commonly occurs in what conditions?**

Post-operative, post-traumatic and burn patients secondary to dehydration and hemolysis secondary to blood transfusions.

❍ **A 22 year-old female with sickle-cell disease presents with fever, shaking chills and jaundice. What is the diagnosis?**

Charcot's triad suggests ascending cholangitis. The precipitating cause is probably pigment stones resulting from chronic hemolysis.

❍ **List the ultrasound findings that are suggestive of acute cholecystitis.**

Formation of gallstones or sludge (in acalculous cholecystitis), thickening of the wall of the gallbladder and the presence of pericholecystic fluid. A dilated common bile duct suggests common duct obstruction.

❍ **Can acalculous cholecystitis perforate?**

Yes. Up to 40% of gallbladder perforations are associated with acalculous cholecystitis.

❍ **A 24 year-old male complains that he has endured two days of rice-water stools, muscle cramps and extreme fatigue. He looks pale, dehydrated and very ill. The patient states that he has just returned from India. What is the diagnosis?**

Cholera. The incidence of cholera in the US is 1/10,000,000. This disease usually develops in persons that have traveled to endemic areas, such as India, Africa, Southeast Asia, southern Europe, Central and South America and the Middle East. Infection occurs by consuming unpurified water, raw fruits and vegetables and undercooked seafood.

❍ **A patient presents with palmar erythema, spider angiomas, testicular atrophy and asterixis. What other signs and symptoms may be exhibited?**

Hematemesis, encephalopathy, hepatomegaly, splenomegaly, jaundice, caput medusa, ascites and gynecomastia may also occur. This patient has cirrhosis.

❍ **A cirrhotic patient vomits bright red blood and has a systolic blood pressure of 90 mm Hg. After aggressive fluid resuscitation with 4 units of packed RBCs and a gastric lavage, his pressure is still 90 mm Hg. What's next?**

Assume a coagulopathy. Transfuse fresh frozen plasma, start a vasopressin or octreotide drip and arrange for an emergent endoscopic evaluation/intervention, usually for sclerotherapy or banding.

❍ **How does the pathology of Crohn's disease differ from that of ulcerative colitis?**

Crohn's is a transmucosal, segmental, granulomatous process, while ulcerative colitis is a mucosal, juxtapositioned, ulcerative process.

❍ **A cirrhotic patient presents with weakness and edema. What electrolyte imbalances might be present?**

Hyponatremia (dilutional or diuretic induced), hypokalemia (from GI losses or diuretics) and hypomagnesemia.

❍ **What diuretic is the optimal choice for cirrhotic patients with ascites?**

Potassium sparing agents. These medications treat the hyperaldosterone state specifically.

❍ **A confused cirrhotic patient enters the hospital. She is afebrile and has asterixis. What should your examination include to determine the precipitant of hepatic encephalopathy?**

Assess her mental status and examine her for localizing neurologic signs suggestive of an occult head injury. Look for dry mucous membranes and a low jugular venous pressure, which are indicative of hypovolemia and azotemia. In addition, check a stool guaiac for GI bleeding. Focused lab testing can pinpoint other causes, including diuretic overuse and hypokalemia, hypoglycemia, anemia, hypoxia and infection. Administer thiamine and folate.

❍ **Aside from fixing the above, what therapy is useful?**

Lactulose. This synthetic disaccharide produces an acidic diarrhea which traps nitrogenous wastes in the gut.

❍ **Which diarrheal illnesses cause fecal leukocytes?**

The usual culprits are shigella, campylobacter and enteroinvasive E. coli. Others include salmonella, yersinia, Vibrio parahaemolyticus and C. difficile. Fecal WBCs are absent in toxigenic and enteropathogenic infection, even with such a virulent organism as Vibrio cholera. Viral and parasitic infections rarely produce fecal WBCs.

❍ **What is the most common cause of bacterial diarrhea?**

E. coli (enteroinvasive, enteropathogenic, enterotoxigenic).

❍ **A 73 year-old woman with no prior medical history presents with fever, chills, vomiting, nausea and an acute onset of pain in her left lower quadrant. Her pain becomes worse after she eats and is mildly relieved after a bowel movement. Upon physical examination, you note that she has guarding, rebound tenderness and a tender, firm, non-mobile mass in the left lower quadrant. What is the most likely diagnosis?**

Diverticulitis.

❍ **If there is associated bleeding with the diverticuli, where is the most likely etiology?**

The right side of the colon. Fifty percent of bleeding episodes originate in this area even though diverticulitis is more common in the left side.

❍ **T/F: A barium enema is not a good diagnostic test if diverticulitis is suspected.**

True. If a patient is having an acute attack of diverticulitis, the risk of perforation is too great.

❍ **Is diverticulitis the probable diagnosis for a patient with lower abdominal pain and bright red blood per rectum?**

No. Typically diverticulosis bleeds, while diverticulitis doesn't. Diverticular bleeding is usually painless.

❍ **A 40 year-old smoker describes an acute crescendo substernal chest tightness penetrating to his back. Antacids do not relieve the pain. An ECG shows ST changes and his pain resolves 7 to 10 minutes after a nitroglycerin tablet. Is this angina?**

Maybe, although the delayed response to nitrates characterizes "esophageal colic" which is caused by segmental esophageal spasm and is often triggered by reflux.

❍ **What is the appropriate management for an ingested button battery that is in the stomach?**

In asymptomatic patients, repeat radiographs. Endoscopic retrieval is required if symptoms occur or if the battery does not pass the pylorus after 48 hours.

❍ **What is the best way to remove a meat bolus causing esophageal obstruction?**

Endoscopy. IV glucagon may be tried first. Both medications relax esophageal smooth muscle. Meat tenderizer should be avoided.

❍ **Which type of hepatitis is characterized by an SPGT greater than the SGOT?**

Viral hepatitis. The SGPT is usually greater than 1,000.

❍ **Which type of hepatitis is usually contracted through blood transfusions?**

Hepatitis C accounts for 85% of hepatitis infections via this route.

❍ **Which LFTs are associated with a poor prognosis in acute viral hepatitis?**

A total bilirubin > 20 mg/dl and a prolongation of the prothrombin time > 3 seconds. The extent of transaminase elevation is not a useful marker.

❍ **Match the following hepatitis serologies with the correct clinical description.**

1) Anti-HBsAb (+) and HBsAg (-)	a) Ongoing viral replication, highly infectious
2) Anti-HBc IgM (+) and HBsAg (-)	b) Remote infection, not infectious
3) Anti-HBc IgG (+) and HBsAg (-)	c) Recent or ongoing infection
4) HBeAg (+)	d) Prior infection or vaccination, not infectious

Answers: (1) d, (2) c, (3) b and (4) a.

❍ **T/F: The d-agent can cause hepatitis D in a patient without active hepatitis B.**

False. The d-agent is an incomplete, "defective" RNA virus that is responsible for hepatitis D. It is an obligate co-virus and requires hepatitis B for replication.

❍ **A patient's groin bulged two days ago. He then developed severe pain with progressive nausea and vomiting. He has a tender mass in his groin. What should you NOT do?**

Don't try to reduce a long-standing, tender, incarcerated hernia. The abdomen is no place for dead bowel.

❍ **What simple test can distinguish between conjugated and unconjugated hyperbilirubinemia?**

A dipstick test for urobilinogen, which reflects conjugated (water soluble) hyperbilirubinemia.

❍ **What is the treatment for intussusception?**

A barium enema is both a diagnostic tool and often curative, i.e., it can reduce the intussusception. If the barium enema is unsuccessful, surgical reduction may be required.

❍ **List four contraindications to the introduction of a nasogastric tube.**

1) Suspected esophageal laceration or perforation
2) Near obstruction due to stricture
3) Esophageal foreign body
4) Severe head trauma with rhinorrhea

❍ **What test should be performed when an elderly patient is suffering from pain that is out of proportion to the physical examination?**

Angiography. This test is the gold standard for diagnosing mesenteric ischemia.

❍ **A KUB suggests a large bowel obstruction. What are the next steps?**

An unprepped sigmoidoscopy to confirm obstruction followed by a barium study to determine the cause. If a pseudo-obstruction is suspected, don't order a barium study because of the possibility of concretion and obstruction. Colonoscopy can be diagnostic as well as therapeutic.

❍ **Pseudo-obstruction is typically caused by medications. What are three classes of drugs that give rise to pseudo-obstruction?**

Anticholinergics, anti-parkinsonian drugs and tricyclic antidepressants.

❍ **What is the most frequent cause of small bowel obstruction?**

Adhesions, followed by incarcerated hernias, are the most common causes of extraluminal obstruction. Gallstones and bezoars are the most common causes of intraluminal obstruction.

❍ **Is a serum amylase test or a lipase test more specific for pancreatitis?**

Lipase.

❍ **Is a nasogastric tube always required for acute pancreatitis?**

No, only if nausea and vomiting are severe. In fact, one study showed that NG tubes contributed to more complications, including aspiration.

❍ **When are antibiotics useful in acute pancreatitis?**

Because pancreatitis is a chemical disease, antibiotics are only useful for treating complications, such as an abscess or sepsis and those cases that are associated with choledocholithiasis.

❍ **What is the most common cause of lower GI perforation?**

Diverticulitis, followed by tumor, colitis, foreign bodies and instrumentation.

❍ **What does burning epigastric pain shooting to the back, hypovolemic shock and a high amylase level suggest?**

A posterior penetration of a gastric ulcer.

❍ **Enteric coated potassium tablets, typhoid, tuberculosis, tumors and a strangulated hernia can all cause what rare process?**

Non-traumatic small bowel perforation.

❍ **What percentage of patients with a perforated viscous have radiographic evidence of a pneumoperitoneum?**

60 to 70%. Therefore, one-third of patients will not have this sign. Maintain the patient in either the upright or the left lateral decubitus position for at least 10 minutes prior to taking x-rays.

❍ **After a high-speed motor vehicle accident, an unrestrained driver develops abdominal and chest pain radiating to the neck. An upper chest film shows left-sided pleural fluid. What gastroesophageal catastrophe might have occurred?**

Impact against a steering wheel can result in Boerhaave's syndrome with esophageal perforation and mediastinitis.

❍ **What test should be ordered if a perforated esophagus is suspected?**

A water soluble contrast study. In the mean time, start broad spectrum antibiotics and consult a surgeon immediately.

❍ **A former IV drug user with sickle-cell disease and a history of splenectomy presents with unremitting fever, crampy abdominal pain and meningismus. He has no diarrhea but has recently purchased a pet turtle. What bacteria may be the culprit?**

Salmonella typhi, the causative agent of typhoid fever. The infection rate is remarkably high for HIV, asplenic and sickle-cell disease patients. Rose spots occur in 10 to 20% of these cases. Relative bradycardia with a high fever and a low to normal WBC with a pronounced left shift are suggestive findings.

❍ **What is the treatment for the above patient?**

IV fluoroquinolone or ceftriaxone. Check blood cultures for the presence of bacteremia. Avoid anti-motility agents.

❍ **What are some indications for surgery in a bleeding ulcer?**

A visible vessel in the ulcer bed, more than 6 units of blood transfused in 24 hours or more than 3 to 4 units transfused per day for three days.

❍ **Are "stress ulcers" a surgical problem?**

Typically not. The diffuse gastric bleeding that results from CNS tumors, head trauma, burns, sepsis, shock, steroids, aspirin or alcohol is usually mucosal and can be life threatening. However, this condition can usually be managed medically. Endoscopic diagnosis is key.

❍ **What medical conditions are related to an increased incidence of peptic ulcers?**

COPD, cirrhosis and chronic renal failure.

❍ **Where is the most common location of a perforated peptic ulcer?**

The anterior surface of the duodenum or pylorus and the lesser curvature of the stomach.

❍ **What are two endocrine problems that can cause peptic ulcer disease?**

Zollinger-Ellison syndrome and hyperparathyroidism (hypercalcemia).

❍ **Should you be concerned when administering cimetidine to a wheezing, anticoagulated patient with a seizure disorder?**

Yes. By decreasing blood flow to the liver and competing with the drug eliminating cytochrome P-450 system, cimetidine can increase the levels of theophylline, warfarin and phenytoin, as well as diazepam, propranolol and lidocaine.

❍ **A patient with new diarrhea and abdominal pain has been on antibiotics for sinusitis for two weeks. What might be revealed by sigmoidoscopy?**

Yellowish superficial plaques. This finding is indicative of pseudomembranous colitis. Stool samples will be positive for the C. difficile toxin.

❍ **What is the treatment for pseudomembranous colitis?**

Oral metronidazole (preferred) or vancomycin.

❍ **An ascitic patient has a fever but no localizing signs or symptoms of infection. He also has a normal WBC. Because you know that spontaneous bacterial peritonitis (SBP) can be an occult disease, you perform an abdominal paracentesis. What amount of WBCs in the ascitic fluid suggests SBP?**

WBC > $250/mm^3$. Also perform a Gram's stain and culture of the ascitic fluid.

❍ **What organism is usually responsible for causing SBP?**

E. coli. Streptococcus pneumoniae is second.

❍ **A patient with chronic and occasionally bloody diarrhea develops severe diarrhea and abdominal pain with marked distention. What "can't miss" diagnosis do these signs suggest?**

Toxic megacolon. This condition is a life threatening complication of ulcerative colitis.

❍ **What is the most common cause of pancreatitis?**

Alcohol and gallstones.

❍ **What are some other causes of pancreatitis?**

Surgery, trauma, post-ERCP, viral and mycoplasma infections, hypertriglyceridemia, vasculitis, drugs, penetrating peptic ulcer, anatomic abnormalities about the ampulla of Vater, hyperparathyroidism, end stage renal disease and organ transplantation.

❍ **What are some of the drugs known to cause pancreatitis?**

Sulfonamides, estrogens, tetracyclines, pentamidine, azathioprine, thiazides, furosemide and valproic acid.

❍ **What are some of the infectious causes of pancreatitis?**
Mumps, viral hepatitis, Coxsackie virus group B and mycoplasma.

❍ **What are the pathological spectra in acute pancreatitis?**

From edematous pancreatitis (mild cases) to necrotizing pancreatitis (severe cases). Hemorrhagic pancreatitis may evolve from either of them.

❍ **What is the most common lipid profile that may result in pancreatitis?**

Type V lipid profile, which is characterized by marked hypertriglyceridemia (usually levels > 1000 mg/dl).

❍ **What are the laboratory abnormalities in pancreatitis?**

Leukocytosis, hemoconcentration followed by anemia, hyperglycemia, prerenal azotemia, hypoxemia, hyperamylasemia and LFT abnormalities.

❍ **What is the role of abdominal ultrasound in pancreatitis?**

Less sensitive than CT. Useful for detection of biliary obstruction and progression of pseudocysts.

❍ **What is the role of CT scanning?**

Useful in diagnosis, severity assessment, detection of complications, aspiration guide and drainage of collections.

❍ **What are the simplified Glasgow prognostic criteria in pancreatitis?**

Age > 55 years, WBCs > 15,000, glucose > 180 mg/dl, LDH > 600, BUN > 45 mg/dl, calcium < 8 mg/dl, albumin < 32 gm/l, arterial PO_2 < 60 mmHg.

❍ **What is a pancreatic pseudocyst?**

Collection of necrotic tissue, fluid and blood that develops without a true capsule. It develops over a period of 1 to 4 weeks.

❍ **What is the treatment for pancreatic pseudocysts?**

Initial therapy is to wait for regression (4 to 6 weeks). If no improvement or superinfection occurs, surgical drainage or excision is required.

❍ **What are the complications of pseudocyst?**

Infection, perforation and hemorrhage.

❍ **What are the most common causes of colonic obstruction?**

Cancer, then diverticulitis followed by volvulus.

❍ **In a patient with pancreatitis, what complications are suggested by symptoms that last longer than a week or an abdominal mass with leukocytosis?**

Pancreatic abscess or pseudocyst.

❍ **Match the diarrheal syndrome with the culprit:**

(1) Aeromonas hydrophilia	**___Diarrhea after eating fried rice at a Chinese buffet.**
(2) Bacillus cereus	**___Diarrhea followed by thigh myalgia, perioral dysesthesia and pruritus.**
(3) Campylobacter	**___ Profuse, foul-smelling diarrhea with bloating and cramps after a fishing trip.**
(4) Clostridium difficile	**___Bloody diarrhea and fever in a child.**
(5) Clostridium perfringens	**___Acute dysentery, fever and pseudoappendicitis.**
(6) Vibrio parahaemolyticus	**___Rice water diarrhea without fever or constitutional symptoms.**
(7) Staphylococcus aureus	**___Diarrhea from raw seafood.**
(8) Yersinia	**___Diarrhea from contaminated meat without nausea or vomiting.**
(9) Giardia	**___Diarrhea due to antibiotic associated enterocolitis.**
(10) Ciguatera toxin	**___Diarrhea (enterocolitis) associated with ham, eggs and mayonnaise**

(Answers: 2, 10, 9, 3, 8, 1, 6, 5, 4, 7)

❍ **What are the indications for the surgical removal of a GI foreign body?**

Obstruction, perforation, toxic properties and shape such that the object will not pass safely.

❍ **What is abdominal compartment syndrome?**

Increased pressure within the confined anatomical space of the abdomen that may impair end organ perfusion and physiologic function.

❍ **What is the most common cause of intra-abdominal compartment syndrome?**

Coagulopathy with post-operative intra-abdominal hemorrhage.

❍ **What is the treatment for leaking ascites following major surgery?**

Return to the operating room for repair of fascial dehiscence.

❍ **What is the difference between fascial dehiscence and evisceration?**

Facial dehiscence involves separation of the closed fascia with or without evisceration of the bowel. Evisceration is a surgical emergency.

❍ **What is the most common cause of fascial dehiscence?**

Intra-abdominal sepsis.

❍ **Forty eight hours post-operatively, a patient develops severe pain about his midline wound, skin bullae, crepitus and irregular blanching at the wound margins with a fever of 104. What is the most likely diagnosis?**

Clostridial gas gangrene.

❍ **What is the treatment for patients who present with the sudden onset of inability to swallow food, liquids or saliva?**

Esophagoscopy to confirm esophageal obstruction, with endoscopic removal of the impacted food or foreign body. Food is the most common obstructing foreign body in the esophagus.

❍ **What are the common radiographic signs suggestive of esophageal perforation?**

Mediastinal air, pneumothorax, pleural effusion and subcutaneous emphysema.

❍ **What is the most appropriate initial therapy for a patient with bleeding esophageal varices?**

Octreotide (somatostatin analogue) infusion. Vasopressin along with nitroglycerin (to offset the coronary vasoconstriction caused by vasopressin) can be used if this is unavailable. Any coagulation defect must be corrected.

❍ **What are the other non-surgical options for bleeding esophageal varices that do not respond to somatostatin infusion?**

Placement of Sengstaken-Blakemore tube, sclerotherapy or banding of varices and transjugular intrahepatic portosystemic shunting.

❍ **What should the early treatment of a bleeding gastric or duodenal ulcer include?**

Therapeutic endoscopy with attempted sclerotherapy or electrocautery. Patients with a visible vessel in the ulcer crater are at highest risk for rebleeding and should be considered for surgery.

❍ **What patients should undergo surgical therapy for bleeding ulcer disease?**

Patients with significant transfusion requirements, patients who rebleed following attempted non-operative therapy and patients with limited physiologic reserves who cannot tolerate repeated insults.

❍ **Four days following placement of a percutaneous endoscopic gastrostomy tube a patient develops sudden onset of fever, chills, tachycardia and hypotension. Physical exam shows abdominal distention and plain films show a large amount of free air. The most likely cause is?**

Gastric leakage due to necrosis.

❍ **What is gastric tonometry?**

Measurement of regional pCO_2 and intramucosal pH, usually via a nasogastric catheter. These values are used to estimate the adequacy of perfusion of the gut.

❍ **What is the incidence of early small bowel obstruction (within thirty days) in patients following laparotomy?**

About 1 to 3%. The most common cause is adhesions.

❍ **What is the treatment for early small bowel obstruction (within thirty days) in patients following laparotomy?**

Nasogastric decompression unless there are signs of ischemia or strangulation.

❍ **What is the most feared complication following duodenal surgery?**

Duodenal fistula with intra-abdominal sepsis.

❍ **What is the risk of tube feeding a patient with an ileus?**

Massive small bowel necrosis. This unusual complication is seen primarily in critically ill patients and has an unclear etiology.

❍ **Are toxic megacolon and fulminant colitis the same thing?**

No. Toxic megacolon refers to colonic dilation superimposed upon fulminant colitis.

❍ **What is the most common cause of toxic megacolon?**

The most common cause is ulcerative colitis, although other causes include Crohn's disease, amebic colitis, shigella or salmonella infection, pseudomembranous colitis, ischemic bowel disease, mucosal ulcerative colitis, cytomegalovirus infection and anti-cancer chemotherapy.

❍ **What procedure should a patient with a bowel obstruction and sigmoid volvulus undergo?**

Attempted colonoscopic decompression, either with a rigid or flexible endoscope. If this is unsuccessful the patient will require laparotomy with sigmoid colectomy.

❍ **What procedure should a patient with a bowel obstruction and cecal volvulus undergo?**

Laparotomy and right hemicolectomy.

❍ **What intravenous antibiotic is effective in treating Clostridium difficile associated with an ileus?**

Metronidazole.

❍ **What is the appropriate surgical therapy for toxic Clostridium difficile colitis?**

Total colectomy with end ileostomy.

❍ **What are the most common causes of lower GI hemorrhage?**

Diverticulosis and angiodysplasia.

❍ **What is the appropriate workup for patients with lower GI bleeding?**

Appropriate treatment of lower GI bleeding requires localization of the bleeding site. This is usually accomplished by a bleeding scan, with subsequent angiography if the bleeding scan fails to localize. Angiography requires the patient to be bleeding at least 0.5 cc/min., where a bleeding scan can detect bleeding at much lower rates. Colonoscopy may be helpful, but it is usually difficult to visualize the bleeding site secondary to luminal blood.

❍ **What is the most common colonic site for massive lower GI bleeding?**

The right colon.

❍ **What is the appropriate surgical procedure for persistent occult massive lower GI bleeding?**

Total colectomy with ileoproctostomy or end ileostomy.

❍ **Why is angiographic embolization a poor choice for treatment of lower GI bleeding?**

The bleeding vessels are end arteries. Embolization would likely cause necrosis.

❍ **What percentage of fulminant hepatic failure is due to acetaminophen?**

In the U.S., about 10% are due to acetaminophen ingestion and another 10% are due to other drugs such as isoniazid, halogenated anesthetics, phenytoin, propylthiouracil and sulfonamides.

❍ **What does the workup in patients with suspected acalculous cholecystitis include?**

Ultrasound or morphine augmented HIDA scan.

❍ **What is the treatment for acalculous cholecystitis?**

Cholecystectomy, because of the high incidence of gallbladder necrosis. Surgical or percutaneous cholecystostomy can be performed before necrosis develops.

❍ **What disease is suggested by Grey-Turner's sign (flank ecchymosis) and Cullen's sign (periumbilical ecchymosis)?**

Severe necrotizing pancreatitis with retroperitoneal hemorrhage.

❍ **What complications of acute pancreatitis may require surgery?**

Pancreatis abscess, necrosis, persistent pseudocyst, fistula or hemorrhage.

❍ **Five days following splenectomy for trauma a patient is diagnosed with a subphrenic abscess. Fluid from a percutaneous drainage reveals the amylase to be 48,000. What is the diagnosis?**

Pancreatic fistula. The tail of the pancreas was likely injured during the splenectomy.

❍ **What are the symptoms of overwhelming post splenectomy infection (OPSI)?**

Brief prodrome of mild fever and nonspecific symptoms followed by overwhelming septic shock.

❍ **What are the most common organisms implicated in cases of OPSI?**

Streptococcus pneumoniae (50-90%), Haemophilus influenzae and meningococcus.

❍ **What is the lifetime risk for OPSI following splenectomy?**

It has been estimated as 5%. It is higher in children than adults.

❍ **T/F: Patients who undergo splenectomy do not require pneumococcal vaccine.**

False.

❍ **A patient admitted to the ICU for shock describes terrible abdominal pain out of proportion to their physical exam. What is the most likely diagnosis?**

Intestinal infarction.

❍ **Following infrarenal aortic replacement for aneurysmal disease, a patient becomes hypotensive with worsening abdominal distention. What is the next appropriate step?**

Immediate return to the operating room for repair of vascular suture line dehiscence.

❍ **A patient with a type B thoracic aortic aneurysm admitted to the ICU for medical treatment develops oliguria, increased fluid requirements and acute abdominal pain 24 hours later. What is the most likely explanation?**

Extension of the dissection with compromise of intestinal perfusion.

❍ **What are the common symptoms of acute pancreatitis?**
Epigastric abdominal pain radiating to the back associated with nausea and vomiting.

❍ **Does acute pancreatitis commonly progress to chronic pancreatitis?**

Only rarely.

❍ **T/F: Acute pancreatitis may be the result of occult biliary microlithiasis or biliary sludge.**

True.

❍ **What is the mechanism of necrosis and vascular damage in acute pancreatitis?**

Autodigestion of the pancreas by various proteolytic and lipolytic enzymes.

❍ **T/F: Normal amylase levels rule out pancreatitis.**

False.

❍ **What else may cause hyperamylasemia besides pancreatitis?**

Pancreatic pseudocyst, pancreatic trauma, pancreatic carcinoma, ERCP, perforated duodenal ulcer, mesenteric infarction, renal failure, intestinal obstruction, salivary gland conditions, ovarian disorders, prostate tumors, DKA and macroamylasemia.

❍ **Does the level of amylase elevation correlate with severity?**

No.

❍ **Match the following hepatotoxic drugs with the correct toxic syndrome:**

(1) Halothane, methyldopa, isoniazid.	**___chronic active hepatitis and cirrhosis.**
(2) Anabolic steroids, oral contraceptives, oral hypoglycemics, erythromycin estolate.	**___massive hepatic necrosis.**
(3) Carbon tetrachloride, acetaminophen, Amanita mushrooms.	**___acute hepatitis.**
(4) Vinyl chloride, arsenic.	**___steatosis, hepatocellular necrosis.**
(5) Ethanol.	**___cholestatic jaundice.**

(Answer: 4, 3, 1, 5, 2)

❍ **What might the abdominal films reveal on a patient with appendicitis?**

Sentinel loops with air fluid levels in the RLQ, a gas filled appendix or a fecalith.

❍ **What is the most common cause of appendicitis?**

Fecaliths. Fecaliths are found in 40% of uncomplicated appendicitis cases, 65% of cases involving gangrenous appendices that have not ruptured and in 90% of cases involving ruptured appendices. Other causes of appendicitis include lymphoid tissue hypertrophy, inspissated barium, foreign bodies and strictures.

❍ **How does retrocecal appendicitis most commonly present?**

Dysuria, poorly localized abdominal pain, anorexia, nausea, vomiting, diarrhea and mild fever.

❍ **Differentiate between reducible, incarcerated, strangulated, Richter and complete hernias.**

Reducible: The contents of the hernia sac return to the abdomen spontaneously or with slight pressure.
Incarcerated: The contents of the hernia sac are irreducible and cannot be returned to the abdomen.
Strangulated: The sac and its contents turn gangrenous.
Richter: Only part of the hernia sac and its contents becomes strangulated. This hernia may spontaneously reduce and be overlooked.
Complete: An inguinal hernia that passes all the way into the scrotum.

❍ **Is mesenteric ischemia more serious in the small or large bowel?**

The small bowel. Embolization in the superior mesenteric artery effects the entire small bowel. Embolization to the large bowel is not as serious due to collateral circulation to the large bowel.

GENITOURINARY PEARLS

Trust only movement. Life happens at the level of events not of words. Trust movement.
Alfred Adler

❍ **What is the most common infectious cause of the hemolytic uremic syndrome?**

E. coli (O157:H7).

❍ **What is the diagnostic triad for HUS?**

Microangiopathic anemia, acute renal failure and thrombocytopenia.

❍ **What is the prognosis for patients with acute renal failure secondary to HUS?**

Over 90% survival with many patients eventually recovering normal renal function.

❍ **What is the role of corticosteroids in the treatment of HUS?**

None.

❍ **What are the pulmonary manifestations of chronic renal disease?**

Pulmonary edema, pleural effusions, uremic pleuritis, metastatic calcifications, urinothorax, pO_2 reduction during hemodialysis and atelectasis associated with peritoneal dialysis.

❍ **What is the mechanism for pO_2 reduction during hemodialysis?**

The primary mechanism is hypoventilation due to decreased CO_2 production that is associated with the oxidation of acetate. Secondarily, complement is activated resulting in leukocyte and platelet aggregation, which alters V/Q.

❍ **A patient with polyuria, low urine osmolality and high serum osmolality is given vasopressin. No change in osmolality is noted. Which type of diabetes insipidus (DI) does she have?**

Nephrogenic. The distal renal tubules are refractory to antidiuretic hormone.

❍ **What are the indications for emergency hemodialysis?**

Elevated potassium with ECG changes, decreased pH, pericarditis, mental status changes and severe volume overload.

❍ **How is the fractional excretion of sodium (FENa) calculated?**

FENa = [(Una / Pna) / (Ucr / Pcr)] x 100.

❍ **What is the most reliable test for differentiation of acute oliguric renal failure from prerenal azotemia?**

FENa, which is greater than 2% in acute renal failure and less than 1% in prerenal azotemia.

❍ **What are the major adverse effects of intravenous radiocontrast given to diabetic patients?**

Acute tubular necrosis, worsening of CHF, precipitation of angina pectoris and allergic reactions.

❍ **What is the etiology of acute renal failure seen a few weeks after cardiac catheterization?**

Cholesterol emboli syndrome.

❍ **What treatments are used to ameliorate bleeding in a uremic patient?**

Dialysis, DDAVP, cryoprecipitate or platelet transfusions.

❍ **What medications are likely to cause acute renal failure with interstitial nephritis?**

Beta-lactam antibiotics, cimetidine, NSAIDs, phenytoin and rifampin.

❍ **What are the most common cause of acute renal failure seen after repair of an abdominal aneurysm?**

Acute tubular necrosis due to aortic cross clamping.

❍ **What glomerular diseases are likely to recur in the allograft of transplant patients?**

Focal glomerulosclerosis and membranoproliferative glomerulonephritis have a high incidence of recurrence.

❍ **What medications may be associated with hemolytic uremic syndrome?**

Mitomycin, estrogens and cyclosporine.

❍ **What is the therapy of choice for a patient with chronic renal failure and pericarditis?**

Dialysis.

❍ **What are the causes of advanced chronic renal failure and large kidneys?**

Amyloidosis, polycystic kidney disease, diabetic nephropathy, HIV nephropathy and multiple myeloma.

❍ **What does acute renal failure in a patient with alcoholic cirrhosis and a urine sodium of less than 10 suggest?**

Pre-renal azotemia or hepatorenal syndrome.

❍ **Acute renal failure caused by Wegener's granulomatosis responds best to what treatment?**

This is usually a rapidly progressive glomerulonephritis and responds to high dose steroids and cyclophosphamide.

❍ **What does total and persistent anuria with renal failure suggest?**

Obstruction.

❍ **Aminoglycosides are likely to cause what type of acute renal failure?**

Non-oliguric acute tubular necrosis (ATN).

❍ **A renal biopsy in a patient with acute renal failure, hematuria and red cell casts will most likely reveal what lesion?**

A proliferative glomerulonephritis, usually with crescents.

❍ **Anemia of chronic renal failure is likely to respond to what agent?**

Erythropoietin.

❍ **What are the most common etiologies of chronic renal failure leading to dialysis in the U.S.?**

Hypertensive and diabetic renal disease.

❍ **What are the first line oral phosphate binders used in CRF?**

Calcium carbonate and calcium acetate. Aluminum containing agents are best avoided.

❍ **What co-morbid factors are likely to increase the risk of contrast induced ATN?**

Azotemia, diabetic nephropathy, CHF, multiple myeloma and dehydration.

❍ **What are the causes of high levels of PTH in CRF?**

Hyperphosphatemia, hypocalcemia due to deficiency of vitamin D and parathyroid receptor resistance.

❍ **What is the etiology of CRF associated with cerebral berry aneurysms?**

Adult polycystic kidney disease is associated with cerebral berry aneurysms.

❍ **What medications have been proven to decrease the mortality in ATN?**

None.

❍ **What are some long term complications seen with the use of aluminum containing phosphate binders?**

Aluminum induced osteomalacia, anemia and rarely dementia.

❍ **What is the major therapy used to treat allergic interstitial nephritis not responding to discontinuation of the causative medication?**

Corticosteroids.

❍ **Sudden ARF, seen after initiation of ACE inhibitors, should prompt a work up for what disease?**

ACE inhibitors are likely to cause ARF in patients with bilateral renal artery stenosis or renal artery stenosis in a solitary kidney.

❍ **What type of ARF is usually seen with rhabdomyolysis?**

Acute tubular necrosis.

❍ **What is suggested by chronic renal failure with hypertension, small shrunken kidneys and gout at an early age?**

Lead nephropathy.

❍ **What pathology is usually seen in patients with nephrotic syndrome and AIDS?**

Focal segmental glomerulosclerosis.

❍ **What factors predispose to acute papillary necrosis?**

Analgesic abuse, sickle cell disease, diabetes mellitus and alcoholism.

❍ **What renal toxicity is seen with amphotericin B?**

Tubulointerstitial disease with a distal hypokalemic renal tubular acidosis and hypomagnesemia.

❍ **What is the mechanism of cocaine induced ARF?**

Rhabdomyolysis induced ATN and acute hypertensive nephropathy.

❍ **What are the major complications seen after placement of percutaneous venous catheters for hemodialysis or CVVH?**

Bleeding, local infection and bacteremia. Pneumothorax and venous stenosis may occur with a subclavian catheter.

❍ **What is the most common cause of acute renal failure?**

Acute tubular necrosis. This occurs after toxic or ischemic renal injuries.

❍ **What is Fournier's gangrene?**

Fournier's gangrene is a polymicrobial infection of the subcutaneous tissue of the perineum characterized by widespread tissue necrosis. Treatment consists of broad-spectrum parenteral antibiotics and immediate surgical debridement.

❍ **What clinical findings are seen with acute glomerulonephritis (GN)?**

1) Oliguria
2) Hypertension
3) Urine sediment containing RBCs, WBCs, protein and RBC casts
4) Edema

❍ **What is the most common cause of post-infectious GN?**

Post streptococcal Group A beta-hemolytic glomerulonephritis. The GN is caused by immune complex deposition in glomeruli. Most patients completely recover normal renal function, spontaneously, within a few weeks.

❍ **What syndrome is characterized by an anti-glomerular basement membrane antibody induced GN that is preceded by pulmonary hemorrhage and hemoptysis?**

Goodpasture's syndrome.

❍ **What are some causes of false positive hematuria?**

Food coloring, beets, paprika, rifampin, phenothiazine, phenytoin, myoglobin or menstruation.

❍ **A urinalysis reveals RBC casts and dysmorphic RBCs. What is the probable origin of hematuria?**

Glomerulus.

❍ **What are the admission criteria for patients with renal calculi?**

Infection with concurrent obstruction, a solitary kidney and complete obstruction, renal insufficiency, uncontrolled pain, intractable emesis or large stones. Only 10% of stones > 6 mm pass spontaneously.

❍ **What is the most common cause of nephrotic syndrome in children? In adults?**

Children: Minimal change disease. Adults: Idiopathic glomerulonephritis.

❍ **What are some common nephrotoxic agents?**

Aminoglycoside, NSAIDs, contrast dye and myoglobin.

❍ **What is the definition of oliguria? Of anuria?**

Oliguria: Urine output < 500 ml/day
Anuria: Urine output < 100 ml/day

❍ **When is a retrograde urethrogram necessary to evaluate a patient with a penile fracture?**

Patients with hematuria, blood at the urethral meatus or the inability to void should undergo this procedure to rule out a urethral injury. A penile fracture is rupture of the corpus cavernosum with tearing of the tunica albuginea. It occurs as a result of a blunt trauma to the erect penis. Urethral injury occurs in approximately 10% of patients with a penile fracture.

❍ **What is the initial treatment for priapism?**

Terbutaline subcutaneously.

❍ **What are the causative organisms of prostatitis?**

E. coli (80%), klebsiella, enterobacter, proteus and pseudomonas.

❍ **What is the anatomical approach to ARF?**

Ask whether the site is pre-, intra-, or post-renal. Pre-renal is due to hypovolemia, intra-renal is mostly due to ATN or toxins and post-renal is due to obstruction.

❍ **What is the most common cause of intrinsic (intra-) renal failure?**

Acute tubular necrosis (80 to 90%), resulting from an ischemic injury (the most common cause of ATN) or from a nephrotoxic agent. Less frequent causes of intrinsic renal failure (10 to 20%) include vasculitis, malignant hypertension, acute GN or allergic interstitial nephritis.

❍ **What abnormal ultrasound findings suggest chronic renal failure?**

Kidneys < 9 cm in length. A difference in length between the two kidneys of > 1.5 cm suggests unilateral kidney disease. Kidneys with a small or absent renal cortex are also indicative of chronic renal failure.

❍ **If a urine dipstick is positive for blood, but a urine analysis is negative for RBCs, what is the probable disease?**

Rhabdomyolysis. Severe muscle damage results in free myoglobin in blood. Very high levels lead to acute renal failure.

❍ **What is the most common form of lupus nephritis?**

Diffuse proliferative nephritis (WHO class IV). This is also the most severe form.

❍ **What is the most common manifestation of Goodpasture's disease?**

Hemoptysis. These patients usually develop pulmonary hemorrhage before any signs of renal failure develop.

❍ **What is the diagnostic triad of the nephrotic syndrome?**

Edema, hyperlipidemia and proteinuria with hypoproteinemia.

❍ **How is renal tubular acidosis (RTA) classified?**

Into one of three types:

Type I - distal RTA
Type II - proximal RTA
Type IV - mineralocorticoid deficiency
There is no type III.

❍ **Which isolated form of RTA will be most likely to lead to renal failure?**

Distal (Type I), though most cases of Type I RTA have an excellent prognosis.

❍ **What two common medications can induce nephrogenic diabetes insipidus?**

Lithium and amphotericin B.

❍ **What are some clinical findings in acute glomerulonephritis (GN)?**

Hematuria, proteinuria, oliguria or anuria, edema and hypertension.

❍ **Mention some diseases that cause glomerular dysfunction (skip this one if you are in a hurry!).**

Goodpasture's syndrome - pulmonary hemorrhage with hemoptysis followed by anti-glomerular basement membrane antibody induced glomerulonephritis.

Post-infectious GN - most common post-streptococcal (group A, ß- hemolytic) infection but may follow other infections with GN secondary to immune complex deposits in glomeruli.

Polyarteritis nodosa (PAN) - a systemic necrotizing vasculitis affecting primarily medium and small caliber arteries particularly at bifurcations and branchings. PAN occurs from infancy to old age with a peak incidence near age 60. 90% of patients with PAN develop renal involvement.

Systemic lupus erythematosus - Autoimmune disorder resulting, in part, in necrotizing vasculitis of primarily small vessels complicated by direct immunoglobulin deposits in glomeruli.

Henoch-Schönlein purpura (HSP) - another systemic necrotizing vasculitis of small vessels with renal presentation of nephritic syndrome. Associated with GI symptoms and lower extremity rash.

Hemolytic uremic syndrome (HUS) - microangiopathic hemolytic anemia, thrombocytopenia and renal dysfunction with rapid onset in children about 1 week after gastroenteritis or upper respiratory tract infection. May occur in adults. Acute renal failure develops in ~ 60% of children with HUS, most of which resolve in weeks with only supportive therapy.

Thrombotic thrombocytopenic purpura (TTP) - closely related to HUS with higher occurrence in young adults and associated with fever, more neurologic problems and less renal involvement, usually with hematuria and proteinuria. The prognosis of TTP is much worse than HUS. Treatment is with plasma exchange and corticosteroids. Platelet transfusions are to be avoided.

❍ **What is the antihypertensive of choice in patient with chronic diabetic nephropathy?**

Angiotensin converting enzyme inhibitors are the preferred agents.

❍ **What do patient's with sickle cell trait most commonly present with?**

Hematuria and decreased urine concentrating ability.

NEUROLOGY PEARLS

Logic is the art of going wrong with confidence.
Joseph Wood Krutch

❍ **A patient with closed head trauma has clear fluid leaking from his nares. How do you distinguish between excessive nasal secretions and a CSF leak?**

By checking the fluid for the presence of glucose. Glucose will be present in CSF but not nasal secretions.

❍ **What is the mechanism for the development of a subdural empyema?**

Subdural empyemas occur most often as a sequelae of chronic sinusitis. There may be direct extension of bacterial pathogens from sinus cavities that are contiguous with the CNS or from septic venous thromboses. Subdural empyemas may also occur on first presentation or after several days of therapy in patients with bacterial meningitis

❍ **Which procedure is more sensitive to detect subarachnoid hemorrhage - a lumbar puncture or CT scan of the head?**

A lumbar puncture is a more sensitive procedure than CT to detect subarachnoid hemorrhage, as it can detect small amounts of blood in the subarachnoid space. An atraumatic lumbar puncture that is bloody, but does not "clear" (the number of RBCs in the first tube is not greater than that in the last tube) is suggestive of a subarachnoid hemorrhage.

❍ **What drugs are thought to be associated with the development of benign intracranial hypertension (pseudotumor cerebri)?**

Antibiotics, such as tetracycline, minocycline, penicillin, gentamicin, oral contraceptives, steroids, NSAIDs such as indomethacin, thyroid hormone and lithium carbonate.

❍ **What signs are associated with increased intracranial pressure?**

Headache, nausea, emesis, papilledema, systemic hypertension, bradycardia, irregular respiratory pattern and paralysis of upward gaze (setting sun sign).

❍ **What is the treatment of choice for brain tumor edema?**

Dexamethasone.

❍ **What is the most common cause of cerebrospinal fluid (CSF) leak?**

Basilar skull fractures.

❍ **What measures assist in decreasing ICP?**

Elevation of the head of the bed to 30 degrees, intermittent drainage of CSF, hyperventilation and osmotic diuresis.

❍ **What are the neurological signs of cerebellar abscesses?**

Horizontal nystagmus when looking towards the side of the lesion, ipsilateral dysmetria and ataxia.

❍ **What is the appropriate empiric antibiotic therapy for a spinal epidural abscess?**

A penicillinase-resistant penicillin such as nafcillin or oxacillin.

❍ **What radiographic feature of the vertebral body endplates is useful in differentiating metastatic lesions from infectious osteomyelitis.**

Tumors tend to "respect" the endplates whereas infections often destroy the endplate and involve the disc space.

❍ **What ECG changes are seen with brain injuries?**

T wave and ST segment changes.

❍ **What are "pontine pupils?"**

Pinpoint but reactive pupils secondary to injury of the sympathetic fibers descending through the tegmentum.

❍ **What is the incidence of seizures in patients with traumatic intracranial hematomas?**

As high as 30 to 36%.

❍ **What are the most common causes of worsened neurological deficit that occurs later in the course of traumatic spinal cord injury?**

Post-traumatic syrinx formation and persistent spinal cord compression.

❍ **What percentage of patients with anterior cord syndromes regain the ability to walk without assistance?**

Fewer than 50%.

❍ **T/F: Severe traumatic brain injury patients should be routinely hyperventilated.**

False.

❍ **What symptoms related to lumbar disc herniation are indications for emergency surgery?**

Urinary retention, perineal numbness and motor weakness of more than a single nerve root.

❍ **What are potential causes of delayed neurological deterioration in patients following intracranial aneurysm rupture?**

Bleeding, vasospasm, hydrocephalus and seizures.

❍ **What spinal abnormality is seen in rheumatoid arthritis?**

Atlanto-axial subluxation.

❍ **What signs and symptoms characterize benign intracranial hypertension?**

Headache, blurred vision, pulsatile tinnitus, vertigo, hearing loss and papilledema.

❍ **What are the major sources of brain abscesses?**

Direct extension from middle ear, mastoid and sinus infections, hematogenous spread and trauma.

❍ **Bilateral facial paralysis associated with progressive ascending motor neuropathy of the lower extremities and elevated cerebrospinal fluid protein is characteristic of what clinical entity?**

Guillain-Barre syndrome.

❍ **A patient with a history of lung cancer presents with a seizure and a ring enhancing lesion on CT of the brain. Examination reveals a new heart murmur in an otherwise normal patient with normal vital signs and no history of fever. What is the most likely diagnosis?**

Bacterial endocarditis.

❍ **What is the most common congenital vascular abnormality of the CNS?**

Intracranial aneurysms.

❍ **A patient presents to the ER with a sudden severe headache. CT scan of the brain is normal. What further test should be performed?**

Lumbar puncture.

❍ **A patient is admitted to the critical care unit with the diagnosis of a subarachnoid hemorrhage secondary to an intracranial aneurysm. What complications may occur?**

More hemorrhage, hydrocephalus, seizure and cerebral vasospasm.

❍ **What clinical findings occur in grade 4 subarachnoid hemorrhage?**

Stupor, hemiparesis and posturing.

❍ **Why is there a higher incidence of complete neurologic loss with thoracic fractures than with cervical or lumbar fractures?**

The thoracic spinal canal has the least cross-sectional area for the spinal cord, thus allowing less room for movement of the cord. Furthermore, since the thoracic spine is so strong, a thoracic spine injury is the result of a tremendous force of injury. In addition, the blood supply to the thoracic cord has more of a watershed distribution than the other regions.

❍ **What is the difference between epidural and subdural hematomas as seen on an axial CT scan view?**

Epidural hematomas are lens-shaped because spread of the hemorrhage is contained by the tight adherence of the dura to the skull, while subdural hematomas are more concave.

❍ **T/F: Excessive hyperventilation in a patient with a head injury may cause brain ischemia and edema.**

True.

❍ **What is cerebral perfusion pressure and what does it signify?**

CPP = MAP - ICP where MAP equals mean arterial pressure. CPP represents the pressure required to push blood from the arterial tree to the venous tree in the intracranial space.

❍ **A 76 year old male is referred to you for evaluation of urinary incontinence. During the examination you note that he has trouble ambulating. Upon further questioning you find that he has had increasing gait difficulty for several months that is associated with incontinence. He has no back pain or other neurologic findings. In addition, you note some memory loss and history of a subarachnoid hemorrhage 15 years ago. You order a head CT that shows ventriculomegaly out of proportion to brain atrophy. What is the most likely diagnosis?**

Normal pressure hydrocephalus (NPH).

❍ **A multiple trauma patient is sleepy and confused after a transient loss of consciousness at the time of injury. The only external sign of injury is a seatbelt/shoulder-strap bruise on the chest and neck. Initial head CT and neck x-rays are normal. The patient deteriorates over the next 12 hours from purposeful movement of all extremities to left hemiplegia. Repeat CT still reveals no obvious focal abnormalities. What is the most likely diagnosis?**

Vascular injury to the carotid artery contralateral to the hemiparesis.

❍ **An elderly man is involved in an MVA. The circumstances of the accident are unclear. After appropriate evaluation and resuscitation he is found to have a small basal ganglia hemorrhage that the radiologist describes as unusual for trauma. What is the most likely explanation for this patient's injury?**

The patient most likely had a cerebral infarct that preceded the MVA.

❍ **A multiple trauma patient is transferred to your facility with a history of head injury. The patient arrives intubated and sedated because he had a seizure prior to transport and was given 20 mg of IV diazepam. The patient now starts to seize again. What is the appropriate treatment?**

Phenytoin.

❍ **What is the role of lumbar puncture in the treatment of increased ICP?**

In general it is contraindicated. It may lead to cerebellar or temporal herniation. An exception is for the treatment of pseudotumor cerebri.

❍ **A trauma patient is found to have a significant acute subdural hematoma by CT scan. What is the appropriate treatment?**

Emergency craniotomy.

❍ **A 35 year old female presents with a right hemisphere TIA. Evaluation reveals angiographic narrowing of the right internal carotid artery. The radiologist describes the appearance as a string of beads. What is the most like cause of the lesion?**

Fibromuscular dysplasia.

❍ **An older gentleman presents with acute right sided hemiparesis and mild aphasia that has improved since arrival to the emergency room. Angiography reveals complete occlusion of the left internal carotid artery. What is the appropriate management?**

Surgical intervention should be delayed for days to weeks since the symptoms are resolving. Furthermore, complete occlusion is not usually amenable to surgical intervention unless it is a hyperacute event. Intra-arterial thrombolytics are being evaluated as possible treatments for acute thrombotic events.

❍ **What is a type II odontoid fracture?**

A fracture between the dens and the body of C2. It is considered unstable and usually requires surgical intervention due to its poor vascular supply.

❍ **A patient presents with foot drop and back pain. What is the diagnostic test of choice?**

MRI. CT myelography can be used as an alternative or adjunctive study.

❍ **What disc level most likely herniated in the above patient?**

L4-5.

❍ **What is a far lateral lumbar disc herniation?**

A far lateral disc herniation implies that the herniated material is more on the posterolateral aspect of the disc space, within the lateral foramen.

❍ **What nerve root exits at the L4-5 level?**

The L4 root.

❍ **A 39 year old male presents to the emergency room after shoveling snow and complains of acute onset of severe low back pain such that he cannot stand upright. Evaluation reveals bilateral weakness of the feet on dorsiflexion, loss of sensation on the inner thighs and perineal regions and a distended bladder. What is the most likely diagnosis?**

Cauda equina syndrome.

❍ **What is the appropriate treatment for the above patient?**

Emergent surgical decompression with removal of the disc fragment(s).

❍ **T/F: The presence of a pacemaker is a contraindication to MRI scanning.**

True.

❍ **What is the etiology of vasospasm following subarachnoid hemorrhage?**

Contraction of the smooth muscle cells in the cerebral vasculature secondary to breakdown of red blood cells and release of hemoglobin into the CSF.

❍ **A 54 year old hypertensive male stopped his anti-hypertensive medication one week ago. He now presents with sudden onset of left hemiparesis and decreased level of consciousness. What is the most likely location of his intracerebral hemorrhage?**

The right putamen.

❍ **What is the most common cause of hemorrhage in the non-hypertensive elderly patient?**

Amyloid angiopathy.

❍ **What is the appropriate treatment for an intracranial arteriovenous malformation?**

Surgical resection is the gold standard of treatment. However, newer therapies, including embolization, filling the malformation with glue or particulate matter and radiosurgery are being investigated.

❍ **What organisms are most commonly implicated in subdural empyemas?**

Staphylococci and streptococci.

❍ **What is the window of opportunity for intravenous tPA administration following CVA?**

Three hours.

❍ **What is the mechanism of diffuse axonal injury?**

Rotation of the brain within the skull secondary to sudden deceleration.

❍ **What is the earliest sign of central herniation?**

Decreased level of consciousness.

❍ **What are the physical findings indicative of a basilar skull fracture?**

Periorbital and perimastoid ecchymosis. Patients may also suffer hearing loss, anosmia and CSF leaks.

❍ **What is the most common source of bleeding from an epidural hematoma?**

Laceration of the middle meningeal artery.

❍ **What is the source of bleeding from a subdural hematoma?**

Shearing of bridging veins between the dura and brain.

❍ **What is the most common intracranial hemorrhage following head trauma?**

A subarachnoid hemorrhage.

❍ **What are the most common forms of disturbed water balance after traumatic brain injury?**

Diabetes insipidus, the syndrome of inappropriate antidiuretic hormone (SIADH) and cerebral salt wasting.

❍ **What are the characteristics of neurogenic pulmonary edema?**

Rapid onset of decreased lung compliance without elevation of the pulmonary capillary wedge pressure (PCWP), diffuse roentgenographic infiltrates and hypoxemia.

❍ **What is the suspected mechanism of disseminated intravascular coagulation (DIC) associated with severe brain injury?**

Activation of the extrinsic clotting cascade by release of thromboplastin from the injured brain.

❍ **What are the commonly employed surgical interventions for controlling medically refractory intracranial hypertension after trauma?**

Ventriculostomy drainage, hematoma evacuation, partial brain resection and decompressive craniectomy.

❍ **What is the difference in pathogenesis and physiologic treatment of acute versus chronic subdural hematoma?**

An acute subdural hematoma occurs within 3 days of the incident, is the accumulation of blood in the subdural space that causes mass effect and requires a full craniotomy. A chronic subdural hematoma is usually older than 3 weeks and can often be adequately treated with a burr hole.

❍ **In the cervical spine, what nerve root exits at the C4-5 level?**

The C5 root.

❍ **A trauma patient presents with an altered level of consciousness, bilateral periorbital and perimastoid ecchymosis and hemotympanum. What injury do these signs suggest?**

A basilar skull fracture.

❍ **What are the most common locations for hypertensive hemorrhages?**

The basal ganglia, brainstem, cerebellum, cerebrum and thalamus.

❍ **What are the clinical spinal cord syndromes?**

Anterior spinal cord syndrome, central cord syndrome and Brown-Sequard syndrome.

❍ **A trauma patient presents with severe head injury and hypotension. What is the role of the neurosurgeon at this point?**

The neurosurgeon should be available to aid in patient evaluation. However, the initial emphasis is on resuscitation of organ perfusion and oxygenation.

❍ **How can a plain skull x-ray be helpful when evaluating a traumatic epidural hematoma?**

Traumatic epidural hematomas are usually associated with a skull fracture.

❍ **What is the most significant indicator of poor outcome after head injury?**

Hypotension.

❍ **Sudden severe headache, photophobia and a stiff neck are most likely associated with what condition?**

A subarachnoid hemorrhage.

❍ **What is the test of choice for a patient with a suspected subarachnoid hemorrhage?**

CT scan of the head. If CT is negative but suspicion is high, a spinal tap should be performed.

❍ **What is the most important initial treatment for the severely head injured trauma patient?**

Establishing an airway.

❍ **What is the classic presentation of an epidural hematoma?**

Brief loss of consciousness followed by a lucid interval with progressive loss of consciousness.

❍ **What are the common locations for brain contusions?**

The frontal and temporal lobes.

❍ **What is the mechanism of action by which hyperventilation decreases ICP?**

It lowers $PaCO_2$ thus increasing pH and causing vasoconstriction.

❍ **Where are congenital berry aneurysms located?**

In the circle of Willis.

❍ **What is the prognosis for a patient recently diagnosed with amyotrophic lateral sclerosis (ALS)?**

Death 3 to 10 years after the onset of symptoms. ALS, also known as Lou Gehrig's disease, involves a progressive loss of the anterior horn cell function of the motor neurons. No sensory abnormalities are involved, just gradual weakness and atrophy of the muscles.

❍ **Which three bacterial illnesses present with peripheral neurologic findings?**

Botulism, tetanus and diphtheria.

❍ **What are the most common neurologic findings in adult botulism cases?**

Eye and bulbar muscle deficit.

❍ **A patient presents with facial droop on the left and weakness of the right leg. Where is the most likely site of the lesion?**

The brainstem, specifically the left pons.

❍ **A 25 year-old was knocked unconscious for ten seconds while playing touch football one week ago. Since then, he has had intermittent vertigo, nausea, vomiting, blurred vision, headache and malaise. His neurological examination and CT are normal. What is the diagnosis?**

Post-concussive syndrome. Most individuals recover fully over a 2 to 6 week time span. A small percentage of patients with post-concussive syndrome will have persistent deficits.

❍ **Differentiate between decerebrate and decorticate posturing.**

Decerebrate posturing: elbows and legs extended (indicative of a midbrain lesion).
Decorticate posturing: elbows flexed and legs extended (suggesting a thalamic lesion).
Remember: DeCORticate = hands by the heart.

❍ **What happens if light is directed into the eyes of a patient who is in a diabetic coma?**

The pupils will constrict.

❍ **What is the most common cause of subarachnoid hemorrhage?**

Saccular aneurysm.

❍ **What are other common causes of a subarachnoid hemorrhage?**

Rupture of cerebral artery aneurysm and arteriovenous malformation. These patients present with an abrupt, severe headache that can progress to syncope, nausea, vomiting, nuchal rigidity and non-focal neurological findings.

❍ **A 29 year-old intoxicated male presents after having his head pounded into the concrete. The patient had a brief episode of LOC, but was then ambulatory and alert. Now he appears drowsy and just threw up on you. What is the diagnosis?**

Epidural hematoma.

❍ **Which is more common, subdural or epidural hemorrhaging?**

Subdural. Subdural hemorrhage results from tearing of the bridging veins. Bleeding occurs less rapidly because the veins, not arteries, are damaged.

❍ **Differentiate between Korsakoff's psychosis and Wernicke's encephalopathy.**

Korsakoff's psychosis: Inability to process new information, i.e., to form new memories. This is a reversible condition resulting from brain damage induced by a thiamine deficiency that is secondary to chronic alcoholism.

Wernicke's encephalopathy: Also due to an alcohol induced thiamine deficiency. Patients experience decreased muscle coordination, ophthalmoplegia and confusion. The treatment is thiamine.

❍ **A 35 year-old woman with a history of flu-like symptoms one week ago presents with vertigo, nausea and vomiting. No auditory impairment or focal deficits are noted. What is the most likely diagnosis?**

Labyrinthitis or vestibular neuronitis.

❍ **How does bacterial meningitis differ from viral meningitis in terms of the corresponding CSF lab values?**

Bacterial meningitis is associated with low glucose and high protein levels, while viral meningitis will have normal glucose and normal protein levels.

❍ **A patient presents with acute meningitis. When should antibiotics be initiated?**

Immediately. Do not wait for results of the LP. Patients should receive a CT prior to LP only if papilledema, a focal neurological deficit or a suspicion for an intracranial mass lesion exists.

❍ **What is the most worrisome diagnosis of a purpuric, petechial rash in 18 year-old with meningitis?**

Meningococcemia.

❍ **Mononeuropathies are most commonly induced by what?**

Trauma that results in compression or entrapment of the involved nerve.

❍ **A 28 year-old woman complains of a two day history of weakness and tingling in her right arm and leg. She reports a previous episode of right eye pain and blurred vision that resolved over one month, but that occurred two years ago. She also recalls a two week episode of intermittent blurred vision the previous year. What is the diagnosis?**

Presumptive multiple sclerosis. Confirm with MRI and CSF (look for oligoclonal bands).

❍ **A 32 year-old female who complains of periods of weakness, especially when she chews her food. She also presents with ptosis, diplopia and dysarthria. Her muscles weaken with repetitive exercise. What test confirms the diagnosis of myasthenia gravis?**

Administration of exogenous anticholinesterase. Myasthenia gravis produces autoimmune antibodies against the acetylcholine receptors in the neuromuscular junction. Administering exogenous anticholinesterase will lead to an increase of acetylcholine and thereby relieve the symptoms.

❍ What is the most common medication associated with neuroleptic malignant syndrome?

Haloperidol. Other drugs, especially antipsychotic medications, are also causative.

❍ **What is the hallmark motor finding in neuroleptic malignant syndrome?**

"Lead pipe" rigidity.

❍ **A patient with a stooped posture, festinating gait (small shuffling steps), mask-like facies, poor balance, slow starting speech, decreased movement, muscular rigidity and a "pill rolling" tremor should be treated with what?**

Dopaminergic agonists, such as amantadine, bromocriptine and levodopa and cholinergic antagonists such as benztropine. Parkinson's syndrome is caused by a loss of dopaminergic cells in the substantia nigra.

❍ **In the US, what animals are most likely to be infected with the rabies virus?**

Bats, skunks and raccoons. Dogs are the usual carriers in developing countries.

❍ **Are rabies transmitted via a rat bite?**

No, rodents do not carry the virus.

❍ **Do individuals infected with the rabies virus really foam at the mouth?**

Yes, hypersalivation is one of the symptoms of furious rabies, along with hyperactivity, fear of water, hyperventilation, aerophobia and autonomic instability. Patients with paralytic rabies develop either ascending paralysis or paralysis that affects one or more limbs individually. Rabies is 100% fatal once symptoms are exhibited.

❍ **What artery is most commonly involved in stroke?**

Middle cerebral artery.

❍ **Unilateral occlusion of the vertebral-basilar arterial distribution results in what kind of symptoms?**

Ipsilateral cranial nerve abnormalities and contralateral motor and sensory deficits.

❍ **A patient with aphasia most likely had a stroke involving which hemisphere?**

The dominant hemisphere. Patients who stroke in the non-dominant hemisphere have apraxia and sensory neglect.

❍ **What is the most common cause of syncope?**

Vasovagal or simple fainting (50%).

❍ **A 74 year-old male presents with a unilateral burning headache that is worse around his temples and his eye. He also complains of visual disturbances and pain in his jaw after heavy use. Upon examination, you palpate a prominent temporal artery that is very tender. What tests should be run to make a diagnosis?**

Biopsy of the temporal artery. This patient most likely has temporal arteritis or giant cell arteritis. A sedimentation rate of over 50 mm/hr suggests this diagnosis.

❍ **For the following clinical presentations, identify which are associated with peripheral vertigo or with central vertigo.**
1) Intense spinning, nausea, hearing loss and diaphoresis
2) Swaying worse with movement, tinnitus and acute onset
3) Unidirectional nystagmus inhibited by ocular fixation and fatigable
4) Mild vertigo, diplopia and ataxia
5) Multidirectional nystagmus not inhibited by ocular fixation and non-fatigable

Answers: peripheral vertigo: (1), (2) and (3), central vertigo: (4) and (5).

❍ **How are upper motor neuron (UMN) lesions of CN VII (facial nerve) distinguished from peripheral lesions?**

Peripheral: Frontalis muscle is not spared.

❍ **Which vitamin should be given routinely during the treatment of tuberculous meningitis?**

Isoniazid can induce a peripheral neuropathy, which can be prevented by the co-administration of vitamin B6.

❍ **What are the three most common predisposing factors in the formation of a brain abscess?**

Cyanotic heart disease, otitis and sinusitis.

❍ **What is the most common cranial neuropathy seen in borreliosis (Lyme disease)?**

Unilateral or bilateral facial palsy. Less frequently, the VIII cranial nerve can also be affected.

❍ **What is the characteristic EEG abnormality seen with subacute sclerosing panencephalitis (SSPE)?**

SSPE is a chronic encephalitis caused by an atypical infection by measles virus. It presents with marked personality changes and a dementia that is characterized by aphasia, apraxia and agnosia. Myoclonic jerks are common and eye findings such as chorioretinitis are seen. The EEG consists of pseudo-periodic EEG complexes.

❍ **Which is the cranial nerve most affected in pseudotumor cerebri?**

Cranial nerve IV can be involved with clinical signs of diplopia. Other findings include decreased visual acuity and restricted peripheral fields with enlargement of the blind spot.

❍ **What systemic diseases can be associated with Moyamoya disease?**

Moyamoya disease ('puff of smoke') refers to the generous fragile collaterals that form due to slowly progressive stenosis and obliteration of the large vessels of the brain. It can be seen in association with sickle cell disease, neurofibromatosis, tuberous sclerosis, chronic basilar meningitis, irradiation and homocystinuria.

❍ **Why is a family history of deafness important in evaluating a patient with episodes of sudden loss of consciousness?**

Jervell-Lange-Nielsen syndrome is associated with prolonged Q-T and neurosensory hearing loss. Prolonged Q-T syndromes must be identified because they can lead to sudden death.

❍ **Ophthalmoplegic migraine affects which cranial nerve?**

Cranial nerve III.

❍ **What was the risk of symptomatic intracranial hemorrhage in patients who receive t-PA?**

Six percent. The risk of fatal intracranial hemorrhage is 3 percent.

❍ **What is the single most important modifiable risk factor for stroke?**

Hypertension.

❍ **When is maximal cerebrospinal fluid xanthochromia observed after subarachnoid hemorrhage?**

48 hours.

❍ **Which of the following signs is not part of the classic Wallenberg syndrome: nystagmus, Horner's syndrome, contralateral hemiparesis, ipsilateral ataxia, contralateral loss of pain and temperature sense.**

Hemiparesis.

❍ **What is the usual localization of the pure sensory stroke?**

Thalamus.

❍ **Rank the following vascular malformations in order of risk of hemorrhage: arteriovenous malformation, capillary telangiectasia, cavernous malformation and venous angioma.**

1) arteriovenous malformation, 2) cavernous malformation, 3) capillary telangiectasia, 4) venous angioma.

❍ **What disorder presents with ischemic and hemorrhagic stroke associated with progressive occlusion of arteries at the Circle of Willis?**

Moyamoya disease.

❍ **What arterial disorder is characterized by the pathological findings of smooth muscle hyperplasia or thinning, elastic fiber destruction, fibrous tissue proliferation and arterial wall disorganization?**

Fibromuscular dysplasia.

❍ **Which of the following laboratory findings are not seen in antiphospholipid antibody syndrome: positive ANA, false-positive VDRL, decreased PTT, lupus anticoagulant, anti-cardiolipin antibody?**

Decreased PTT.

❍ **What recently discovered condition causes activated protein C resistance and a hypercoagulable state?**

The factor V Leiden mutation.

❍ **Which viral infection classically causes a delayed stroke syndrome?**

Herpes zoster.

❍ **What potential adverse effect requires monitoring in patients treated with ticlopidine?**

Neutropenia.

❍ **A head trauma patient develops hyponatremia. What criteria would diagnose SIADH?**

The criteria are: 1) Hyponatremia with a normal or mildly increased extracellular fluid volume, 2) elevated urinary osmolarity (>200 mOsm), 3) elevated urine sodium (>20 mEq/L), 4) no adrenal, thyroid or renal disease.

❍ **How is SIADH distinguished from cerebral salt wasting syndrome?**

In cerebral salt wasting syndrome urinary sodium loss persists despite fluid restriction and there is a normal or reduced extracellular fluid volume.

❍ **What are the clinical features of myxedema coma?**

Non-pitting edema, hypothermia, bradycardia, dry skin and brittle hair.

❍ **What are the neurological causes of diabetes insipidus?**

Lesions of the hypothalamus or pituitary caused by post-operative edema, head trauma, sarcoid, lymphoma, craniopharyngioma, pituitary adenoma and metastatic tumors.

❍ **What are the clinical features of an epidural abscess?**

Spinal tenderness, fever, radicular pain, myelopathy, elevated CSF protein and CSF pleocytosis.

❍ **What is the treatment of epidural abscess?**

Immediate laminectomy, drainage of the abscess and antibiotic therapy. A delay may result in permanent myelopathy.

❍ **What are the clinical features of H. simplex encephalitis?**

Personality changes, fever, headache, delirium followed by coma, focal or generalized seizures, aphasia and focal motor symptoms.

❍ **What are the CSF, EEG and MRI findings in H. simplex encephalitis?**

CSF shows elevated protein, mononuclear pleocytosis, normal glucose and often red cells. H. simplex DNA may be detected in CSF by PCR testing. EEG shows periodic temporal lobe sharp wave complexes. MRI shows lesions in the medial temporal lobe, insula, inferior-medial frontal lobes and cingulate gyrus.

❍ **What drug is used to treat H. simplex encephalitis?**

Acyclovir.

❍ **What drug will reduce the risk of vasospasm following subarachnoid hemorrhage?**

Nimodipine.

❍ **What are the causes of cerebral hemorrhage?**

Trauma, hypertension, ruptured aneurysms, cerebral amyloid angiopathy, vascular malformations, hemorrhage into a tumor (e.g., melanoma, choriocarcinoma, renal cell carcinoma), anticoagulant use, hemophilia, thrombocytopenia, stimulant drugs (e.g., amphetamines, cocaine, phenylpropanolamine) and vasculitis (e.g., Wegener's granulomatosis).

❍ **What is the drug treatment for convulsive status epilepticus?**

Lorazepam followed by phenytoin are the initial drugs.

❍ **What are the clinical features of spinal cord compression from metastatic cancer?**

Localized spinal tenderness, radicular pain, sensory level, paraparesis or quadriparesis, bowel or bladder incontinence, brisk deep tendon reflexes, upgoing plantar reflexes and spasticity.

❍ **What is the treatment for acute spinal cord compression from metastatic cancer?**

Usually with high dose corticosteroids and radiation therapy. Surgical therapy is used instead of radiation therapy if the primary cancer type is unknown, the tumor is radioresistant, spinal instability or the patient has received the maximum radiation dose.

❍ **What are the features of neuroleptic malignant syndrome?**

The features are altered mental status, fever, rigidity, irregular pulse, irregular blood pressure, tachycardia, diaphoresis and elevated CPK.

❍ **What is the treatment for neuroleptic malignant syndrome?**

Immediate withdrawal of the neuroleptic drug. Sinemet, bromocriptine or dantrolene are used.

❍ **What are the features of botulism infection?**

History of recent ingestion of home canned or prepared foods, followed by sudden onset of diplopia, dysphagia, muscle weakness, dry mouth, fixed dilated pupils and respiratory paralysis.

❍ **What is the medical treatment of confirmed botulism?**

Botulism antitoxin.

❍ **What are the features of hypertensive encephalopathy?**

Diastolic blood pressure usually over 130 torr, papilledema and altered mental status.

❍ **What are the earliest clinical features of uncal herniation?**

Uncal herniation begins with a unilateral enlarged pupil and a sluggish pupillary light reaction.

❍ **What is the Cushing reflex?**

Elevation in blood pressure and reduction in pulse that follows an increase in intracranial pressure. It is a brainstem mediated reflex.

❍ **What are the clinical criteria for the diagnosis of brain death?**

The criteria are: (1) coma is present from a known cause, (2) reversible causes of coma such as hypothermia (temperature $< 32^{o}$ C) or drug intoxication have been excluded and (3) there is no clinical evidence of brain or brainstem function.

❍ **What is the initial therapy for acute MS?**

High dose IV methylprednisolone.

❍ **Are there any predisposing factors to Guillain-Barre Syndrome (GBS)?**

Viral infection, gastrointestinal infection, immunization or surgery often precedes the neurological symptoms by 5 days to 3 weeks.

❍ **Can Guillain-Barre Syndrome (GBS) involve respiratory muscles quickly?**

Yes. It can start as rapidly progressing symmetric weakness, facial paresis, oropharyngeal and respiratory paresis, loss of DTRs and impaired sensation in the hands and feet.

❍ **When do GBS symptoms "level off"?**

After several days to three weeks.

❍ **Does early treatment with IVIG or plasmapheresis accelerate recovery in GBS?**

Yes. It also diminishes the incidence of long-term neurologic disability.

❍ **Does activity of the disease correlate with the appearance of serum antibodies to peripheral nerve myelin?**

Yes.

❍ **Is there any increase in CSF cells in GBS?**

Usually not. Occasionally 10 to 100 monocytes. Protein is usually increased.

❍ **Can GBS be fatal?**

Yes. Especially with autonomic dysfunction, but very uncommonly.

❍ **What is the differential diagnosis of GBS?**

1- Porphyria (normal CSF protein, mental symptoms, recurrent abdominal crises, onset after exposure to drugs like barbiturates)
2- AIDS
3- Hypophosphatemia
4- Toxic neuropathies (hexane, thallium, arsenic)
5- Botulism

❍ **What is the difference between dysarthria and aphasia?**

Dysarthria is a disorder of speech, a motor function. Aphasia is a disorder of language, a higher cortical function.

❍ **What are the typical features of transient global amnesia?**

Abrupt onset of amnesia that spares personal identity, resolves within 24 hours, has no other neurologic deficits and occurs typically between ages 50 and 70.

❍ **What characterizes delirium?**

Delirium is characterized by rapid onset, fluctuations in alertness and level of consciousness and reversibility over hours to days with correction of the underlying toxic or metabolic disturbance. Asterixis, tremulousness and a diffusely slow EEG may accompany delirium.

❍ **Are all dementias progressive?**

No. For example, a single closed head injury may cause a non-progressive dementia.

❍ **Headache, altered mentation, seizures and an EEG showing periodic lateralizing epileptiform discharges suggest what diagnosis?**

Herpes simplex encephalitis.

❍ **What is the characteristic triad of normal pressure hydrocephalus?**

Dementia, incontinence and a gait apraxia (often described as a "magnetic" gait due to difficulty picking up the feet).

❍ **A rapidly progressive dementia with myoclonus and periodic sharp wave EEG discharges suggest what diagnosis?**

Creutzfeldt-Jakob disease.

O How does the new variant Creutzfeldt-Jakob disease (CJD) differ from sporadic CJD?

New variant CJD has a younger age of onset (2nd to 4th decade), early psychiatric symptoms, prominent ataxia, a longer duration of symptoms and no periodic EEG discharges. Less than 30 cases have been reported, primarily in Great Britain, where concerns about transmission from cattle with bovine spongiform encephalopathy have been raised.

O The post-concussive syndrome includes what symptoms?

Headaches, dizziness, impaired memory and concentration, irritability and depression.

O What are some presynaptic disorders of neuromuscular transmission?

Botulism is caused by a toxin made by Clostridium botulinum, found in improperly canned foods. Botulinum toxin impairs release of acetylcholine at neuromuscular junctions resulting in oculomotor weakness, dysphagia and ultimately respiratory paralysis and death. Infantile botulism often comes from ingestion of spores in raw honey and results in weak feeding, weak cries and flaccid paralysis.

Black widow spider venom promotes presynaptic release of acetylcholine, resulting in depletion of neurotransmitter, muscle spasm followed by weakness.

Lambert-Eaton myasthenic syndrome is a paraneoplastic disorder usually related to small cell carcinoma of the lung resulting in proximal muscle weakness. Antibodies against presynaptic calcium channels block calcium entry into the presynaptic site, inhibiting release. Repetitive stimulation or exercise causes accumulation of presynaptic calcium, facilitation of release and transiently improved strength/reflexes.

Tetanus toxin blocks release of inhibitory neurotransmitters at the spinal level, resulting in persistent activation of antagonist muscle groups, muscle spasms and rigidity, especially of the masseter muscles (trismus) and lip retraction (risus sardonicus).

O What is myasthenia gravis?

Myasthenia gravis (MG) is an autoimmune disorder in which antibodies attack the postsynaptic end plate, resulting in focal (especially oculomotor) or generalized weakness that is worse after exercise. MG is associated with thymoma (15%) or thymic hypertrophy (50%) and most patients benefit from thymectomy. The diagnosis is aided by single fiber EMG studies, in which the pairing of muscle fiber action potentials show increased jitter (fluctuation in the timing of paired firing).

O What drugs act at the neuromuscular junction?

D-Tubocurarine (curare) is a nicotinic AChR antagonist that binds to the receptor and prevents channel opening. It is used as a non-depolarizing neuromuscular blocker in general anesthesia.

Succinylcholine binds to and persistently activates nAChRs, resulting in depolarization blockade and paralysis. It is also used for induction of general anesthesia. Neither agent depresses mental status.

Anticholinesterases (neostigmine, pyridostigmine) prolong the duration of ACh in the synaptic cleft and are used in the treatment of MG. The Tensilon (edrophonium) test is an anticholinesterase challenge that usually improves strength (or ptosis) rapidly but briefly in untreated patients.

Alpha-bungarotoxin, a snake venom, binds to and blocks nAChRs.

O A 25 year old presents with a history of being knocked unconscious for 10 seconds while playing touch football one week ago. Since then he has felt malaise, intermittent vertigo, nausea,

vomiting, blurred vision and a headache. Neuro exam and CT are normal. What is the most likely diagnosis?

Post-traumatic vertigo. Expect recovery to normal over 2 to 6 weeks.

❍ **How are seizures categorized?**

Lots of ways, but clinically important dichotomies include focal seizures, which affect one area of one hemisphere or generalized, those seizures that act bilaterally. Another important distinction is between simple seizures (without impairment of consciousness) and complex (with decreased consciousness or loss of consciousness).

❍ **What are the essentials of the initial emergency management of seizures?**

As always, attend to the "ABCs" first. Spontaneous ventilation is absent during the tonic phase of a tonic-clonic seizure and is unpredictably present during the clonic phase. Anticonvulsant therapy may further impair central respiratory function.

❍ **What is the circulatory response to generalized seizure?**

There is usually striking sympathetic autonomic outflow with hypertension and tachycardia.

❍ **What is the next step in managing this seizing patient?**

Make sure the patient is not hypoglycemic, a common and easily treatable cause of seizures. Use a test strip if available or treat empirically if not.

❍ **Do seizures cause brain injury?**

Evidence from animal studies suggests that generalized tonic-clonic seizures may cause irreversible neuronal damage. Less certain is the harm that may be caused by focal seizures. It is certainly safest to assume that generalized seizures lasting longer than 10 minutes may well have important adverse long term consequences for the patient and treat them aggressively.

❍ **What is the initial therapy for seizures?**

The most popular initial therapy is diazepam. Lorazepam is also usually effective and provides a longer duration of anticonvulsant action. Both drugs may cause hypotension and respiratory depression.

❍ **What is "status epilepticus"?**

Seizures continuing unabated for 15 to 30 minutes or more is a common operational definition of status epilepticus. Failure to return to a normal level of consciousness between episodic seizure activity over any period of time is also considered to be status epilepticus.

❍ **What's the significance of status epilepticus?**

With status epilepticus, more significant complications become likely. These include hyperthermia from the muscle activity of the continuing seizure, metabolic acidosis and hypoxia and hypercarbia from respiratory compromise.

❍ **What are the common causes of status epilepticus?**

Failure of patient with epilepsy to take medications

Meningitis
Hyponatremia and other metabolic abnormalities
Brain tumors
Stroke (infarct or hemorrhage)
Alcohol withdrawal

❍ **What is the next step if benzodiazepines do not halt the seizures?**

Phenytoin is given. Even if the seizures stop with the benzodiazepine therapy, load with phenytoin to prevent recurrence of seizures when the relatively short-acting initial therapy wears off.

❍ **What drug should be tried if phenytoin (or fosphenytoin) fail to stop the seizures?**

If the patient continues to have seizure activity despite benzodiazepine and phenytoin treatment, then most authorities would next add phenobarbital IV.

❍ **What is the last maneuver in the attempt to stop an episode of status epilepticus?**

General anesthesia is the remaining therapeutic option. Thiopental or pentobarbital can be used. Watch for hypotension.

❍ **What other type of general anesthesia can be used?**

Inhalational anesthesia using isoflurane has been used successfully in this situation. With either type of general anesthesia, remember that full neuromuscular blockade mandates continuous EEG monitoring. It is generally appropriate to maintain general anesthesia for 12 to 24 hours, then lighten the anesthetic level and observe for recurrence of seizures. Continue at least phenytoin and phenobarbital during the anesthetic.

❍ **What type of seizure is most commonly associated with metabolic abnormalities?**

The classic generalized tonic-clonic seizure.

❍ **An elderly patient presenting to the emergency department with seizures has persistent diffuse background slowing on EEG. What is the differential diagnosis?**

Diffuse background showing EEG suggests a more diffuse process such as metabolic derangements, a generalized infection such as encephalitis or a toxic ingestion.

❍ **What toxic ingestions are associated with seizures?**

<u>Theophylline</u> overdose causes CNS excitability and seizures. These seizures are usually focal rather than generalized. With acute ingestions, the seizures are usually brief and resolve spontaneously without medical intervention. Seizures occurring after chronic overdose may persist and not respond to usual drug interventions.

Hemodialysis or charcoal hemoperfusion is an option in patients with status epilepticus associated with high blood levels of aminophylline.

<u>Tricyclic antidepressant</u> overdosage is associated with seizures. These may be myoclonic jerks or generalized convulsions. Impaired level of consciousness is typically associated with blood levels of tricyclics high enough to cause seizures.

<u>Lidocaine, cocaine and other local anesthetics</u> can also produce seizures. These are usually of brief duration and self-limited. When they are not, the usual supportive care and conventional anticonvulsant therapy can be expected to produce satisfactory outcomes.

Isoniazid seizures are characterized by intractability to the usual anti-seizure medications. Pyridoxine is the drug of choice.

❍ **A 52 year old known alcoholic male presents to the emergency department with repeated seizures. What is the differential diagnosis?**

It is the same as for any other patient. Alcohol ingestion per se is not thought to promote seizures. Withdrawal from alcohol can produce seizures ("rum fits") from 8 to 48 hours after cessation of or decreasing the rate of alcohol intake. Seizures associated with alcohol withdrawal usually are brief generalized tonic-clonic and limited to a single episode. Less commonly, status epilepticus occurs in alcohol withdrawal. Many alcoholics with seizures have an underlying structural (traumatic) basis for their seizures.

Extraordinary alcohol ingestion can be associated with hypoglycemia, which can be severe enough to cause seizures.

❍ **Describe the symptoms and signs of myasthenia gravis.**

Weakness and fatigability with ptosis, diplopia and blurred vision are the initial symptoms most patients. Bulbar muscle weakness is also common with dysarthria and dysphagia.

❍ **Describe the presenting symptoms of botulism poisoning.**

Botulism poisoning often presents with ocular bulbar deficits. Symmetrical descending weakness, usually with no sensory abnormalities, classically develops. Commonly associated symptoms include dysphagia, dry mouth, diplopia, and dysarthria. Deep tendon reflexes may be decreased or absent.

❍ **Describe a patient with tick paralysis.**

A rapid progressive ascending paralysis that develops over one to two days. First symptoms occur in the extremities and trunk and move to bulbar musculature. It is almost identical to Guillain-Barré Syndrome.

❍ **Under what conditions does neurogenic pulmonary edema occur?**

Neurogenic pulmonary edema is commonly associated with increased intracranial pressure. It is commonly seen with head trauma, subarachnoid hemorrhage and seizures.

❍ **How many minutes of cerebral anoxia will result in irreversible brain injury?**

Over 8 minutes.

❍ **Which artery is most likely to be compressed in transtentorial herniation of the temporal lobe?**

Posterior cerebral artery.

❍ **What is the most useful study to assess for shunt malfunction?**

CT is the most useful study to assess for shunt malfunction and ideally the scan should be compared to the patient's previous scan. It should be remembered that the ventricles do not always dilate and patients with large ventricles and a small cortical mantle may also show no change.

❍ **What is the most common cause of shunt malfunction?**

Obstruction is the most common cause of shunt malfunction. The most common site of obstruction is at the proximal end of the shunt as it becomes occluded with choroid plexus, ependymal cells, glial tissue, brain debris, fibrin or blood.

❍ **What is the most common organism accounting for VP shunt infections?**

The organisms most frequently implicated in shunt infections are the staphylococci. Approximately 40% are caused by Staphylococcus epidermidis and 20% by Staphylococcus aureus. Other organisms include streptococci, enterococci, gram-negative rods and yeast.

❍ **What is the most common time course for a shunt infection to manifest following shunt insertion?**

The majority of infections occur in the first two months following implantation. Following insertion the shunt becomes covered with a glycocalyx which serves as a binding site for bacteria.

❍ **What is the BEST indication for assisted ventilation in a 70 kg patient with Guillian-Barre syndrome?**

Abnormal blood gases are a late finding in patients with GBS or other neuromuscular syndromes and bedside pulmonary functions including forced vital capacity (FVC) are the most sensitive.

❍ **What is the gold standard for monitoring ICP?**

Ventricular catheter.

❍ **A 14 year old patient who is now 48 hours following resection of a medulloblastoma who had been receiving a continuos fentanyl and midazolam infusion was successfully extubated this AM. You are called to his bedside for dilated pupils, sweating, goose flesh, rhinorrhea, tachycardia and muscle twitching. What is the most likely explanation for these findings?**

Opioid withdrawal.

A helpful mnemonic to recall the signs and symptoms of withdrawal is:

W: Wakefulness
I: Irritability
T: Tremulousness/Temperature instability (Fevers)
H: Hyperactivity/hyperreflexia
D: Diarrhea and diaphoresis
R: Respiratory distress/rhinorrhea
A: Apnea/autonomic dysfunction
W: Weight loss
A: Alkalosis
L: Lacrimation

INFECTIOUS DISEASE PEARLS

"Nobody will fly for a thousand years!"
Wilbur Wright, 1901, in a fit of despair.

❍ **What cell wall inhibitor antibiotic does not cross react in patients who are allergic to penicillin?**

Aztreonam.

❍ **What infectious agents may cause myositis?**

Infectious causes of myositis are usually viral in origin and include Influenza A and Coxsackie virus, types A and B. Muscle abscesses due to Staphylococcus aureus and trichinosis are unusual causes.

❍ **What class of bacteria is most commonly isolated from brain abscesses that are secondary to chronic sinusitis or otitis?**

Anaerobes.

❍ **In a patient with a chest x-ray typical of tuberculosis, the PPD is negative. A repeat PPD after two weeks is still negative. A panel of skin tests is placed and all of them prove to be positive. Does this rule out tuberculosis as a cause of the chest x-ray abnormality?**

No. Patients with tuberculosis can be selectively anergic. If TB is suspected, one must continue to maintain a high index of suspicion for that disease. Other more aggressive approaches will need to be taken to prove the diagnosis such as gastric washings, bronchoscopy or lung biopsy.

❍ **What are some of the most convenient ways to make the diagnosis of Mycoplasma pneumonia?**

The gold standard for diagnosis is a 4 fold rise in the complement fixation titer between the acute and convalescent sera. A single titer of 1:128 or greater for either cold agglutinins or the complement fixation antibody in the right clinical setting is highly suggestive of active disease.

❍ **How is the diagnosis of histoplasmosis made?**

By culture or staining from sputum, bronchoalveolar lavage or tissue and by a positive serology.

❍ **How is the diagnosis of coccidioidomycosis made?**

By culture or staining of sputum, bronchoalveolar lavage or tissue and by a positive serology.

❍ **How does one diagnose invasive aspergillosis?**

By biopsy.

❍ **What is the most common complication of AIDS?**

Pneumocystis carinii pneumonia (PCP). Kaposi's sarcoma is the second most common.

❍ **What organisms are most commonly responsible for overwhelming postsplenectomy sepsis?**

Pneumococci, meningococci, E. coli, H. influenzae, staphylococci and streptococci.

❍ **Contrast pneumonia due to Mycoplasma with pneumonia due to pneumococcus.**

	S. pneumoniae	M. pneumoniae
Prodrome	Uncommon	Mild fever, malaise, cough, headache
Onset	Rapid	Gradual
Severe respiratory symptoms	Tachypnea, cough, occasionally pleuritic pain	Uncommon
Associated findings	High fever	Exanthem, arthritis, GI complaints, neurologic complications
Pleural effusion	Occasionally	Rarely
Lab	Leukocytosis	WBC normal or slight elevation
Treatment	Penicillin	Erythromycin

❍ **Describe the skin lesions associated with a Pseudomonas aeruginosa infection.**

Pale, erythematous lesions, 1 cm in size, with an ulcerated necrotic center.

❍ **What signs indicate an HIV positive patient is at increased risk for opportunistic infections as PCP?**

An absolute CD-4 count of less than 200 and a CD-4 lymphocytic percentage of less than 20.

❍ **History of contact with mammals or birds may suggest infection by what organisms?**

Coxiella burnetii (Q fever), Brucella species or Chlamydia psittaci.

❍ **A nosocomial cluster of cases post-operatively may be caused by what organisms?**

Legionella or mycobacterium species.

❍ **Hantavirus occurs most commonly in what geographic location?**

Southwestern US, especially in areas with deer mice.

❍ **The initial therapy for PCP includes which antibiotics?**

Trimethoprim-sulfamethoxazole (preferred) or pentamidine.

❍ **What other medication should be prescribed to a patient with PCP?**

Corticosteroids, when the pO_2 is < 70 mmHg or A-a gradient is > 35 mmHg.

❍ **What three findings should be present to consider a sputum sample adequate?**

1) > 25 PMNs
2) < 10 squamous epithelial cells per low-powered field
3) A predominant bacterial organism

❍ **A 56 year-old smoker with COPD presents with chills, fever, green sputum and extreme shortness of breath. CXR shows a right lower lobe pneumonia. What is expected from the sputum culture?**

Haemophilus influenzae. This organism is generally found in COPD patients who develop pneumonia and bronchitis. The two other common organisms in COPD patients are Streptococcus pneumoniae and Moraxella catarrhalis.

❍ **Match the pneumonia with the treatment.**

1) Klebsiella pneumoniae	**a) Erythromycin, azithromycin or clarithromycin**
2) Streptococcus pneumoniae	**b) Penicillin G**
3) Legionella pneumophila	**c) Cefuroxime**
4) Haemophilus influenzae	**d) Erythromycin and rifampin**
5) Mycoplasma species	

Answer: 1) c, 2) b, 3) d, 4) c, 5) a.

❍ **A 67 year-old alcoholic was found in an alley, covered in his own vomit and beer. Upon examination, he is shaking, has a fever of 103.5° F and is coughing up currant jelly sputum. What is the most likely diagnosis?**

Pneumonia induced by Klebsiella pneumoniae. This is a likely etiology in alcoholics, the elderly, the very young and immunocompromised patients. Other gram-negative bacteria, such as E. coli and other Enterobacteriaceae, may cause pneumonia in alcoholics.

❍ **A 23 year-old male presents with a dry cough, malaise, fever and a sore throat that developed in the past two weeks. What is the most likely diagnosis?**

Mycoplasma pneumonia. This condition usually has a slow onset and occurs in the young. Treat the patient with erythromycin, azithromycin or clarithromycin.

❍ **What are the extrapulmonary manifestations of mycoplasma?**

Erythema multiforme, pericarditis, GI and CNS disease.

❍ **What agent used for the prevention of stress ulcers in ICU patients is associated with the lowest risk of nosocomial pneumonia?**

Sucralfate.

❍ **What is the definition of nosocomial pneumonia?**

Pneumonia occurring in patients who have been hospitalized for at least 72 hours.

❍ **Which lung segments are most often the sites of lung abscess formation?**

The posterior segments of the upper lobes and superior segments of the lower lobes.

❍ **What is the single most important risk factor for hospital acquired bacterial pneumonia?**

Endotracheal intubation.

❍ **What three roentgenographic findings are associated with a poor outcome in patients with pneumonia?**

Multiple lobe involvement, pleural effusion and cavitation.

❍ **What two new macrolide antibiotics offer broad coverage of the following common causes of community acquired pneumonia: Streptococcus pneumoniae, Hemophilus influenzae, Legionella pneumophila, Moraxella catarrhalis and Mycoplasma pneumoniae?**

Azithromycin and clarithromycin.

❍ **What common type of community acquired pneumonia is typically spread by aspiration of microdroplets from common water supplies?**

Legionnaire's disease.

❍ **What is the most common etiologic agent of atypical pneumonia?**

Mycoplasma pneumoniae.

❍ **What is considered to be the second most common cause of atypical pneumonia?**

Chlamydia pneumoniae.

❍ **What is the most important risk factor for Moraxella catarrhalis pneumonia?**

Chronic obstructive lung disease.

❍ **T/F: Penicillin is effective in this treatment of pneumonia due to Moraxella catarrhalis.**

False.

❍ **What category of bacteria is most important in hospital acquired pneumonia?**

Gram negative bacilli and Staphylococcus aureus.

❍ **Are any extrapulmonary manifestations specific for the diagnosis of Legionnaire's disease?**

No.

❍ **What is the treatment of choice for Legionella pneumonia?**

Erythromycin +/- rifampin.

❍ **What is the leading identifiable cause of acute community acquired pneumonia in adults?**

Streptococcus pneumoniae.

❍ **Among patients with cystic fibrosis, what bacteria are seen with increased frequency as causes of pneumonia?**

Pseudomonas aeruginosa and Staphylococcus aureus.

❍ **What is the most common cause of community acquired pneumonia among alcoholic patients?**

Streptococcus pneumoniae.

❍ **Which other bacteria are seen with increased frequency as causes of pneumonia among alcoholic patients?**

Klebsiella pneumoniae and Hemophilus influenzae.

❍ **Which microaerophilic bacterium can produce lung abscesses and sinus tracts that drain yellow-brown material resembling sulfur granules?**

Actinomycosis.

❍ **What fungus has a propensity to colonize a pre-existing pulmonary cavity?**

Aspergillus.

❍ **What pulmonary fungal infection grows in soil, is endemic to the Mississippi River basin and rarely results in symptoms?**

Histoplasmosis.

❍ **What fungus is endemic to the deserts of the southwestern United States, produces a granulomatous tissue reaction and can cause the triad of pneumonitis, erythema nodosum and arthralgias known as "valley fever"?**

Coccidioidomycosis.

❍ **What ubiquitous protozoan is responsible for a diffuse interstitial pneumonitis in immunocompromised patients?**

Pneumocystis carinii.

❍ **What are the signs and symptoms of Lyme disease, stages I to III?**

Stage I: Erythema chronicum migrans, malaise, fatigue, headache, arthralgias, fever and chills.
Stage II: Neurologic and cardiac symptoms include headache, meningoencephalitis, facial nerve palsy, radiculoneuropathy, ophthalmitis and 1°, 2° and 3° AV blocks.
Stage III: Arthritis (knee > shoulder > elbow > TMJ > ankle > wrist > hip > hands > feet).

❍ **What kind of tick transmits Rocky Mountain spotted fever (RMSF)?**

The female andersoni tick. It transmits Rickettsia rickettsii.

❍ **What is the most common symptom in RMSF?**

Headache occurs in 90% of patients.

❍ **Describe the rash of RMSF.**

It is a macular rash, 2 to 6 mm in diameter, located on the wrists and palms and spreads to the soles and trunk.

❍ **What tick transmits Lyme disease?**

The Ixodes dammini tick.

❍ **Describe the skin lesion seen in Lyme disease.**

A large distinct circular skin lesion called erythema chronicum migrans. It is an annular erythematous lesion with central clearing.

❍ **Describe a patient with tick paralysis.**

Bulbar paralysis, ascending flaccid paralysis, paresthesias of hands and feet, symmetric loss of deep tendon reflexes and respiratory paralysis.

❍ **What agent is usually responsible for the onset of endemic encephalitis?**

Arbovirus.

❍ **What is the most common source of gram-negative infections in patients with septic shock?**

The urinary tract.

❍ **An HIV-positive patient presents with a history of weight loss, diarrhea, fever, anorexia and malaise. She is also dyspneic. Lab studies reveal abnormal LFTs and anemia. What is the most likely diagnosis?**

Mycobacterium avium-intracellulare. Lab confirmation is made by an acid fast stain or culture.

❍ **What is the most common cause of focal encephalitis in AIDS patients?**

Toxoplasmosis. Symptoms include focal neurologic deficits, headache, fever, altered mental status and seizures. Ring enhancing-lesions are evident on CT.

❍ **What are the signs and symptoms of CNS cryptococcal infection in an AIDS patient?**

Headache, depression, lightheadedness, seizures and cranial nerve palsies. The diagnosis is confirmed by an India ink prep, fungal culture or by testing for the presence of cryptococcal antigens in the CSF.

❍ **What is the presentation of an AIDS patient with tuberculous meningitis?**

Fever, meningismus, headache, seizures, focal neurologic deficits and altered mental status.

❍ **What is the most common opportunistic infection in AIDS patients?**

PCP. Symptoms may include a non-productive cough and dyspnea. A chest x-ray may reveal diffuse interstitial infiltrates or it may be negative. Although Gallium scanning is more sensitive, false positives occur. Initial treatment is with TMP-SMX. Pentamidine is an alternative.

❍ **What is the most common gastrointestinal complaint in AIDS patients?**

Diarrhea. Cryptosporidium and Isospora are common causes of prolonged watery diarrhea.

❍ **A patient is infected with Treponema pallidum. What is the treatment?**

The treatment depends upon the stage of the infection. Primary and secondary syphilis are treated with benzathine penicillin G IM x 1 or doxycycline po. Tertiary syphilis is treated with benzathine penicillin G IM x 3.

❍ **What causes tetanus?**

Clostridium tetani. This organism is a gram positive rod. It produces tetanospasmin, an endotoxin, which causes the disinhibition of the motor and autonomic nervous systems.

❍ **What is the incubation period of tetanus?**

Hours to over one month. The shorter the incubation period, the more severe the disease. Most patients who contract tetanus in the US are over 50 years old.

❍ **What is the most common presentation of tetanus?**

Generalized pain and stiffness in the trunk and jaw muscles. Trismus develops and results in risus sardonicus, i.e., a sardonic smile.

❍ **Which cranial nerve is most commonly involved in cephalic tetanus?**

Cephalic tetanus usually occurs after injuries to the head and typically involves the seventh cranial nerve.

❍ **Outline the treatment for tetanus.**

Respiratory: Ventilatory support when needed.
Immunotherapy: Human tetanus immune globulin will neutralize circulating tetanospasmin and toxin in the wound. However, it will not neutralize toxin fixed in the nervous system.
Antibiotics: Penicillin G is the drug of choice.
Muscle rigidity: Diazepam, morphine and dantrolene.
Autonomic dysfunction: Deep sedation and magnesium sulfate.

❍ **A patient presents with fever, dyspnea, cough, hemoptysis and eosinophilia. What is the likely diagnosis?**

Ascaris lumbricoides. This helminth is a roundworm. The treatment is with mebendazole.

❍ **What is the pathophysiology of rabies?**

Infection occurs within the myocytes for the first 48 to 96 hours. It then spreads across the motor endplate and ascends and replicates along the peripheral nervous system and into the dorsal root ganglia, spinal cord and CNS. From the gray matter, the virus spreads by peripheral nerves to tissues of the organ systems.

❍ **What is the characteristic histologic finding associated with rabies?**

Eosinophilic intracellular lesions within the CNS neurons, called Negri bodies, are the sites of CNS viral replication. Although these lesions occur in 75% of rabies cases and are pathognomonic for rabies, their absence does not eliminate the possibility of rabies.

❍ **What are the signs and symptoms of rabies?**

Incubation period of 12 to 700 days with an average of 20 to 90 days. Initial signs and systems are fever, headache, malaise, anorexia, sore throat, nausea, cough and pain or paresthesias at the bite site.

In the CNS stage, agitation, restlessness, altered mental status, painful bulbar and peripheral muscular spasms, bulbar or focal motor paresis and opisthotonos are exhibited. 20% develop ascending, symmetric flaccid and areflexic paralysis. Hypersensitivity to water and sensory stimuli including light, touch and noise may occur.

The progressive stage includes lucid and confused intervals with hyperpyrexia, lacrimation, salivation and mydriasis, along with brainstem dysfunction, hyperreflexia and extensor plantar response.

The final stage includes coma, convulsions and apnea, followed by death between the fourth and seventh day for the untreated patient.

❍ **How is rabies treated?**

Wound care includes debridement and irrigation. The wound must not be closed primarily. Rabies immune globulin, half at wound site and half in the deltoid muscle, should be administered. The rabies vaccine, HDCV, is given IM on days 0, 3, 7, 14 and 28.

❍ **A patient presents has a 40° C fever and an erythematous, macular and blanching rash, which becomes deep red, dusky, papular and petechial. The patient is vomiting and has a headache, myalgias and cough. Where did the rash begin?**

Rocky Mountain spotted fever (RMSF) rash typically begins on the flexor surfaces of the ankles and wrists and spreads in a centripetal manner.

❍ **Which test confirms RMSF?**

Immunofluorescent antibody staining of a skin biopsy or serology.

❍ **Which antibiotics are prescribed for the treatment of RMSF?**

Doxycycline is preferred, chloramphenicol is an alternative. Antibiotic therapy should not be withheld pending serologic confirmation.

❍ **What lab findings are expected in a patient with malaria?**

Normochromic normocytic anemia, a normal or depressed leukocyte count, thrombocytopenia, an elevated sedimentation rate, azotemia, elevated LFTs, hyponatremia, hypoglycemia and a false positive VDRL.

❍ **How is malaria diagnosed?**

Visualization of parasites on Giemsa stained blood smears. In early infection, especially with P. falciparum, parasitized erythrocytes may be sequestered and undetectable.

❍ **Which two diseases are transmitted by the deer tick, Ixodes dammini?**

Lyme disease and babesiosis.

❍ **How do patients present with Babesiosis?**

Intermittent fever, splenomegaly, jaundice and hemolysis. The disease may be fatal in patients without spleens. Treatment is with clindamycin and quinine.

❍ **What is the most frequently transmitted tick borne disease?**

Lyme disease. The causative agent is the spirochete Borrelia burgdorferi.

❍ **When are patients most likely to acquire Lyme disease?**

Late spring to late summer with the highest incidence in July.

❍ **How is Lyme disease diagnosed?**

By serology.

❍ **What is the treatment for Lyme disease?**

This depends on the stage and type of infection. Stage I is treated with doxycycline or amoxicillin. Stage II is treated with IV ceftriaxone (for carditis and meningitis) or doxycycline or amoxicillin for an isolated and mild facial nerve palsy. The arthritis of stage III is treated with doxycycline, amoxicillin or IV ceftriaxone.

❍ **Which type of paralysis does tick paralysis cause?**

Ascending paralysis. The venom that causes the paralysis is probably a neurotoxin. A conduction block at the peripheral motor nerve prevents the release of acetylcholine at the neuromuscular junction. Forty-three species of ticks have been implicated as causative agents.

❍ **What is the most common sign of tularemia?**

Lymphadenopathy, usually cervical in children and inguinal in adults. It is caused by Francisella tularensis and is transmitted by the vectors Dermacentor variabilis and Amblyomma americanum.

❍ **A patient presents with sudden onset of fever, lethargy, a retro-orbital headache, myalgias, anorexia, nausea and vomiting. She is extremely photophobic. The patient has been on a camping trip in Wyoming. What tick-borne disease might cause these symptoms?**

Colorado tick fever caused by a virus of the genus Orbivirus. The vector is the tick D. andersoni. The disease is self-limited and treatment is supportive.

❍ **What is the most common cause of cellulitis?**

Streptococcus pyogenes. Staphylococcus aureus can also cause cellulitis, though it is generally less severe and more often associated with an open wound.

❍ **What is the most common cause of cutaneous abscesses?**

Staphylococcus aureus.

❍ **Which bite is more prone to infections – dog or cat?**

Cat.

❍ **What is the probable cause of an animal bite infection arising that develops in less than 24 hours? More than 48 hours?**

Less than 24 hours: Pasteurella multocida or streptococci. More than 48 hours: Staphylococcus aureus.

❍ **What is the most common cause of gas gangrene?**

Clostridium perfringens.

❍ **What pathophysiologic process is suggested by infiltrates in the posterior segment of the upper lobes or the apical segment of the lower lobes?**

Aspiration.

❍ **What degree of leukocytosis is considered a risk factor for poor outcome among patients with bacterial pneumonia?**

Greater than 30,000 cells/mm^3.

❍ **What degree of leukopenia is considered a risk factor for poor outcome among patients with bacterial pneumonia?**

Less than 4000 cells/mm^3.

❍ **What bacteria are associated with pneumonia following influenza?**

Streptococcus pneumoniae, Staphylococcus aureus and Haemophilus influenzae.

❍ **In addition to Streptococcus pneumoniae, what other bacteria are associated with acute, lobar pneumonia in adults?**

Haemophilus influenzae, Staphylococcus aureus, Klebsiella pneumoniae and Streptococcus pyogenes.

❍ **How long before elective splenectomy should the pneumococcal vaccine be administered in order to achieve an adequate antibody response?**

Two weeks or more.

❍ **What two underlying medical conditions are associated with Haemophilus influenzae pneumonia?**

Chronic obstructive lung disease and HIV infection.

❍ **What category of bacteria is most important in community acquired aspiration pneumonia?**

Anaerobic.

❍ **What is the antibiotic of choice for patients with community acquired aspiration pneumonia?**

Clindamycin.

❍ **What antibiotic has been consistently effective against penicillin resistant Streptococcus pneumoniae?**

Vancomycin.

❍ **Can infection with penicillin resistant Streptococcus pneumoniae be recognized on clinical grounds?**

No.

❍ **Of the following organisms, which is commonly spread by person-to-person contact: Legionella pneumoniae or Mycoplasma pneumoniae?**

Mycoplasma pneumoniae.

❍ **Is single antibiotic therapy typically effective in the treatment of Klebsiella pneumoniae?**

Yes.

❍ **What is the most common cause of community acquired bacterial pneumonia among patients infected with HIV?**

Streptococcus pneumoniae.

❍ **Besides pneumococcus, what other organisms that cause bacterial pneumonia appear to occur with increased frequency among patients infected with HIV?**

Haemophilus influenzae and Pseudomonas aeruginosa.

❍ **What are the two most important risk factors for the development of anaerobic lung abscess?**

Poor oral hygiene and a predisposition toward aspiration.

❍ **Which lung is most often the site of anaerobic lung abscess formation?**

The right lung.

❍ **Which lung segments are most common sites of abscess formation?**

The posterior segments of the upper lobe and the superior segments of the lower lobes.

❍ **What are the characteristic findings on sputum gram stain in cases of anaerobic lung abscess?**

Numerous polymorphonuclear cells and both gram positive and gram negative bacteria of various morphologies.

❍ **What anaerobic respiratory infection is associated with slowly enlarging pulmonary infiltrates, pleural effusions, rib destruction and fistula formation?**

Actinomycosis.

❍ **What are the indications for drainage of a pleural effusion associated with pneumonia?**

Positive gram stain or culture, the presence of gross pus, pleural fluid glucose less than 40 mg/dl or fluid pH less than 7.0.

❍ **An air-fluid level in the pleural space suggests what pathologic process?**

Bronchopleural fistula.

❍ **What are the two most important routes of transmission of nosocomial bacterial pneumonia?**

Person-to-person transmission via healthcare workers and contaminated ventilator tubing.

❍ **How may stress ulcer prophylaxis in ICU patients contribute to the development of nosocomial pneumonia?**

By raising the gastric pH and increasing bacterial colonization.

❍ **What are the usual CSF findings in bacterial meningitis?**

Neutrophilic pleocytosis, increased protein, hypoglycorrhachia (CSF glucose <50% of serum glucose). Bacterial antigens may be positive.

❍ **What are the CSF findings in viral meningitis?**

Lymphocytic pleocytosis, normal (or slightly elevated) protein and normal glucose.

❍ **What are the CSF characteristics of tuberculous meningitis?**

Lymphocytic pleocytosis, high protein and low glucose.

❍ **What is the management of herpes simplex encephalitis?**

Early treatment with acyclovir, anticonvulsants for seizures and general supportive care.

❍ **Is the vasculitis that is seen in syphilis, a large or a small vessel disease?**

Both. Large vessel (Heubner arteritis) is caused by adventitial lymphocytic proliferation of large vessels and is commonly seen in late meningovascular syphilis. The small vessel (Nissl-Alzheimer) vasculitis is the dominant vasculitic pattern seen in paretic neurosyphilis.

❍ **What is the recommended treatment for neurosyphilis?**

Intravenous penicillin G.

❍ **What complication may arise from aggressive treatment of neurosyphilis with penicillin?**

Jarisch-Herxheimer reaction. It is due to a release of endotoxin when large numbers of spirochetes are lysed during penicillin treatment and consists of mild fever, malaise, headache, arthralgia and may produce a temporary worsening of the neurological status.

❍ **At which stage of Lyme disease does neurological involvement occur?**

The second and third stages. 2nd stage - cranial neuropathies and meningitis. 3rd stage - encephalitis and a variety of CNS manifestations including stroke like syndromes, extrapyramidal and cerebellar involvement.

❍ **Which is the vector responsible for the transmission of Lyme disease?**

The deer tick, Ixodes dammini.

❍ **What historical feature should be sought in a patient in whom a neurological involvement from Lyme disease is being considered?**

History of erythema chronicum migrans (ECM), which is present in 60 to 80% of patients early in the disease.

❍ **What is Weil's disease?**

Weil's syndrome is the less common variety of leptospirosis, with icterus, marked hepatic and renal involvement and a bleeding diasthesis. Hence the name leptospirosis-ictero-hemorrhagica.

❍ **What is the most common neurological feature of leptospirosis?**

Aseptic meningitis (present in over 50%).

❍ **What clinical feature of leptospirosis sets it apart from other infections of the nervous system and hints at the diagnosis?**

Hemorrhagic complications. These are not uncommon and intraparenchymal and subarachnoid hemorrhages have been reported.

❍ **What are the neurological features of brucellosis?**

Mainly a chronic meningitis and the vascular complications thereof. Cranial neuropathies, demyelination and mycotic aneurysms may occur.

❍ **How is brucellosis spread?**

By ingestion of contaminated milk and milk products. It may also be spread by contact with an infected animal (usually cattle).

❍ **What are the characteristic features of cerebral amebiasis and what is the pathogenic organism?**

Cerebral amebiasis is usually a secondary infection and patients often have intestinal or hepatic amebiasis. The causative organism is Entamoeba histolytica. The clinical features are that of intracerebral abscesses causing focal neurological signs. The frontal lobe and basal nucleus are common sites of abscess formation.

❍ **What are the differences between cerebral amebiasis and primary amebic meningoencephalitis?**

The former is caused by E. Histolytica and is usually a secondary infection. The latter is caused by the free-living Naegleria species. This organism causes an acute meningoencephalitis.

❍ **What pathological findings are seen in the brain biopsy of toxoplasma encephalitis?**

Tachyzoites around necrotic lesions.

❍ **What is the current recommended treatment for intracranial toxoplasmosis in HIV disease?**

Combination therapy with sulfadiazine, pyrimethamine and folinic acid.

❍ **What is the commonest cause of meningitis in HIV disease?**

Cryptococcus.

❍ **Which amongst the following is responsible for subacute sclerosing panencephalitis (SSPE). Paramyxoviruses, enteroviruses or polyomaviruses?**

It is caused by the measles virus, which belongs to the morbillivirus subgroup of the paramyxoviruses.

❍ **What are characteristic findings in the cerebrospinal fluid in SSPE?**

Normal cells and glucose. Normal to raised protein content, positive oligoclonal bands and a raised titer of measles antibody. The measles specific antibody index is greater than 10.

❍ **What are infectious causes of paraparesis?**

Syphilis, tuberculosis with Pott's disease of the spine, leptospirosis and Varicella zoster.

❍ **What is the single most helpful antemortem test for supportive diagnosis of Creutzfeldt-Jakob disease (CJD)?**

EEG, which demonstrates 1 to 2 cycles per second triphasic sharp waves superimposed on a depressed background. They are usually asymmetrical and slow with advancing disease.

❍ **How is botulism contracted and what are the principal clinical features?**

It is contracted by consumption of contaminated foods, by injury from non-sterile objects (wound botulism) and in infants from intestinal colonization by Clostridium botulinum (lack of normal intestinal flora permit this colonization). The clinical features are that of a descending paralysis with ophthalmoplegia, bulbar and somatic palsy.

❍ **Is the motor paralysis induced by botulinum toxin reversible?**

Yes, but slowly, as axons must be regenerated.

❍ **What condition resembles Guillain-Barre syndrome by causing a symmetric paralysis and often results in miraculous improvement within a day?**

Tick paralysis, which results in an ascending paralysis within a few days of attack by the tick Dermacentor (hard tick). This releases a toxin in its saliva, which is responsible for the neuromuscular blockade. Within hours after tick removal, the weakness begins to resolve.

❍ **What is the cause of Sydenham's chorea and what are the principal clinical features?**

This is caused by an immunological cross-reaction after group A streptococcus infections. The development often occurs several months after the acute infection. It is characterized by development of involuntary choreiform movements that may be unilateral and remits spontaneously. There are also associated behavioral changes that may reach the severity of obsessive compulsive disorder.

❍ **What is epidemic pleurodynia (Bornholm’s disease)?**

An upper respiratory tract infection followed by pleuritic chest pain and tender muscles.

❍ **What organism is responsible for causing Bornholm's disease?**

Coxsackie group B.

❍ **What are the neurological manifestations of poliomyelitis?**

Spinal poliomyelitis, bulbar poliomyelitis and the encephalitic form, in descending order of frequency.

❍ **What are the CSF characteristics of polio?**

In the acute stages, it is associated with a lymphocytic pleocytosis, elevated protein and normal glucose. There may be a neutrophilic response very early in the disease. Chronic residual polio has normal CSF.

❍ **What are the best drugs to use against cytomegalovirus?**

Ganciclovir and foscarnet.

❍ **What is the most common cause of infectious arthritis in patients with sickle cell disease? What joint is most commonly affected?**

Staphylococcus aureus remains the most common cause, as in otherwise healthy children. However, salmonella is more commonly seen in septic arthritis in children with hemoglobinopathies. The hip is most commonly affected.

❍ **Why should a patient with suspected idiopathic thrombocytopenic purpura (ITP) be tested for HIV?**

Because thrombocytopenia may be the presenting sign for HIV infection.

❍ **How do viral meningitis and bacterial meningitis differ with regards to CSF pressure? CSF leukocytes? CSF glucose?**

The pressure in bacterial infection is increased, whereas it is normal or slightly increased in viral meningitis. The leukocytosis is greater than 1000 (up to 60K) in bacterial and rarely over 1000 in viral meningitis. The glucose concentration is decreased in bacterial meningitis and is generally normal in viral.

❍ **Why do so many patients with meningitis become hyponatremic?**

A majority of patients with this disease develop some degree of SIADH.

❍ **Which cephalosporins are effective against Listeria monocytogenes?**

None. That is why ampicillin is usually added to the antibiotic regimen when infection with this organism is a possibility.

❍ **A patient is diagnosed with impetigo due to group A streptococcus. What sequelae may occur?**

Acute post-streptococcal glomerulonephritis. It will not lead to rheumatic fever, however.

❍ **What is the drug of choice for meningococcal disease?**

Aqueous penicillin G is the ideal, though patients can be started effectively on empiric cefotaxime or ceftriaxone for suspected cases.

❍ **What is the most common cause of aseptic meningitis?**

Enteroviruses.

❍ **Clinically, how can you distinguish orbital cellulitis from periorbital cellulitis?**

Extra-ocular muscle dysfunction, decreased pupillary reflexes, decreased visual acuity and change in globe position are seen only in orbital cellulitis.

❍ **Does trismus more commonly occur with a peritonsillar abscess or peritonsillar cellulitis?**

Peritonsillar abscess.

❍ **Why does therapy for TB take several months, when other infections usually clear in a matter of days?**

Because the mycobacterium divide very slowly and have a long dormant phase, during which time they are not responsive to medications.

❍ **What are the organisms most commonly thought to be associated with Guillain-Barre Disease?**

CMV, EBV, coxsackie virus, Campylobacter jejuni and Mycoplasma pneumoniae.

❍ **What CSF protein and WBC findings occur in Guillain-Barre?**

An increase in cerebrospinal fluid protein without a corresponding increase in cerebrospinal fluid white cells.

❍ **Patients with HIV infections who go on to develop AIDS are most commonly infected with what organisms?**

Pneumocystis carinii, cytomegalovirus, candida, aspergillus, nocardia, cryptococcus and mycobacteria.

❍ **What is the evaluation for candida of the lung?**

Fresh sputum or transtracheal aspirate should reveal yeast and pseudohyphae. A tissue exam is necessary to demonstrate invasion versus colonization.

❍ **What is the most common infectious disease problem in patients with lupus that are not on steroid therapy?**

Urinary tract infections and urosepsis.

❍ **What rapid diagnostic test is now available to diagnose herpes simplex virus encephalitis in patients of all ages and how reliable is it?**

HSV polymerase chain reaction (PCR) on cerebrospinal fluid is considered to be highly sensitive and specific in the diagnosis of HSV encephalitis.

❍ **What are the most common organisms found in human bite wounds?**

Staphylococcus aureus, streptococcus and Eikenella corrodens. Anaerobes are also commonly seen.

❍ **Pasteurella multocida infection from an animal bite is best treated with which antibiotic?**

Penicillin.

❍ **A patient who develops encephalitis following a near drowning episode is most likely to be infected with what organism?**

Acanthamoeba. Granulomatous amebic encephalitis may also be seen to occur in patients with systemic lupus erythematosus, AIDS, steroids or lymphoreticular malignancies.

❍ **What two common urinary pathogens do not give a positive urine nitrate test?**

Enterococcus and Staphylococcus saprophyticus. Acinetobacter also fails to give a positive urine nitrate test.

❍ **What are the most common organisms isolated from dog and cat bites?**

Pasteurella multocida, Staphylococcus aureus, Staphylococcus intermedius and anaerobic streptococci. Much less common, but particularly dangerous in immunocompromised or asplenic patients, is Capnocytophaga canimorsus.

❍ **What is the most common infectious disease complication of both measles and influenza?**

Pneumococcal pneumonia.

❍ **Which rickettsial infection is most common in the United States?**

Rocky Mountain spotted fever, caused by Rickettsia rickettsii.

❍ **What prophylactic intravenous antibiotic should be given systemically to burn victims?**

None. Prophylactic antibiotics are given topically.

❍ **On Tuesday you are driving home from work in rural California and pass a dead squirrel. On Wednesday, taking a different route, you pass two more dead squirrels. The following morning you see a twenty-six year old male with enlarged tender lymphadenitis and a 105° F fever. What illness do you suspect?**

Cases of human plague (Yersinia pestis) are sometimes heralded by squirrel die-offs. A squirrel die-off occurs when the organism is introduced into a highly susceptible mammalian population, causing a high mortality rate among infected animals. This is referred to as epizootic plague.

❍ **One day after a previously healthy adult has been admitted to the hospital after an accidental overdose of oral iron, she appears to become septic. What is the most likely organism causing her sepsis?**

Yersinia enterocolitica. The growth of Y. enterocolitica appears to be enhanced after exposure to excess iron.

❍ **Helicobacter pylori have been isolated from the gastric antrum in what percentage of patients with duodenal ulcer disease?**

Nearly 100%. When the organism is treated with an antibiotic effective against H. pylori, the relapse rate is approximately 20%.

❍ **What is the outcome of empiric antimicrobial therapy for patients with post-operative peritonitis?**

Post-operative peritonitis is associated with high mortality rate. A recent study evaluated empiric antibiotic therapy given to 100 consecutive patients at their first reoperation for peritonitis occurring after elective surgery. The average time frame for re-operation was 10 +/- 8 days and was most commonly due to suture line leakage and bowel perforations.

Empiric treatment was deemed inadequate by culture in 56% of those on 2 drug therapy and 41% of patients who received 3 drug therapy. Despite appropriate changes made in the antibiotic regimens at 48 hours (guided by sensitivity results), those patients whose initial empiric treatment was inadequate had significantly higher length of stay, number of subsequent re-operations and mortality rate than those whose initial treatment was adequate. Fungal peritonitis, present in 23% of patients, was associated with an especially high mortality rate, of 61%.

❍ **What treatment is recommended for patients with severe Clostridium difficile colitis with associated ileus?**

Oral metronidazole is recommended first line regimen for mild to moderate cases of Clostridium difficile colitis, due to its similar efficacy to oral vancomycin and significantly lower cost.

In patients with significant ileus, intravenous metronidazole is recommended as bactericidal levels may still be attained in the colon. Oral treatment should be given simultaneously with vancomycin by nasogastric tube. Vancomycin is preferred over oral metronidazole in these circumstances as metronidazole is highly absorbed by the small intestine, whereas oral vancomycin is poorly absorbed and more likely to reach the target in the large bowel. Intravenous vancomycin does not have significant excretion into the gastrointestinal tract.

❍ **What are the CDC recommendations to help limit the spread of vancomycin resistance?**

The CDC recommends that vancomycin be given only for specific indications including:

Infections due to beta-lactam resistant gram positive bacteria.
Severe or life threatening antibiotic associated colitis unresponsive to metronidazole.
Endocarditis prophylaxis per American Heart Association guidelines.
Prophylactic use for prosthetic joint implantation in hospitals where there is a known prevalence of methicillin resistant staphylococcus aureus and epidermis.
Significant beta lactam allergy.

Empiric use should be limited to suspected prosthetic valve infections, suspected MRSA infections and meningitis treatment in areas with a high incidence of penicillin resistant Streptococcus pneumoniae.

❍ **What criteria are used to make the diagnosis of empyema?**

Classically, empyema fluid has a pH of less than 7.00, glucose of less than 40 mg/dl and elevated LDH levels greater than 1000 mg/dl. The pleural fluid WBC count is not a good criterion. Chest tube drainage is indicated for pleural fluid samples meeting these criteria (the LDH criterion by itself is controversial), those that are grossly purulent, those with a large number of organisms seen on gram stain and those with a positive culture. Patients with marginal values of pH between 7.00 and 7.20 may be observed on empiric therapy and re-tapped within 24 hours.

❍ **What is the microbiological spectrum of Imipenem?**

Imipenem, a carbapenem, is a different type of beta-lactam antibiotic, which has activity against a broad spectrum of microorganisms, including streptococci, Staphylococcus aureus and epidermidis, most enterobacteriaceae, Pseudomonas aeruginosa, anaerobes, and (including Bacteroides fragilis). It causes lysis of bacterial cells by binding to the penicillin binding proteins of both gram negative and gram positive bacteria. It is resistant to most beta-lactamase, penicillinase and cephalosporinase.

❍ **T/F: Fluconazole is effective against Candida albicans.**

True.

❍ **T/F: Fluconazole is effective against Candida krusei and lusitaniae and Torulopsis glabrata.**

False. There is a high rate of resistance of these organisms against fluconazole.

❍ **What is the epidemiology of Listeria monocytogenes?**

Listeria monocytogenes is a gram positive aerobic bacillus that has been found in soil, water, sewage and in animal feed and silage. It caused both epidemic and sporadic disease. The portal of entry is felt to be the gastrointestinal tract. Epidemics have been traced to contaminated milk and cheese products, vegetable products such as cole slaw and shellfish and raw fish. Listeriosis preferentially strikes pregnant women, newborns, the elderly and the immunocompromised, especially those with impaired T-cell immunity, such as transplant recipients.

❍ **What are the clinical features of patients with Listeria monocytogenes infection?**

Pregnant women present with a different syndrome than nonpregnant patients. Pregnant patients develop a flu-like illness, GI symptoms, amnionitis and rarely, meningitis.

Nonpregnant patients present with meningitis 30 to 55% of the time. Other presentations include sepsis, meningoencephalitis and brainstem and spinal cord abscesses. The CSF is usually purulent. Unlike other forms of bacterial meningitis, the CSF glucose levels are normal in more than 60% of cases. The organism takes up gram stain poorly and has been misinterpreted as pneumococci or even as gram negative bacteria. Gram stain of the CSF is positive in less than 40% while CSF cultures will usually be positive. Blood cultures will be positive in the majority of patients with listeriosis if there is CNS involvement.

❍ **What is the treatment for Listeria monocytogenes?**

Ampicillin. Gentamicin may be added for synergistic effect.

❍ **How common is Listeria monocytogenes meningitis?**

Listeria monocytogenes has been found to be the fourth most common cause of community acquired meningitis and is responsible for approximately 10% of such cases.

❍ **What is the best method for managing central venous catheters to minimize the risk of infection?**

This remains a controversial area. In one study, three catheter maintenance techniques were compared in a prospective, randomized fashion. The authors found no significant difference in infection rates when comparing weekly guidewire changes, weekly catheter changes with a fresh site and no weekly change. Catheters were also changed in all groups if signs of sepsis, positive blood cultures or inflammation at the insertion site developed.

Other studies have shown an increase in colonization and infection rates directly proportional to the length of time the catheter is in place. Common practice recommendations include routine guidewire changes on a weekly basis, sending the catheter tip for culture. Should the tip grow more than 15 cfu, the catheter is then removed and replaced at a new site. Most do not recommend changing over a guidewire if a catheter infection or sepsis is suspected. Conversion should be made to peripheral access as soon as it is feasible.

❍ What is the significance of a patient who received amphotericin bladder irrigation and has not cleared their urine of candida?

Patients who do not clear the yeast from the urine should be evaluated for urinary tract obstruction with a renal ultrasound. Candidal urine casts are a sign of upper urinary tract involvement. Patients who have infection of the upper tract will require treatment with amphotericin. A patient who is clinically deteriorating and at high risk for systemic infection, such as the neutropenic patient, should be evaluated for the possibility of disseminated candidiasis.

❍ When should consideration be given to surgical drainage in patients with septic arthritis?

Bacterial arthritis is most commonly due to Staphylococcus aureus in adults, although Neisseria gonorrhea is the most likely etiology in adults less than 30 years of age. Besides appropriate antibiotics, repeated needle aspirations is recommended during the first 7 days. Effusions should resolve with appropriate antibiotics and aspiration. Persistent effusions after this period of time imply the need for surgical drainage.

❍ What is the epidemiology of necrotizing fasciitis?

Necrotizing fasciitis is a severe infection distinguished by necrosis of the fascia and subcutaneous tissues, resulting in undermining of the skin. Onset is abrupt and is more common in diabetics, alcoholics and IV drug abusers, usually precipitated by a traumatized area of skin.

❍ What are the clinical findings of necrotizing fasciitis?

Initial physical findings may mimic cellulitis with swollen, very tender, erythematous skin. Unlike cellulitis, the margins are usually not well demarcated and the involved area typically becomes anesthetic due to the destruction of cutaneous nerves by the inflammatory process. Some patients develop subcutaneous gas and grossly necrotic skin or bulla formation. Very high fever and signs of toxicity disproportionate to the physical findings suggest necrotizing fasciitis. The superficial skin findings can be thought of as the tip of the iceberg.

❍ How is necrotizing fasciitis diagnosed?

Early diagnosis, which can be made by biopsy of subcutaneous tissue, fascia and muscle, may help decrease the mortality rate (from up to 50% in the untreated patient).

❍ What is the treatment for necrotizing fasciitis?

Organisms seen with Type I necrotizing fasciitis include streptococci, anaerobes and enterobacteriaceae. These are treated with penicillin/clindamycin/gentamicin. Type II necrotizing fasciitis is caused by invasive group A streptococci, which is popularly referred to as the "flesh-eating bacteria." Penicillin and clindamycin are the agents of choice. Systemic involvement may occur with type II infection, resulting in streptococcal toxic shock syndrome. Assertive surgical debridement is necessary for both types.

❍ What are the clinical features of Rocky Mountain spotted fever?

Patients present with fever, myalgias, headache and gastrointestinal symptoms three days to two weeks after a tick bite. Mental status changes may occur. The disease, caused by Rickettsia rickettsii, is most common between the months of April and October. Rash may not be apparent until several days into the illness and is absent in 10% of cases. It usually begins on the extremities and often involves the palms and soles. The lesions generally begin macular or maculopapular, but then become petechial or purpuric. Most deaths occur in the second week of illness and are usually due to the diagnosis having been missed.

❍ How is Rocky Mountain spotted fever diagnosed?

The diagnosis is presumptive in many cases. Treatment with tetracycline or chloramphenicol should be initiated while awaiting serologic tests, which usually do not become diagnostic until the disease has been present for at least a week. If a rash is present, skin biopsy may confirm the diagnosis earlier.

❍ **What are potential etiologies of brain abscesses in the immunocompromised patient?**

Brain abscesses that occur in the immunocompetent host are most commonly due to contiguous spread from a focus of infection in the paranasal sinuses, chronic otitis media, a hematogenous source or post-surgical. Abscesses that are hematogenous in origin tend to be multiple. The bacterial type reflects the primary source. The immunocompromised host is prone to more exotic organisms, including toxoplasmosis, cryptococcus, Listeria monocytogenes, aspergillus, nocardia and mycobacteria.

❍ **What is the significance of a retropharyngeal infection?**

The retropharynx is bounded by the pharynx anteriorly and the spine posteriorly. Between the retropharyngeal space and the prevertebral space in the "danger space" which extends from the base of the skull to the diaphragm via the posterior mediastinum. The retropharyngeal space may become infected from penetrating injuries or contiguous spread of infection from the lateral pharyngeal space, which can result from tonsillitis, parotitis, mastoiditis and odontogenic infections.

A retropharyngeal space infection may result in acute mediastinitis with a high mortality rate. Meningitis and pericarditis are other potential complications.

❍ **What are the clinical features of a patient with a retropharyngeal space infection?**

Patients generally have fever, dysphagia, neck stiffness and appear systemically ill. Respiratory distress may occur due to compression of the supraglottic structures. Chest pain may be present if the infection has tracked into the mediastinum.

❍ **How is a retropharyngeal space infection diagnosed?**

Diagnosis is suggested by thickening of the retropharyngeal structures on lateral neck films, with the prevertebral fascia being greater than 7 mm in width at the C2 level. CT scanning is diagnostic. Surgical drainage is required.

❍ **What patients are at increased risk for developing sternal wound infections and mediastinitis after cardiac surgery?**

Sternal wound infections occur with an incidence of 1 to 5% after median sternotomy. Patients at increased risk include diabetics, those with bilateral inferior mammary takedowns, re-operations and patients with a low cardiac output state. Responsible microorganisms are predominately Staphylococcus aureus, Staphylococcus epidermidis, pseudomonas species and enterobacteriaceae.

❍ **What are the clinical features in a patient with such an infection?**

Symptoms manifest a week or more post-operatively and include fever, drainage, inability to wean from mechanical ventilation and an unstable sternum. More catastrophic complications related to sternal wound infection include hemorrhage from the heart and great vessels. This may occur by several mechanisms, including right ventricular rupture, suture line leaks at the aortotomy site and vein graft anastomotic leaks.

❍ **How are sternal wound infections managed?**

Sternal wound infections are commonly managed with operative debridement and muscle flaps. Other methods including a "double-catheter irrigation technique" are under evaluation.

❍ **What is the epidemiology of influenza? What are the clinical features of uncomplicated influenza?**

Influenza is responsible for taking approximately 10,000 lives per year, with 80 to 90% of the deaths occuring in patients greater than 65 years of age. Patients present with abrupt onset of fever, chills, myalgia, fatigue, headache and cough. Elderly patients may present with fever and confusion

❍ **What laboratory findings are typical in patients with hantavirus pulmonary syndrome?**

Elevated hematocrits are commonly seen in these patients due to pronounced endothelial dysfunction and capillary leak. Thrombocytopenia is seen in over 75% of patients. Dramatically elevated serum LDH is often present. Diagnosis is confirmed by Western blot or polymerase chain reaction.

❍ **What side effects have been associated with the use of vancomycin?**

Red man syndrome, characterized by flushing of the face, thorax and hypotension, is caused by histamine release and is associated with rapid infusion. It is not considered to be an allergic reaction. Ototoxicity and nephrotoxicity may occur, especially with older preparations of the drug.

❍ **What is Charcot's triad?**

Fever, right upper quadrant pain and jaundice are the three classic signs in patients with acute cholangitis. Biliary decompression, either surgically, via stent placement or percutaneous drainage techniques, is essential in addition to appropriate antibiotic coverage.

❍ **What are the uses and side effects of ganciclovir?**

Ganciclovir is an antiviral agent that is active against all herpes viruses but is an especially potent inhibitor of cytomegalovirus. Ganciclovir causes neutropenia in up to 40% of patients and thrombocytopenia in approximately 20%. AIDS patients are more prone to these effects than transplant patients. Headache, personality changes or confusion may occur. Seizures or coma may occur but are rare. Ganciclovir is carcinogenic and teratogenic. It has also been approved for prevention of CMV disease in transplant patients.

❍ **How are prosthetic valve infections classified?**

Prosthetic valve infections are classified as early (< 2 months post-operative) and late (>2 months post-operative). Both types are very serious infections, although early valve infections tend to have a worse prognosis. Bacteremic patients with new prosthetic valves should be suspected to have endocarditis.

❍ **When do patients with prosthetic valve infections require surgery?**

If annular involvement becomes apparent, the patient requires operative debridement and valve replacement. Antibiotic therapy alone may be curative in cases of late bioprosthetic endocarditis, which is usually valvular in nature. However, many patients require surgery due to serious valvular dysfunction or bulky vegetations. Mechanical valve infections are also around the suture ring. Patients presenting in shock or severe congestive heart failure require emergent surgery.

❍ **What factors increase the likelihood of infectious complications following penetrating abdominal trauma?**

Patients with gunshot wounds are 3 times as likely as those with stab wounds to develop post-operative infections. Hollow viscus injuries have a high risk of post-operative infection, especially colon injuries.

The type of surgical drainage also is a factor, closed suction being preferable to sump drainage and in some cases Penrose drains. The use of gauze packing is associated with a higher risk of perihepatic abscesses.

❍ **What is the significance of persistent vs. recurrent fever during treatment of infective endocarditis?**

A recent series of patients with endocarditis revealed the cause of persistent fever (fever lasting more than one week of initiation of appropriate antibiotic therapy) to be due to extensive cardiac infection in 56% of cases. This complication necessitates cardiac surgery.

Recurrent fever, defined as a fever returning after at least two days of defervescence, was most commonly due to drug hypersensitivity reactions (usually due to beta-lactam antibiotics).

❍ **What is the antimicrobial spectrum of cefepime?**

Cefepime is a "fourth-generation" parenteral cephalosporin with anti-pseudomonal activity and broad activity against both gram negative and gram positive bacteria. Its beta lactamase resistance confers improved efficacy against the enterobacteriaceae, which have become more and more problematic due to their increased resistance to many antibiotics. Cefepime is renally excreted and dialyzable.

❍ **What time after insertion are pulmonary artery catheters considered at high risk to be infected?**

After 72 hours.

❍ **What are the most common organisms involved with line infections?**

Staphylococcus epidermidis and Staphylococcus aureus.

❍ **What is the etiologic agent of Pittsburgh pneumonia?**

Legionella micdadei.

❍ **Of the 14 serogroups of Legionella pneumoniae, how many are detected by the urinary antigen test?**

One (serogroup 1).

❍ **What factors affect the outcome in cases of invasive aspergillosis?**

Patient characteristics associated with a poor response to treatment included persistent neutropenia, no reduction in immunosuppression, diffuse pulmonary disease, recurrent leukemia, major hemoptysis and angioinvasion seen on histological examination.

Treatment factors affecting outcome include a delay in initiating treatment, low dosages of amphotericin, very low serum levels of itraconazole and lack of secondary antifungal prophylaxis during subsequent neutropenic episodes.

Of transplant recipients, heart, lung and renal transplant patients tend to have better outcomes than bone marrow transplant and liver transplant patients.

Site of infection affects outcome - cerebral aspergillosis has a 99% mortality and pulmonary aspergillosis has an 86% mortality. Invasive rhinosinusitis, which occurs mostly in bone marrow transplant recipients and leukemic patients, has a better outcome with a mortality rate of 66%.

❍ **Which antibiotics are recommended as adjunctive therapies in combination with macrolides (erythromycin, azithromycin or clarithromycin) in the treatment of legionellosis?**

Rifampin or ciprofloxacin.

❍ **Which of the above antibiotics is the treatment of choice in transplant patients with legionellosis?**

Ciprofloxacin, since both macrolides and rifampin interact pharmacologically with immunosuppressive agents, such as tacrolimus.

❍ **Rifampin has bactericidal activity against which microorganisms?**

Besides TB, it is an effective agent against coagulase positive and negative staphylococci. Rifampin is also effective against some gram negative organisms, especially after exposure to Neisseria meningitidis. It is commonly used as an adjunct against legionella. Unfortunately, bacteria rapidly develop resistance to rifampin. Thus, with the exception of short term prophylactic treatment protocols, rifampin is limited to an adjunctive mode.

❍ **Which drugs have shown promise in the treatment of Mycobacterium avium complex (MAC) infections?**

MAC has traditionally been a frustrating disease to treat, due to its resistance to the standard, first line antimycobacterial agents, such as isoniazid and rifampin. Newer regimens, including various combinations of clarithromycin, azithromycin, rifabutin, streptomycin and ethambutol have improved response rates.

❍ **What adverse reactions should you be alert for when using dapsone as salvage therapy for pneumocystis carinii pneumonia?**

Dapsone produces dose dependent hemolysis which is ordinarily of an insignificant degree except in patients with glucose 6-phosphate dehydrogenase deficiency. Patients should be screened for this disorder prior to initiating treatment. Rash is fairly common and usually well tolerated. Bone marrow suppression and mild hyperkalemia is occasionally seen. Methemoglobinemia is very common during treatment with dapsone.

❍ **What is the differential diagnosis of extreme hyperthermia?**

Fevers greater than 106 degrees Fahrenheit (extreme pyrexia) are usually not infectious in nature. Causes include heat stroke, malignant hyperthermia, neuroleptic malignant syndrome, HIV disease, central fevers and drug fever.

❍ **What are the extracutaneous manifestations of chickenpox in the adult?**

Varicella pneumonia occurs in up to 1 out of 400 adult cases of chickenpox. CXR findings include diffuse interstitial or nodular infiltrates. Cough, dyspnea, hemoptysis and respiratory failure may develop. Sputum Tzanck smear may be positive. Encephalitis, myocarditis and hepatitis may also complicate the infection. Treatment is IV acyclovir.

❍ **What constitutes reliable treatment for pneumococcal infections?**

Streptococcus pneumoniae had maintained exquisite sensitivity to penicillin for decades. In the past few years, there has been an increasing incidence of intermediate penicillin resistance as well as the emergence of strains with multiple drug resistance. A majority of isolates in Spain were found to be drug resistant. Resistance is less of a problem in the United States, but has been increasing. The mechanism for intermediate penicillin resistance is related to a mutation that results in a higher concentration of penicillin being necessary to saturate the penicillin binding proteins.

Multiple drug resistance appears to occur via transfer of genetic material from other species of bacteria. Many strains are resistant to penicillin, erythromycin, sulfa drugs, cephalosporins and tetracycline. This can be quite problematic, especially in the treatment of meningitis, where antibiotic selection is also limited by a drug's ability to obtain sufficient concentrations in the CSF. At the present time, the drug resistant strains are still susceptible to vancomycin and at least in vitro to chloramphenicol.

❍ **What are the classic chest x-ray findings of Klebsiella pneumonia?**

Lobar pneumonia with the "bulging fissure" sign. Patients are often alcoholics or have other underlying chronic lung disease and may produce "currant-jelly" sputum.

❍ **How does a subphrenic abscess present?**

It follows surgery for a ruptured viscus, cholecystitis or penetrating abdominal wound. Patients may complain of right upper quadrant or shoulder pain in addition to fever and chills. Subphrenic abscesses occur far more commonly on the right. The chest x-ray typically reveals an elevated hemidiaphragm and may show a pleural effusion or an air/fluid level below the diaphragm in more advanced cases. CT is diagnostic.

❍ **What is the treatment for influenza?**

Amantadine or rimantadine should ideally be initiated within 48 to 72 hours from the onset of symptoms. Complicating bacterial pneumonias are common, especially Streptococcal pneumoniae and Staphylococcus aureus and need to be specifically treated as well.

❍ **What mechanism is felt to be responsible for the association of aminoglycoside and muscle weakness?**

Aminoglycosides can prevent calcium uptake into the presynaptic membrane at the neuromuscular junction, which can inhibit acetylcholine release. They also can blunt the effects of acetylcholine at the postsynaptic membrane.

The likelihood of muscle weakness is increased in patients who have received neuromuscular blockers, in patients who have muscle disorders or are hypocalcemic or hypomagnesemic. Calcium channel blockers may potentiate this effect.

❍ **How is ventilator associated pneumonia diagnosed?**

Clinical signs that are ordinarily suggestive of pneumonia, including the presence of fever, elevated white blood cell count, worsening oxygenation, progression of pulmonary infiltrates and presence of organisms on sputum culture, are unreliable markers for the diagnosis of ventilator associated pneumonia.

The First International Consensus Conference on Clinical Investigation of Ventilator-associated Pneumonia recommended bacterial counts of 10 to the fourth cfu per ml as a criteria to distinguish colonization from infection with bronchoalveolar lavage (BAL) samples. The specificity of BAL samples, however have been somewhat inferior to protected specimen brushing (PSB) in most studies. Bacterial growth of greater than 10 to the third cfu per ml on quantitative culture has been recommended as the criterion of significance for PSB.

Recovery of greater than 1% squamous epithelial cells in a centrifuged BAL sample was an accurate predictor of contamination with oropharyngeal secretions. Neutrophil predominance in BAL samples is present with pneumonia but is not a specific finding. The Consensus Conference recommended the combination of PSB and BAL as the most accurate diagnostic technique. These tests, however, are often confounded when the patient is already on antibiotic treatment.

❍ **What adverse reactions may be seen with amphotericin infusion?**

Release of tumor necrosis factor has been postulated to cause the fever, rigors and a drop in blood pressure commonly seen with administration of Amphotericin B. Hypotension occurs frequently in debilitated patients, especially in the early stages of treatment. This is the reason why a 1mg test dose is given prior to a full daily treatment dose. True allergic reactions to Amphotericin B are uncommon.

❍ **What is an effective method to clean one's stethoscope?**

Isopropyl alcohol swabs significantly reduces bacterial loads on the stethoscope. Soap and water are ineffective.

❍ **What is the likelihood for a bronchoalveolar lavage sample to contain cytomegalovirus in the presence of HIV disease?**

Lavage samples frequently are culture positive for cytomegalovirus (CMV) in AIDS patients, regardless of the presence or absence of pulmonary symptomatology. CMV is uncommonly a pulmonary pathogen in this population. Those patients with significant CMV pulmonary disease almost always have extremely low CD4 counts.

❍ **What is the sensitivity of two dimensional transesophageal echocardiography in detecting vegetations?**

95%.

❍ **Who is at high risk for developing endocarditis?**

People with prosthetic heart valves, previous episodes of endocarditis, complex congenital heart disease and surgically constructed systemic pulmonic shunts.

❍ **Who is at moderate risk for developing endocarditis?**

Moderate risk factors include acquired valvular dysfunction, hypertrophic cardiomyopathy and uncorrected congenital conditions. These latter conditions include patent ductus arteriosus, ventricular septal defect, primum atrial septal defect, coarctation of the aorta and bicuspid aortic valve.

❍ **What procedures increase the risk for developing bacterial endocarditis?**

Procedures of the dental oral, respiratory, gastrointestinal and genitourinary tracts and vaginal delivery.

❍ **What is the appropriate prophylaxis for these procedures?**

Depending upon the nature of the procedure, amoxicillin, ampicillin, gentamicin, clindamycin or a combination of these antibiotics.

❍ **What is the clinical picture of a myocardial abscess?**

Low grade fevers, chills, leukocytosis, conduction system abnormalities and nonspecific ECG changes.

❍ **What is streptococcal toxic shock syndrome?**

The recent emergence of highly virulent strains of Group A Streptococcus pyogenes has been associated with severe invasive disease that may cause multiorgan failure. This fulminant process may be precipitated by seemingly minor trauma to skin or mucosal surfaces and is rarely associated with streptococcal pharyngitis. Exotoxin production by these strains has been implicated as the cause of tissue injury, which often includes organ failure, ARDS and necrotizing fasciitis. Patients with prior exposure to streptococcal M proteins are relatively protected from this syndrome.

A definite case includes isolation of group A streptococci from a normally sterile site (e.g., blood, CSF, pleural or peritoneal fluid) and the presence of hypotension or shock plus at least two of the following signs: renal impairment, disseminated intravascular coagulation, abnormal liver function, ARDS, erythematous rash with or without desquamation and soft tissue necrosis (e.g., necrotizing fasciitis, myositis or gangrene).

A probable case has group A streptococcus isolated from a normally nonsterile site (eg, pharynx, skin and sputum), in addition to hypotension, shock and at least two of the above listed signs.

❍ **What are risk factors for developing sinusitis in the intensive care unit?**

Nasally intubated patients develop sinusitis with an incidence from 2 to 25%. This complication is related to trauma, edema and obstruction of drainage from the ostia in the lateral nasal wall. Trauma patients with facial fractures, patients with limited head mobility and those who require nasal packing and nasogastric tubes are especially prone.

❍ **What is the clinical scenario in which sinusitis occurs in the ICU?**

Though sinusitis develops relatively early after nasal intubation, the diagnosis may not be readily apparent, as it is often not accompanied by purulent nasal drainage. Most typically patients present with fever and leukocytosis and may progress to sepsis.

❍ **How is sinusitis that occurs in the ICU diagnosed and treated?**

Sinus CT scans will confirm the diagnosis, but antral taps for gram stain and culture are recommended to guide treatment. Unlike community acquired sinusitis, Staphylococcus aureus and gram negative rods are the most common organisms. Polymicrobial infections are frequently seen. Removal of any foreign body is necessary. Phenylephrine nasal drops decrease edema and promote drainage. Some patients require repeated antral lavage. Patients who are nasotracheally intubated should be reintubated orally.

❍ **What are the characteristics of drug fever?**

Patients with a drug related fever often will appear relatively well, despite a high temperature. Usual temperatures are in the range of 102 to 104 degrees Fahrenheit, though low grade and extreme elevations may also be seen. Sustained fevers and a relative bradycardia are typical. Besides antibiotics, other common causes of drug fever include amphotericin, procainamide, salicylates, barbiturates, phenytoin, quinidine and interferon. Drug fever is not always accompanied by rash.

❍ **Who is especially at risk for developing meningococcal disease?**

Neisseria meningitidis, a gram-negative diplococcus, classically strikes children and young adults, especially military recruits and those in crowded living conditions. The reservoir of the meningococcus is in the nasopharynx of asymptomatic carriers. Congenital deficiencies of complement, especially terminal complement components C5 to C9 or properdin, impact an increased risk of developing an infection. Acquired complement deficiencies related to nephrotic syndrome, liver disease, systemic lupus erythematosus, as well as asplenia and immunoglobulin deficiencies also result in increased risk.

❍ **Who should receive meningococcal vaccination?**

Vaccination is recommended for patients 2 years of age or older with functional or anatomic asplenia, complement deficiencies and military recruits. The currently available vaccine is tetravalent and contains the polysaccharides groups A, C, Y and W135. There is no effective vaccine available for serogroup type B, which accounts for almost half of the infections in the United States.

❍ **What are the risk factors for developing primary peritonitis?**

Primary peritonitis, also known as spontaneous bacterial peritonitis, is an acute or subacute bacterial infection of the peritoneum unrelated to the usual causes of peritonitis, such as a perforated viscus or intra-abdominal abscess. The vast majority of cases occur in patients with alcoholic cirrhosis, but patients with cirrhosis and ascites from other causes are also predisposed.

❍ **What are the clinical findings and treatment for primary peritonitis?**

Fever and abdominal pain are present in most patients, but peritoneal signs may not be appreciable. Most cirrhotic patients with primary peritonitis will have advanced liver disease and present with coexisting encephalopathy. The most useful findings on analysis of peritoneal fluid include an elevated polymorphonuclear count > 250/mm3. Gram stains of peritoneal fluid are negative in the majority of cases, so empiric treatment should be initiated if there is suspicion. These infections tend to be due to a single organism in most cases, commonly Escherichia coli and Streptococcus pneumoniae, unlike secondary peritonitis which is usually polymicrobial.

❍ **What are the clinical findings of herpes simplex encephalitis?**

Herpes Simplex encephalitis is the most common cause of nonepidemic encephalitis in the United States. Patients will generally present with headache, fever, anosmia, memory or personality changes and a decreased level of consciousness. Focal signs are common, including hemiparesis, seizures or an ataxic gait.

❍ **What is the pathophysiology of HSV encephalitis?**

Unlike the arthropod-borne viruses, which spread to the CNS hematogenously, HSV-1's mode of entry is neuronal, often due to reactivation of latent virus present in the trigeminal ganglia, which sends fibers to the frontal and temporal lobes. This may explain why these sites seem to be preferentially involved. This disease has an extremely high morbidity and mortality.

❍ **How is HSV encephalitis diagnosed and treated?**

Focal findings on electroencephalography may show characteristic periodic spike and slow waves in the temporal zones. MRI and CT may also show abnormalities in these areas. Routine CSF findings are nonspecific. The diagnosis may be made by CSF polymerase chain reaction for HSV. Brain biopsy is useful to help distinguish HSV encephalitis from other potentially treatable syndromes, including bacterial brain abscesses, cryptococcal disease, tuberculosis, toxoplasmosis and malignancies.

IV acyclovir is generally nontoxic and should be instituted empirically and promptly in patients in whom there is a clinical suspicion for Herpes simplex encephalitis.

❍ **What ultrasound findings suggest the diagnosis of acalculous cholecystitis?**

These include thickening of the gallbladder wall > 4 mm, intramural gas, subserosal edema without ascites or a sloughed gallbladder mucosal membrane. The diagnosis can be difficult to make. Gallbladder sludging, wall thickening and hydrops have been found to be common findings in asymptomatic medical intensive care unit patients. The presence of sepsis, new onset jaundice and ultrasound induced Murphy's sign help to confirm the significance of suggestive ultrasound findings.

❍ **What are the risk factors for acalculous cholecystitis?**

Multiple trauma, recent major surgery, critical illness and hyperalimentation.

❍ **How is acalculous cholecystitis treated?**

Percutaneous cholecystostomy, laparoscopic cholecystectomy or traditional cholecystectomy.

❍ **Which antibiotics are most frequently implicated as precipitants for Stevens-Johnson syndrome?**

Stevens-Johnson syndrome or erythema multiforme major, is a serious hypersensitivity reaction that presents with a generalized vesiculobullous eruption of the skin, mouth, eyes and genitals. Many drugs have been identified as triggering this reaction, but the most common antibiotics are the sulfa drugs and the penicillins. Stevens-Johnson syndrome has also been seen in patients with recent mycoplasma infections.

❍ **What causes toxic shock syndrome (TSS)?**

An exotoxin derived from certain strains of Staphylococcus aureus. Other organisms that cause toxic shock syndrome are group A streptococci, Pseudomonas aeruginosa and Streptococcus pneumoniae. Tampons, IUD's, septic abortions, sponges, soft tissue abscesses, osteomyelitis, nasal packing and postpartum infections all can house these organisms.

❍ **What dermatological changes occur with TSS?**

Initially, the patient will have a blanching erythematous rash that lasts for 3 days. After 10 days there will be a desquamation of the palms and soles.

❍ **What are the criteria for the diagnosis of TSS?**

All of the following must be present: $T > 38.9^{\circ}$ C (102° F), rash, systolic BP < 90 orthostasis, involvement of 3 or more organ systems (GI, renal, musculoskeletal, mucosal, hepatic, hematologic or CNS) and negative serologic tests for diseases such as RMSF, hepatitis B, measles, leptospirosis and syphilis.

❍ **How should a patient with TSS be treated?**

Fluids, vasopressor support, vaginal irrigation with iodine or saline and anti-staphylococcal penicillin or cephalosporin with anti-beta-lactamase activity. Rifampin should be considered to eliminate the carrier state.

❍ **Which factors may contribute to a false-negative TST (TB skin test)?**

Viral infections (measles, mumps, chickenpox, HIV) and live virus vaccination.
Bacterial (typhoid fever, typhus, overwhelming TB).
Advanced renal disease.
Severe malnutrition.
Decreased immunity (steroids, sarcoidosis, Hodgkin's, lymphoma and chronic lymphatic leukemia).
Advanced age.
Errors in application, reading and documentation.

❍ **Which medical conditions increase the risk of TB disease?**

HIV infection.

Substance abuse.
CXR findings suggestive of previous TB (in a person inadequately treated).
Diabetes mellitus.
Silicosis.
Low body weight (10% or more below the ideal).
Cancer of the head and neck.
Hematologic and reticuloendothelial diseases.
End-stage renal disease.
Intestinal bypass or gastrectomy.
Chronic malabsorption syndromes.
Prolonged corticosteroid therapy.
Other immunosuppressive therapy.

❍ **T/F: A negative TST "rules-out" TB in an HIV-negative patient.**

False. In miliary disease 50% are TST negative and in pulmonary TB probably <10%.

❍ **What CXR findings are associated with primary versus reactivated TB?**

Primary: normal, air space consolidation in any segment of the lung (more often in middle or lower lung zone), hilar or paratracheal lymph node enlargement, most often seen in infants and children.

Reactivated: focal air space consolidation, linear densities connecting to the ipsilateral hilum and cavitation. Most often seen in apical or posterior segment of the upper lobes or in the superior segment of the lower lobes.

❍ **What are the CXR findings in TB associated with HIV infected patients?**

Early in HIV infection TB presents radiographically as typical reactivation disease. In advanced HIV disease, lower lung zone or diffuse infiltrates and adenopathy are more frequent while cavitation is less often seen.

❍ **T/F: The CXR pattern of "fibrosis" in the upper lobes is adequate to rule out active TB.**

False. Disease activity is determined by microbiological studies.

❍ **Which diseases can mimic TB?**

Nocardiosis, melioidosis, paragonimiasis.
Ankylosing spondylitis.
Sarcoidosis, berylliosis.
Lymphoma, cancer.
Klebsiella, aspergillus.

❍ **Which form of extrapulmonary TB is considered the most infectious?**

Laryngeal TB produces the highest number of contacts. It probably reflects extensive pulmonary cavitary TB with spillover to the larynx.

❍ **What biochemical abnormalities can be seen in active TB?**

Anemia, leukocytosis with neutrophilia, lymphopenia, monocytopenia, thrombocytosis, increased ESR, ferritin or B12, abnormal RBC folic acid, increased LFTs, hyponatremia and hypoalbuminemia.

❍ **What are the intrathoracic complications of TB?**

Pneumothorax, endobronchial stenosis, bronchiectasis, empyema, mycetoma, hemorrhage, Rasmussen's aneurysm (dilated vessel in the wall of an old TB cavity) and broncholithiasis.

❍ **What are the extrapulmonary manifestations of TB?**

Miliary, genitourinary, skeletal, CNS tuberculoma, meningitis, abdominal (any intra-abdominal organ), pericardial and pleural disease.

❍ **What are the treatment options for pulmonary TB?**

6 month regimen: INH, RIF (rifampin), PZA (pyrazinamide), EMB (ethambutol) or SM (streptomycin) daily for 2 months followed by 4 months of INH and RIF. If low prevalence (<4%) of INH resistance, then can drop EMB or SM from regimen. Alternatively, the initial 4 drugs can be given daily for 2 weeks followed by 6 weeks of direct observation of the same drugs twice per week. Subsequently, complete the course with twice weekly INH and RIF for 4 months. The third 6 month regimen is the same four drugs three times weekly for 6 months.

9 month regimen: nine months of daily INH and RIF or 1-2 months of daily INH and RIF followed by 7-8 months of twice-weekly dosing. EMB or SM should be given in the first 2 months if INH resistance is not known to be < 4%.

HIV-related disease: the six month regimen may be used for a total of 9 months or at least 6 months after culture conversion.

❍ **What is the therapy for extrapulmonary TB?**

Generally, the same regimen as for pulmonary TB with the following exception. Bone and joint TB, miliary TB or TB meningitis in children should be treated for 12 months. Corticosteroids are beneficial in pericarditis, CNS tuberculomas and meningitis.

❍ **What are surgical indications for TB treatment?**

Decortication for "trapped lung"/fibrothorax.
Lobectomy/pneumonectomy for cavitary multidrug resistant TB on a weak or failing regimen.
Drainage for empyema or pericardial effusion.
Drainage for a large pleural effusion with midline shift or symptoms.
Mycobacteria other than tuberculosis cervical lymph node resection (95% cure rate).

❍ **What are the clinical scenarios of M. avium complex (MAC)?**

Colonization of the oral cavity and upper respiratory tract (without disease).
Upper lobe cavities (mostly in male smokers with COPD).
Bronchiectasis and small reticulonodular infiltrates in elderly women.
Disseminated disease and mycobacteremia in HIV-patients.

❍ **Which non-tuberculosis mycobacteria (NTMs) are commonly implicated in pulmonary disease?**

MAC, M. kansasii, M. abscessus, M. xenopi and M. malmoense.

❍ **What is the treatment for M. kansasii pulmonary disease?**

INH, RIF and ETH for 18 months because of a high relapse rate.

❍ **What is the most common clinical presentation of tuberculous meningitis?**

Symptoms are generally chronic or subacute in nature, although the occasional patient may present with fulminant meningitis. Typically, intermittent headaches and low-grade fevers progress to persistent headache, lethargy, nausea and vomiting and altered mental status. A gelatinous mass may ultimately extend to encase the base of the brain, optic chiasm, floor of the third ventricle and may surround the spinal cord. Invasion of vessels may result in cerebral infection. Obstructive hydrocephalus may also occur. The majority of patients will have an extrameningeal site of tuberculosis present. The propensity for tuberculosis to involve the basilar aspects of the subarachnoid space accounts for the cranial nerve palsies seen in some patients.

❍ **What are the diagnostic tests in tuberculous meningitis?**

CT or MRI may reveal tuberculomas or basilar enhancement. Traditional teaching is that the CSF will show hypoglycorrhachia, with the glucose being less than 45 mg/dl. This is present in only a minority of cases. Cell counts may range from 0 to 1500, usually with a lymphocytic predominance. Earlier on, polymorphonuclear leukocytes may predominate. CSF protein is usually moderately elevated. AFB stains are positive only one third of the time with a single lumbar puncture, but the yield increases to 87% after four lumbar punctures.

❍ **What is the treatment for tuberculous meningitis?**

Four drug therapy with INH, rifampin, pyrazinamide and ethambutol. Steroids have been recommended.

❍ **What organisms constitute the M. avium complex?**

M. avium, M. intracellulare and M. scrofulaceum.

❍ **T/F: TB may mimic the atypical pneumonia syndrome (as stereotyped by a Mycoplasma pneumoniae infection).**

True.

❍ **What are the most common microbes in patients with life threatening community acquired pneumonia (admitted to the ICU from the community)?**

Pneumococcus and legionella.

❍ **What are the signs and symptoms of diphtheria infection?**

Infection is heralded by acute onset of exudative pharyngitis, high fever and malaise. A pseudomembrane may form in the oropharynx with possible respiratory compromise. A circulating exotoxin has direct effects on the heart, kidneys and nervous system. Diphtheria infection may lead to paralysis of the intrinsic and extrinsic eye muscles.

❍ **What is the most common cause of endocarditis in IV drug abusers?**

Staphylococcus aureus, most commonly involving the tricuspid valve.

❍ **What does the India ink test stain for?**

Cryptococcus neoformans.

❍ **What strain of influenza is more common in adults? In children?**

Adults: Influenza A. Children: Influenza B.

❍ **What strain of influenza is most virulent?**

Influenza A.

❍ **A 34 year-old female presents with a maculopapular rash on her palms and soles. She complains of headaches and general weakness. On examination, you find she has multiple condyloma lata and lymphadenopathy. What is the diagnosis?**

Secondary syphilis. This develops 6 to 9 weeks after the syphilitic chancre, which will have resolved by this time. If it goes untreated, tertiary syphilis will develop. This can affect all the tissues in the body, including the CNS and the heart. Treatment is with penicillin.

HEMATOLOGY AND ONCOLOGY PEARLS

"Nature does nothing without a purpose."
Aristotle

❍ **What are the pulmonary manifestations of sickle cell disease?**

Acute chest syndrome, bacterial pneumonia, cor pulmonale, reduction in DLCO, reduced static lung volumes and a right shifted oxygen dissociation curve.

❍ **What is the mechanism for the acute chest syndrome?**

Microvascular occlusion by sickle cells which ultimately results in alveolar wall destruction and subsequent fibrosis.

❍ **What is the treatment for a severe case of acute chest syndrome?**

Exchange transfusion.

❍ **What are the common pathogens causing pneumonia in sickle cell patients?**

S. pneumoniae, H. influenzae, alpha-hemolytic streptococcus and salmonella.

❍ **What is the hyperleukocytosis syndrome?**

Vascular occlusion due to high numbers of circulating leukemic cells. Pulmonary manifestations include hypoxemia, dyspnea, infiltrates and fever in the absence of infection. The treatment is emergent leukapheresis.

❍ **What is the cutoff for platelets before lung biopsy can be performed?**

50,000 or more platelets for biopsy.

❍ **What are the pulmonary manifestations of amyloidosis?**

Tracheobronchial submucosal amyloidosis (discrete or diffuse), nodular or diffuse parenchymal involvement and pleural effusion.

❍ **T/F: Most episodes of transfusion associated acute lung injury are caused by donor antibodics reacting with recipient neutrophil or HLA antigens.**

True.

❍ **What are the pulmonary manifestations of polycythemia?**

Pulmonary vascular sludging related to hyperviscosity and pulmonary hemorrhage related to an increased bleeding tendency.

❍ **What is the differential diagnosis of pulmonary infiltrates in patients with hematological malignancies?**

Infection, treatment related (radiation, chemotherapy), hemorrhage, malignant infiltration and hyperleukocytosis.

❍ **What is pseudohypoxemia?**

Hypoxemia from consumption of oxygen by cells in blood during transport, as can occur with hyperleukocytosis.

❍ **What is the acute chest syndrome in sickle cell lung disease?**

Fever, chest pain, leukocytosis and pulmonary infiltrates. The major dilemma is in distinguishing infarction from pneumonia. Fat embolism is a less common cause.

❍ **What is sickle cell chronic lung disease?**

It is thought to be the result of years of uncontrolled and often asymptomatic sickling and is characterized by pulmonary hypertension, cor pulmonale and ventilatory defects.

❍ **What is the most common cause of pneumonia in sickle cell disease?**

Streptococcus pneumoniae.

❍ **A SICU trauma patient is noted to be oozing from multiple wound sites. What tests and accompanying results would be consistent with disseminated intravascular coagulopathy (DIC)?**

Decreased platelet count, elevated prothrombin time, elevated activated partial thromboplastin time, decreased fibrinogen, elevated fibrin degradation products and presence of D-dimers.

❍ **What four types of blood loss indicate a bleeding disorder?**

1) Spontaneous bleeding from many sites
2) Bleeding from non-traumatic sites
3) Delayed bleeding several hours after trauma
4) Bleeding into deep tissues or joints

❍ **What common drugs have been implicated in acquired bleeding disorders?**

Ethanol, ASA, NSAIDs, warfarin and antibiotics.

❍ **Mucocutaneous bleeding, including petechiae, ecchymoses, epistaxis, GI, GU and menorrhagia, indicate what coagulation abnormalities?**

Qualitative or quantitative platelet disorders.

❍ **Delayed bleeding and bleeding into joints or potential spaces, such as the retroperitoneum, suggests what type of bleeding disorder?**

Coagulation factor deficiency.

❍ **What is primary hemostasis?**

The platelet interaction with the vascular subendothelium that results in the formation of a platelet plug at the site of injury.

❍ **What four components are required for primary hemostasis?**

1) Normal vascular subendothelium (collagen)
2) Functional platelets
3) Normal Von Willebrand factor (connects the platelet to the endothelium via glycoprotein Ib)
4) Normal fibrinogen (connects platelets to each other via glycoprotein IIb-IIIa)

❍ **What is the end product of secondary hemostasis (coagulation cascade)?**

Cross-linked fibrin.

❍ **What mechanism limits the size of the fibrin clots that are formed?**

The fibrinolytic system.

❍ **What is the principal physiologic activator of the fibrinolytic system?**

Tissue plasminogen activator (tPA). Endothelial cells release tPA, which converts plasminogen, absorbed in the fibrin clot, to plasmin. Plasmin degrades fibrinogen and fibrin monomer into fibrin degradation products (FDPs) and cross-linked fibrin into D-dimers.

❍ **Below what platelet count is spontaneous hemorrhage likely to occur?**

$< 10{,}000/mm^3$.

❍ **It is generally agreed that most patients with active bleeding and platelet counts $< 50{,}000/mm^3$ should receive platelet transfusion. How much will the platelet count be raised for each unit of platelets infused?**

5,000 to $10{,}000/mm^3$.

❍ **What patients with thrombocytopenia are unlikely to respond to platelet infusions?**

Those with platelet antibodies (ITP).

❍ **How can an overdose of warfarin be treated? What are the advantages and disadvantages of each treatment?**

Fresh frozen plasma (FFP) or vitamin K. If there are no signs of bleeding, temporary discontinuation may be all that is necessary.
FPP advantages: Rapid repletion of coagulation factors and control of hemorrhage.
FPP disadvantages: Volume overload, possible viral transmission.
Vitamin K advantages: Ease of administration.
Vitamin K disadvantages: Possible anaphylaxis when given IV. Delayed onset of 12 to 24 hours. Effects may last up to 2 weeks, making anticoagulation of the patient difficult or impossible.

❍ **What is the only coagulation factor not synthesized by hepatocytes?**

Factor VIII.

❍ **Which four hemostatic alterations are seen in patients with liver disease?**

1) Decreased protein synthesis leading to coagulation factor deficiency
2) Thrombocytopenia
3) Increased fibrinolysis
4) Vitamin K deficiency

❍ **What five treatments are available to bleeding patients with liver disease?**

1) Transfusion with RBCs (maintains hemodynamic stability)
2) Vitamin K
3) Fresh frozen plasma
4) Platelet transfusion
5) DDAVP (Desmopressin)

❍ **What hemostasis test is most often prolonged in patients with uremia?**

Bleeding time.

❍ **What treatment options are available to patients with renal failure and coagulopathy?**

1) Dialysis
2) Optimize hematocrit (erythropoietin or transfusion with RBCs)
3) DDAVP
4) Conjugated estrogens
5) Cryoprecipitate and platelet transfusions if hemorrhage is life threatening

❍ **What are the clinical complications of DIC?**

Bleeding, thrombosis and purpura fulminans.

❍ **Which laboratory studies are most helpful in diagnosing DIC?**

1) PT and PTT (prolonged)
2) Platelet count (usually low)
3) Fibrinogen level (low)
4) Presence of D-dimers

❍ **What are the most common hemostatic abnormalities in patients infected with HIV?**

Thrombocytopenia and acquired circulating anticoagulants (causes prolongation of aPTT).

❍ **What is the pentad of thrombotic thrombocytopenic purpura (TTP)?**

1) Fever
2) Thrombocytopenia
3) Neurologic symptoms
4) Renal insufficiency
5) Microangiopathic hemolytic anemia

❍ **What is the most common inherited bleeding disorder?**

Von Willebrand's disease.

❍ **Seventy to eighty percent of patients with Von Willebrand's disease have type I. What is the current approved mode of therapy for bleeding in these patients?**

DDAVP.

❍ **What is the most common hemoglobin variant?**

Hemoglobin S (valine substituted for glutamic acid in the sixth position on the beta chain).

❍ **Which clinical crises are seen in patients with sickle-cell disease?**

1) Vasoocclusive (thrombotic)
2) Hematologic (sequestration and aplastic)
3) Infectious

❍ **Which is the most common type of sickle-cell crisis?**

Vaso-occlusive.

❍ **What percentage of patients with sickle-cell disease have gallstones?**

75%.

❍ **What are the mainstays of therapy for a patient with vaso-occlusive sickle-cell crisis?**

1) Hydration
2) Analgesia
3) Oxygen
4) Cardiac monitoring (if patient has history of cardiac disease or is having chest pain)
5) Blood transfusion in patients with severe anemia
6) Exchange transfusion for severe acute chest syndrome

❍ **What is the most commonly encountered sickle hemoglobin variant?**

Sickle-cell trait.

❍ **What is the most common human enzyme defect?**

Glucose-6-phosphate dehydrogenase (G-6-PD) deficiency.

❍ **What drugs should be avoided in patients with G-6-PD deficiency?**

1) Drugs that induce oxidation
2) Sulfa
3) Antimalarials
4) Pyridium
5) Nitrofurantoin

❍ **What is the most useful test to ascertain hemolysis and a normal marrow response?**

The reticulocyte count.

❍ **What is the most common clinical presentation of TTP (thrombotic thrombocytopenic purpura)?**

Neurologic symptoms including headache, confusion, cranial nerve palsies, coma and seizures.

❍ **What is the most common worldwide cause of hemolytic anemia?**

Malaria.

❍ **What components of whole blood are used for transfusion?**

1) RBCs
2) Platelets
3) Plasma
4) Cryoprecipitate

❍ **How much will the infusion of 1 unit of RBCs raise the hemoglobin and hematocrit in a 70-kg patient?**

Hemoglobin: 1 g/dl. Hematocrit: 3%.

❍ **What are the five contents of cryoprecipitate?**

1) Factor VIIIC
2) Von Willebrand factor
3) Fibrinogen
4) Factor XIII
5) Fibronectin

❍ **What is the first step in treating all immediate transfusion reactions?**

Stop the transfusion.

❍ **What infection carries the highest risk for transmission by blood transfusion?**

Hepatitis C.

❍ **What is the current recommended emergency replacement therapy for massive hemorrhage?**

Type-specific, uncrossmatched blood. Type O negative, which may be immediately life saving in certain situations, carries the risk of life threatening transfusion reactions.

❍ **In current practice, what blood components are routinely infused along with RBCs in a patient receiving a massive transfusion?**

None. The practice of prophylactically using platelet transfusion and fresh frozen plasma is costly and unwarranted.

❍ **What is the only crystalloid fluid compatible with RBCs?**

Normal saline.

❍ **What condition should be suspected in a patient with multiple myeloma who presents with paraplegia and urinary incontinence?**

Acute spinal cord compression. This condition occurs primarily with multiple myeloma and lymphoma and it is also encountered with carcinomas of the lung, breast and prostate.

❍ **What are the two most common neoplasms that cause pericardial effusion and tamponade?**

Carcinoma of the lung and breast.

❍ **A 48 year-old male smoker presents with a headache, swelling of the face and arms and a feeling of fullness in his face and neck. He is noted to have JVD upon physical examination and papilledema upon funduscopic examination. What is the most likely diagnosis?**

Superior vena cava syndrome.

❍ **What is the most common cause of hyperviscosity syndrome?**

Waldenstrom's macroglobulinemia (IgM myeloma).

❍ **What should be considered in a patient who presents in a coma and has anemia and Rouleaux formation on the peripheral blood smear?**

Hyperviscosity syndrome.

❍ **What are the major causes of GI bleeding in cancer patients?**

Hemorrhagic gastritis and peptic ulcer disease.

❍ **What are the vitamin K dependent factors of the clotting cascade?**

X, IX, VII and II. Remember 1972.

❍ **An adult patient sustains a major head injury. He also suffers from classic hemophilia. What treatment should be given?**

Give factor VIII.

❍ **What is Von Willebrand's disease?**

An autosomal dominant disorder of platelet function. It causes bleeding from mucosal membranes, menorrhagia and increased bleeding from wounds. Patients with Von Willebrand's disease have less (or dysfunctional) Von Willebrand's factor.

❍ **What is Von Willebrand's factor?**

Von Willebrand's factor is a plasma protein secreted by endothelial cells and serves two functions: 1) it is required for platelets to adhere to collagen at the site of vascular injury, which is the initial step in forming a hemostatic plug. 2) it forms complexes in plasma with factor VIII, which are required to maintain normal factor VIII levels.

❍ **What is appropriate initial treatment for a life threatening level of hypercalcemia of 16 mg per deciliter?**

Give the patient 0.9 NS at 5 to 10 liters per day. After attaining euvolemia, administer furosemide. Additional therapy includes pamidronate, glucocorticoids, mithramycin or calcitonin.

❍ What factors are deficient in classic hemophilia, Christmas disease and Von Willebrand's disease, respectively?

Classic hemophilia:	Factor VIII
Christmas disease:	Factor IX
Willebrand's disease:	Factor VIIIc and Von Willebrand's cofactor

❍ What pathway involves factors VIII and IX?

Intrinsic pathway.

❍ What effect does deficiency of factors VIII and IX have on PT and on PTT?

Deficiency leads to an increase in PTT.

❍ What pathway does the PT measure? What factor is unique to this pathway?

Extrinsic pathway. Factor VII.

❍ Can hemophilia A be clinically distinguished from hemophilia B?

No.

❍ What blood product is given when the coagulation abnormality is unknown?

Fresh frozen plasma.

❍ What agent can be used to treat mild hemophilia A and Von Willebrand's disease type 1?

DDAVP induces a rise in factor VIII levels.

❍ Where does esophageal cancer most commonly metastasize?

Lungs, liver and bones.

❍ Which types of cancer metastasize to bone?

Prostate, thyroid, breast, lung and kidney.

❍ What is the most common type of brain tumor in adults?

Glioblastoma multiforme (40%). Meningiomas account for 15 to 20% and metastatic tumors account for 5 to 10%.

❍ Pheochromocytomas produce what compounds?

Catecholamines. This group of chemicals result in hypertension, perspiration, palpitations, anxiety and weight loss.

❍ If vanillylmandelic acid, normetanephrine and metanephrine are detected in the urine, what is the likely cause?

Pheochromocytoma.

❍ **What is the rule of "tens" for pheochromocytomas?**

10% are malignant, 10% are multiple or bilateral, 10% are extra-adrenal, 10% occur in children, 10% recur after surgical removal and 10% are familial.

❍ **What are the three major proteins that inhibit clotting?**

Antithrombin III, Protein C and Protein S.

❍ **What does deficiency of antithrombin III, protein C or protein S increase the risk of?**

Venous thrombosis.

❍ **Why should warfarin, as an initial treatment for venous thrombosis secondary to protein C deficiency, be avoided?**

It may, by inhibiting the synthesis of protein C, lead to paradoxical hypercoagulability. This is prevented by the use of heparin.

❍ **What is the most important aspect of treating DIC?**

Correcting the underlying disorder (usually septic shock).

❍ **What is the characteristic bone marrow finding in idiopathic thrombocytopenic purpura (ITP)?**

Increased or normal megakaryocytes.

❍ **What are the potential treatment modalities for ITP?**

Corticosteroids, gammaglobulin, plasmapheresis and splenectomy.

❍ **What are the typical signs and symptoms of central nervous system infarction secondary to sickle cell vaso-occlusion?**

Mild, fleeting TIA-like symptoms, seizures, hemiparesis and coma.

❍ **What is the treatment of central nervous system vaso-occlusive crisis?**

Exchange transfusion.

❍ **What are the signs and symptoms of splenic sequestration crisis?**

Pallor, weakness, lethargy, disorientation, shock, decreased level of consciousness and enlarged spleen.

❍ **What is the treatment of splenic sequestration crisis?**

Rapid infusion of saline and transfusion of red cells.

❍ **In anemia, which way is the oxygen dissociation curve shifted?**

The right (affinity of hemoglobin for oxygen is decreased).

❍ **The most important aspect of the treatment of anemia of chronic disease is:**

Correction of the underlying disorder.

❍ **What are the laboratory findings in iron deficiency anemia?**

Decreased serum ferritin and iron saturation, elevation of TIBC, low MCV and rise in RDW.

❍ **What are the most common sites for bleeding in patients with hemophilia?**

Joints, muscles and subcutaneous tissue.

❍ **What are typical lab findings in Von Willebrand's disease?**

Normal platelet count, normal prothrombin time, normal or increased partial thromboplastin time and increased bleeding time.

❍ **There is simultaneous activation of coagulation and fibrinolysis in what pathologic condition?**

Disseminated intravascular coagulation.

❍ **What is the predominant symptom in DIC?**

Bleeding.

❍ **What are some common ischemic complications of DIC?**

Renal failure, seizures, coma, pulmonary infarction and hemorrhagic necrosis of the skin.

❍ **What are the common lab findings in DIC?**

Decreased platelets, increased PT and PTT, decreased fibrinogen, increased FDP and D-dimers.

❍ **G-6-PD deficiency is prevalent in what ethnic groups?**

Greeks, southern Italians, Sephardic Jews, Filipinos, southern Chinese, African-Americans and Thailanders.

❍ **What does Prothrombin Time (PT) measure? How is it performed?**

PT measures the extrinsic and common pathways of the coagulation system. The time to clot formation is measured after the addition of thromboplastin. If the concentration of factors II, V, VII, and X are significantly lower than usual, the PT will be prolonged.

❍ **What does Activated Partial Thromboplastin Time (aPTT) measure? How is it performed?**

PTT measures the intrinsic and common pathways of the coagulation cascade. After the blood sample is exposed to celite for activation and a reagent is added, the clot formation is measured. When factors II, V, VIII, IX, X, XI, XII or fibrinogen are deficient, the PTT will be prolonged.

❍ **What are the indications for the administration of FFP?**

1-Replacement of isolated factor deficiencies.
2-Reversal of coumadin effect.
3-Treatment of pathological hemorrhage in patients who have received massive transfusion.

4-Use in antithrombin III deficiency.
5-Treatment of immunodeficiencies.

❍ **What are the indications for cryoprecipitate administration?**

For the treatment of congenital or acquired fibrinogen and factor VIII deficiencies. Cryoprecipitate can also be administered prophylactically for nonbleeding perioperative or peripartum patients with congenital fibrinogen deficiencies or for Von Willebrand's disease that is unresponsive to desmopressin (DDAVP).

❍ **What is the most reproducible manifestation of dilutional coagulopathy?**

Thrombocytopenia.

❍ **What is the incidence of hemolytic transfusion reactions (HTR)?**

1 in 33,000 units. The HTR is potentially life threatening and often regarded the most serious complication of transfusions. Fifty one percent of 256 transfusion associated deaths reported to the US Food and Drug Administration between 1976 and 1985 resulted from acute hemolysis following the transfusion of ABO-incompatible blood or plasma.

❍ **What are the types of HTRs and what is the pathophysiology of each one?**

HTRs are divided in two types of reactions: 1) intravascular hemolysis and 2) extravascular hemolysis. Intravascular hemolysis occurs when the antibody coated RBC is destroyed by the activation of the complement system. Extravascular hemolysis destroys antibody coated RBC s via phagocytosis by macrophages in the reticuloendothelial system. In most HTR s, some RBCs are probably destroyed by both mechanisms.

❍ **What is the treatment for HTRs?**

The transfusion should be stopped immediately. The mainstay of treatment is supportive.

❍ **What causes febrile reactions to blood and what is the incidence?**

The febrile reaction is the most common mild transfusion reaction and occurs in 0.5% to 4% of transfusions. It is caused by donor antibodies to antigens on the recipient's WBCs.

❍ **What is transfusion related acute lung injury?**

It is a form of noncardiogenic pulmonary edema, occurring within 2 to 4 hours after a transfusion. This reaction should be suspected in any patient who develops pulmonary edema after a transfusion in which volume overload is thought to be unlikely. Clinical signs of respiratory distress vary from mild dyspnea to severe hypoxia. It usually resolves within 48 hours in response to oxygen, mechanical ventilation and other forms of supportive treatments.

❍ **After a course of chemotherapy, your patient has had a course of fever, neutropenia and granulocytopenia for over a week, despite antibiotic usage. What should you do now?**

Add Amphotericin B for a presumed fungal infection while continuing your search for the source of the infection.

❍ **A patient on chemotherapy for his Burkitt's lymphoma is found to be hyperkalemic, hypocalcemic, hyperphosphatemic and hyperuracemic. What is the presumptive diagnosis?**

Tumor lysis syndrome.

❍ **What are the three phases of type and crossmatch of blood?**

The first phase combines recipient serum and donor cells to test ABO group compatibility at room temperature. It identifies M, N, P and Lewis incompatibilities. This phase takes approximately 5 minutes. The second phase incubates the products from the first phase in albumin at 37°C, enhancing incomplete antibodies. The last phase is the antiglobulin test. Antiglobulin serum is added to the previous incubated test tubes. This phase aids in the detection of incomplete antibodies in Rh, Kell, Duffy and Kidd systems.

❍ **Which solutions are considered incompatible with PRBC?**

Calcium containing solutions should not be added to blood, particularly at slow infusion rates, because small clots may form due to the presence of calcium in excess of the chelating ability of the citrate anticoagulant.

❍ **What are the problems associated with citrate in a massive transfusion?**

Massive transfusions increase citrate levels and decrease ionized calcium levels.

❍ **How does renal papillary necrosis that is secondary to sickle cell vaso-occlusion commonly present?**

Painless hematuria.

❍ **What procedures might be included to treat the type of renal papillary necrosis mentioned in the previous question?**

Intravenous hydration, red blood cell transfusion or exchange transfusion

❍ **What is the most common cause of aplastic crisis in patients with hemolytic anemia?**

Parvovirus B19 infection.

ELECTROLYTE, ACID-BASE AND ENDOCRINE PEARLS

We are here on earth to do good for others. What the others are here for, I don't know.
W.H. Auden

❍ **What is the sodium concentration of some frequently used intravenous fluids?**

Normal saline (0.9% NS)	154 mEq/L
Half normal saline (0.45% NS)	77 mEq/L
3% saline	513 mEq/L
Lactated Ringer (LR)	130 mEq/L
5% dextrose (D5W)	0

❍ **How is osmolality calculated?**

Osmolality = Na (mEq/L) x 2 + glucose (mg/dl)/18 + BUN (mg/dl)/2.8 + any solute (mg/dl)/ (molecular weight of the solute/10)

Ethanol molecular weight = 56

❍ **What is the relationship between serum sodium to water balance?**

Generally, due to renal mechanisms:
Hypernatremia means "too little free water", rather than "too much sodium."
Hyponatremia means "too much free water", rather than "too little sodium."

❍ **How is plasma sodium interpreted in the presence of hyperglycemia?**

High glucose concentration draws water out of cells and dilutes sodium in plasma.
For every 100 mg/dl of glucose above 200 mg/dl the serum sodium is decreased by 1.6 mEq/L.

❍ **What is "pseudohyponatremia"?**

Pseudohyponatremia, also called isotonic hyponatremia, is a laboratory artifact in the presence of severe hyperproteinemia or hyperlipidemia. Plasma sodium is normal.

❍ **What are the symptoms of hyponatremia? At what sodium levels do they present?**

Acute decrease in plasma sodium produces lethargy, nausea, headaches, confusion, weakness, abdominal cramps, vomiting, delirium, seizures and coma. Acutely serum sodium has to drop to around 125 mEq/L for symptoms to be present.

Coma and seizures are seen at sodium levels below 115 mEq/L.
Chronic hyponatremia may be asymptomatic until sodium drops below 115 mEq/L.

❍ **How do you calculate fractional excretion of sodium?**

FENa = (Urine Na x Plasma Creatinine) / (Urine Creatinine x Plasma Na) x 100.

❍ **What diagnostic criteria are necessary for the diagnosis of the syndrome of inappropriate antidiuretic hormone secretion (SIADH)?**

SIADH is a diagnosis of exclusion. The following criteria are necessary:
1. Hypotonicity
2. Euvolemia
3. Absence of renal, thyroid, cardiac or adrenal disease
4. Inappropriately elevated urine osmolality for the level of plasma osmolality
5. Absence of other causes of hyponatremia

❍ **What causes SIADH?**

1. Malignancies (pulmonary, hematologic, pancreatic)
2. Pulmonary disease (tumor, tuberculosis, pneumonia, asthma)
3. CNS disorders (meningitis, trauma, tumors)
4. Drugs (chlorpropamide, oxytocin, vincristine, cytoxan)
5. Post-operative period (pain)

❍ **What findings are diagnostic of diabetes insipidus?**

Large urinary volumes (usually greater than 3 L/ day), dilute urine (osmolality < 300 mOsm/L) specific gravity < 1.010 and hypernatremia.

❍ **How fast should hyponatremia be corrected?**

No faster than 0.5 to 1.0 mEq/L/hour of sodium. The initial goal is to correct to sodium level no higher than 120 to 125 mEq/L

❍ **What is the complication if hyponatremia is corrected too rapidly?**

Central pontine myelinolysis or osmotic demyelinating syndrome. This syndrome can present several days after the treatment of hyponatremia. Symptoms include quadraparesis with swallowing dysfunction, pseudobulbar palsy and inability to speak.

❍ **If 3% normal saline is used for correction of hyponatremia how is the replacement volume calculated?**

Total body water = 60% body weight in kilograms
Salt replacement = (120 - actual serum sodium) x total body water
Volume of hypertonic saline = salt replacement / sodium content of 3% saline

Sodium content of 3% saline is 513 mEq/l.

❍ **How is free water excess calculated in a hyponatremic patient?**

Water excess = present body water - (present body water x present serum sodium / normal serum sodium)

Total body water = 60% body weight in kilograms

❍ **What typical urine sodium value is found with furosemide therapy?**

Sodium ~ 75 mEq/L

❍ **Loss of free water can cause hypernatremia. What are normal insensible losses? How does temperature affect insensible losses?**

Insensible loss averages 500 ml/day. For each 1°F increase in body temperature above 100°F 1000 ml of additional electrolyte free fluid is lost as sweat.

❍ **What is the osmolality of sodium bicarbonate (NaHCO3)?**

One ampoule (50 ml) contains 50 mEq of sodium and 50 mEq of HCO3.
Therefore, one liter would contain 2000 mEq.

❍ **T/F: Renal dose dopamine improves outcome in patients with oliguria.**

False. Renal dose dopamine increases urine output but does not improve renal function.

❍ **What is the mechanism of action of atrial natriuretic peptide (ANP)?**

Sodium overload and retention results in volume overload that distends the atria. Atria then release ANP. ANP increase renal vasodilatation and natriuresis.

❍ **What tests indicate that the kidney is conserving sodium?**

1. Low urinary sodium (< 20 mEq/L).
2. In states of metabolic alkalosis and volume depletion (e.g., vomiting) kidney excretes bicarbonate which pulls sodium along with it. Urinary sodium may be high, despite volume depletion. The urinary chloride will be low in this situation.

❍ **What is normal plasma osmolality?**

Normal plasma osmolality is 285 to 295 mOsm/kg.

❍ **What are the symptoms of hypernatremia?**

Dehydration of brain cells causes lethargy, fatigue, mental status changes, coma, seizures and death. Most adults do not develop symptoms until serum sodium reaches 160 mEq/L.

❍ **What are some causes of hypernatremia?**

1. Diabetes insipidus (central, nephrogenic)
2. Insensible losses (burns, sweating)
3. Osmotic diuresis (mannitol, hyperglycemia)
4. Hypertonic fluid administration

❍ **What mechanism causes hypovolemia to result in a metabolic alkalosis?**

The kidney will resorb sodium and excrete hydrogen ion to maintain intravascular volume. This is under the influence of aldosterone.

❍ **What are the muscular manifestations of hyperkalemia?**

Hyperkalemia partially depolarizes the cell membrane. Patients may present with neuromuscular weakness that may progress to flaccid paralysis and hypoventilation.

❍ **How much potassium is contained in extracellular fluid?**

Approximately 70 mEq.

❍ **What hormones regulate potassium balance?**

Insulin (promotes tissue uptake)
Catecholamines
via beta-receptors (increased cellular uptake)
via alpha-receptors (decreased cellular uptake; hepatic release)
Aldosterone (renal excretion)

❍ **How does acute metabolic acidosis affect serum potassium? Is there a difference between organic and inorganic acidosis?**

Acute inorganic acidosis: plasma potassium increases by 0.8 mEq/l for each 0.1 decline in pH.

Organic acidosis: does not affect potassium.

❍ **How does acute metabolic alkalosis affect serum potassium?**

Plasma potassium falls by 0.3 mEq/L for every 0.1 unit rise in pH.

❍ **How do respiratory acid-base disorders affect plasma potassium?**

Respiratory acid-base imbalances are usually not associated with significant changes in plasma potassium.

❍ **What therapy is available for severe hyperkalemia?**

Calcium - protects against depolarizing effects of hyperkalemia (avoid in simultaneous digitalis toxicity)
Sodium bicarbonate - results in cellular potassium uptake
Beta-adrenergic agonists - promotes cellular uptake
Cation exchange resin - binds potassium in bowel
Loop diuretics - enhance potassium secretion in nephrons
Insulin/glucose - promotes cellular uptake
Dialysis – removes potassium from blood directly

❍ **List some medications that may cause hyperkalemia.**

Non-steroidal anti-inflammatory drugs
Angiotensin converting enzyme inhibitors
Heparin - inhibits adrenal steroidogenesis
Spironolactone - blocks renal mineralocorticoid receptor
Triamterene, amiloride – aldosterone independent effects in tubular potassium secretion

❍ **How does magnesium depletion affect potassium?**

Magnesium depletion is associated with renal potassium wasting, hypocalcemia and hypokalemia.

❍ **How would you estimate the deficit in total body potassium in a patient with plasma potassium of 3 mEq/L? Or 2 mEq/L?**

A decrease in serum potassium from 4 to 3 mmol/L corresponds to a 100 to 200 mEq decrement in total body potassium. Each additional fall of 1 mEq/L in serum potassium represents an additional deficit of 200 to 400 mEq.

❍ **Succinylcholine is a rapid onset depolarizing neuromuscular blocking agent. How does it affect plasma potassium?**

Muscle membrane depolarization results in leakage of potassium producing an average increase of 0.5 to 1.0 mEq/L in serum potassium. However, when succinylcholine depolarizes muscle that has been previously traumatized or denervated (e.g., stroke), large increases in serum potassium can occur causing arrhythmias and cardiac arrest.

❍ **Non-depolarizing neuromuscular blocking agents are frequently used in intensive care units. What is their effect on plasma potassium?**

Non-depolarizing neuromuscular blocking agents do not affect plasma potassium levels.

❍ **What are the hypertensive hypokalemic syndromes?**

Hypertensive hypokalemic syndromes are all associated with glucocorticoid or mineralocorticoid excess, renal potassium wasting and metabolic alkalosis.
They include:
1. Primary hyperaldosteronism (e.g., adrenal adenoma)
2. Secondary hyperaldosteronism (e.g., renal artery stenosis)
3. Cushing's syndrome (e.g., glucocorticoid therapy, ACTH-secreting tumor)

❍ **What is the cause of hyperkalemia in diabetics?**

Cellular uptake of potassium is decreased because of hypoinsulinism. These patients often have hyporeninemic hypoaldosteronism (type IV renal tubular acidosis).

❍ **What mechanism causes hypokalemia to induce a metabolic alkalosis?**

The kidney to will attempt to absorb additional potassium in exchange for hydrogen (lost from blood) in response to hypokalemia.

❍ **What is the mechanism of alveolar hypoventilation (manifested by high PCO_2) in myxedema?**

Depression of the hypoxic and hypercapnic respiratory drive. Respiratory muscle myopathy and phrenic neuropathy are uncommon.

❍ **T/F: Serum sodium is increased in the hyperglycemic patient.**

False. Hyperosmolar extracellular fluid shifts body water from the intracellular to the extracellular space. For each 100 mg/dl increase in glucose, sodium decreases 1.6 mEq/L.

❍ **Osmoreceptors in the hypothalamus control what two primary regulators of water balance?**

Thirst and ADH secretion.

❍ **A patient admitted with one week of persistent vomiting from gastric outlet obstruction is expected to have what acid-base disturbance?**

Non-anion gap metabolic alkalosis associated with hypokalemia.

❍ **What is the most common underlying disorder in respiratory acidosis?**

Alveolar hypoventilation.

❍ **How much sodium is in normal saline?**

154 mEq/L.

❍ **What is the daily fluid requirement for a 70 kg man?**

2500 ml/d.

❍ **What are the clinical manifestations of hyponatremia?**

Weakness, fatigue, muscle cramps, confusion, anorexia, nausea, vomiting, headache, delirium, seizures and coma.

❍ **At what serum sodium level would one expect to see clinical signs and symptoms of acute hyponatremia?**

Approximately 125 mEq/L.

❍ **At what sodium level would one expect signs and symptoms of hypernatremia?**

Approximately 160 mEq/L.

❍ **What are the signs and symptoms of hypernatremia?**

Restlessness, irritability, ataxia, fever, spasms and seizure.

❍ **T/F: Elderly patients may have urine sodium levels that are inappropriately high in the face of decreased renal blood flow.**

True.

❍ **What is the urine sodium level and plasma osmolality in SIADH?**

Urine sodium greater than 20 mEq/L and plasma osmolality less than 290 mOsm/L. The urine osmolality is typically greater than 200 mOsm/L.

❍ **What are the possible reasons for the development of post-operative hypokalemia?**

Intracellular shift secondary to high insulin or β-agonist levels, hypothermia, hemodilution, hyperventilation, alkalosis, on-going diuresis and nasogastric suctioning

❍ **What is the relation between magnesium and potassium?**

Magnesium depletion promotes the loss of potassium in the urine, hence its replacement helps to limit renal potassium wasting. Hypomagnesemia also inhibits sodium-potassium transport resulting in decreased intracellular concentrations of potassium.

❍ **What signs are associated with hypocalcemia?**

Decreased contractility, hypotension, ventricular arrhythmias, muscle spasms, laryngospasm, paresthesias and tetany.

❍ **What are the most common causes of hypernatremia?**

Diabetes insipidus, insensible losses, osmotic diuresis and hypertonic fluid administration.

❍ **What therapy is available for severe hyperkalemia?**

Calcium, sodium bicarbonate, β-adrenergic agonists, cation exchange resins, loop diuretics, insulin and glucose and dialysis. Calcium is contraindicated in cases of hyperkalemia related to digitalis toxicity.

❍ **How is body potassium distributed?**

90% is intracellular (mainly in muscle), 2% is extracellular and the remainder is in bone.

❍ **What are the most common causes of SIADH?**

Malignancies, pulmonary disease, CNS disorders and drugs.

❍ **What is the treatment for diabetes insipidus?**

Vasopressin intravenously or DDAVP intranasally.

❍ **How fast should hyponatremia be corrected?**

No faster than 0.5 to 1.0 mEq/l/hour.

❍ **How is urine osmolality calculated?**

Urine osmolality = 2 x (urinary sodium + urinary potassium) + urine urea nitrogen / 2.8.

❍ **Are the T wave amplitudes heightened or diminished in hyperkalemia? What about the QRS duration?**

The T waves are taller and the QRS is prolonged.

❍ **What ECG abnormalities are associated with hypercalcemia?**

Shortened Q-T interval, bradycardia and heart block.

❍ **At normal body temperature, what is the average daily insensible water loss?**

600 to 900 ml/day or 8 to 12 ml/kg/day.

❍ **What are the consequences of too rapid sodium replacement in hyponatremia?**

Central pontine myelinolysis (quadriplegia, dysarthria and dysphasia).

❍ **What are the common causes of hyperosmolar hyponatremia?**

Hyperglycemia, mannitol and radiologic contrast.

❍ **Patients with asymptomatic hyponatremia are best treated in what manner?**

Free water restriction.

❍ **Urine sodium levels below what value may distinguish extrarenal from renal sodium loss in a patient with hyponatremia?**

20 mEq/L.

❍ **What ECG changes are associated with hyperkalemia?**

Widened QRS and PR interval, peaked T waves, flattened P waves, deep S waves, sine-wave configuration, ventricular tachycardia or fibrillation and asystole.

❍ **Compensation for persistent hypoventilation occurs by what mechanism?**

Resorption of sodium bicarbonate by the kidney.

❍ **What is the role of chromium in human metabolism?**

It promotes insulin action in peripheral tissues.

❍ **Diabetes insipidus infers what tonicity of urine and plasma?**

Dilute urine and hypertonic plasma osmolality.

❍ **What is the major cause of extrarenal potassium depletion?**

Diarrhea.

❍ **What are the clinical manifestations of hypokalemia?**

Arrhythmias, muscle weakness, mental status changes, impaired intestinal peristalsis and predisposition to digitalis toxicity.

❍ **T/F: Beta-blockers raise the serum potassium concentration.**

True. They inhibit uptake of potassium by skeletal muscle.

❍ **What is the main determinant of the osmolarity of the extracellular fluid space?**

Serum sodium concentration.

❍ **How is the sodium deficit calculated?**

Sodium deficit = (normal sodium - observed sodium) x total body water.

❍ **How does hyperglycemia lead to hyponatremia?**

Because glucose stays in the extracellular fluid, hyperglycemia draws water out of the cell into the extracellular fluid. Each 100 mg/dl increase in plasma glucose decreases the serum sodium by 1.6 mEq/L.

❍ **What are the most common causes of hypotonic fluid loss leading to hypernatremia?**

Diarrhea, vomiting, hyperpyrexia and excessive sweating.

❍ **What are the ECG findings of a patient with hypokalemia?**

Flattened T waves, depressed ST segments, prominent U waves, arrhythmias and prolonged QT intervals.

❍ **What is the quickest way to treat hyperkalemia?**

Calcium gluconate (10%) IV.

❍ **What are the causes of hyperkalemia?**

Acidosis, tissue necrosis, hemolysis, blood transfusions, GI bleed, renal failure, Addison's disease, primary hypoaldosteronism, excess oral K^+ intake, RTA Type IV and medications as succinylcholine, beta-blockers, captopril, spironolactone, triamterene, amiloride and high dose penicillin.

❍ **What are the causes of hypocalcemia?**

Shock, sepsis, multiple blood transfusions, hypoparathyroidism, vitamin D deficiency, pancreatitis, hypomagnesemia, alkalosis, fat embolism syndrome, phosphate overload, chronic renal failure, loop diuretics, hypoalbuminemia, tumor lysis syndrome and medications as calcitonin and mithramycin.

❍ **What is the most common cause of hyperkalemia?**

Hemolysis (of lab error variety). Chronic renal failure is the most common cause of "true" hyperkalemia.

❍ **In order of prevalence, what are the three most common causes of hypercalcemia?**

Malignancy, primary hyperparathyroidism and thiazide diuretics.

❍ **What are the signs and symptoms of hypercalcemia?**

The most common gastrointestinal symptoms are anorexia and constipation. Remember:

Stones:	Renal calculi
Bones:	Osteolysis
Abdominal groans:	Peptic ulcer disease and pancreatitis
Psychic overtones:	Psychiatric disorders

❍ **What is the initial treatment for hypercalcemia?**

Restoration of the extracellular fluid with 5 to 10 L of normal saline within 24 hours. After the patient is rehydrated, administer furosemide. Patients with hypercalcemia are dehydrated because high calcium levels interfere with ADH and the ability of the kidney to concentrate urine.

❍ **A patient with a history of alcohol abuse presents after a recent tonic-clonic seizure. What particular electrolyte abnormality should be considered and treated during evaluation?**

Hypomagnesemia.

❍ **What is the most common cause of hyperphosphatemia?**

Acute and chronic renal failure.

❍ **As PCO_2 increases, pH will decrease. Acutely, how much is the pH expected to decrease for every 10 mmHg increase in PCO_2?**

PH decreases by 0.08 units for each 10 mmHg increase in PCO_2.

❍ What is the equation that describes the relation between pH and $[H^+]$ and what are normal values for each?

PH is defined as -Log $[H^+]$. The normal plasma pH is 7.4 and the normal $[H^+] = 40$ nEq/L = 40 nM/L.

❍ What is a buffer?

Buffers are weak acids or bases (proton donor/acceptor) that resist changes in solution pH with addition of acid or base. Buffers are most effective within 1 pH unit above and below their pK (isoelectric point).

❍ What is the equation that describes the relation between pH, HCO_3^- and PCO_2?

The Henderson-Hasselbach equation describes the biologic acid-base relation by examining the CO_2-bicarbonate system, which describes the overall reaction:

$$CO_2 + H_2O \rightarrow H_2CO_3 \rightarrow H^+ + HCO_3^-$$

When CO_2 dissolves in water, formation of H_2CO_3 (carbonic acid) occurs very slowly. Carbonic anhydrase, an enzyme found in erythrocytes and the renal tubules, greatly accelerates the rate of this reaction.

The law of mass action states:

$$Ka = \frac{[H^+][HCO_3^-]}{[H_2CO_3]}$$

The $[H^+]$ in solution can be derived to give the following:

$$[H^+]\ (nEq/L) = \frac{24 * PCO_2}{[HCO_3^-]}$$

❍ What happens to the pH if the [H+] increases from 40 to 80 nEq/L?

The pH falls from 7.40 to 7.10. Each doubling/halving of the $[H^+]$ causes the pH to decrease/increase by 0.3, respectively. Similarly, a change in proton ion concentration of 1 nEq/L causes a change in pH of 0.015 units in the opposite direction.

❍ What is an open buffer system?

An open buffer system describes a state where one member of the buffer pair can exchange with the environment. For example, the bicarbonate system results in the formation of carbon dioxide gas, which is rapidly eliminated by pulmonary ventilation. The advantage of this system is that it allows for rapid adjustment to moment-to-moment changes in acid production.

❍ Why does the kidney excrete fixed acids?

To regenerate HCO_3^-.

❍ What are the major body buffer systems?

In the intravascular space, bicarbonate, hemoglobin, phosphate and plasma proteins are the major buffer systems. The bicarbonate system functions as the proton shuttle carrying carbon dioxide from tissue to lung using the erythrocyte as the transporter and it is the major way in which the body eliminates volatile acid.

In the extravascular space, the major buffers are bicarbonate, phosphate, cellular proteins and bone hydroxyapatite.

❍ What determines the level of PCO_2 in body fluids?

CO_2 homeostasis is determined by relative rates of CO_2 production and removal. The rate of CO_2 production is determined by tissue metabolism. The rate of CO_2 elimination is determined by alveolar ventilation. During a cardiac arrest, no CO_2 is eliminated even if ventilation is adequate.

$$PaCO_2 = \frac{0.86 * VCO_2}{F * (Vt - Vd)}$$

Where VCO_2 is the rate of CO_2 production (ml/min.), Vt is the tidal volume (ml), Vd is the dead space and F is the breathing frequency (breaths/min.).

❍ Regarding CO_2 blood transport, what are the forms of CO_2 carriage and what contribution do they make to the total CO_2 transport?

81% is transported as bicarbonate, 11% as carbamino grouped bound directly to hemoglobin and 8% is dissolved in the plasma.

❍ What are normal and abnormal blood gas values?

VALUE	NORMAL	DECREASED	INCREASED
ARTERIAL BLOOD			
pH	**7.35-7.45**	**<7.35 acidemia**	**>7.45 alkalemia**
$PaCO_2$, mmHg	**40**	**<36 respiratory alkalosis, hyperventilation**	**>44 respiratory acidosis, hypoventilation**
HCO_3^-a, mEq/L	**24**	**<24 metabolic acidosis**	**>24 metabolic alkalosis**
VENOUS BLOOD			
PHv, units	**7.30-7.35**		
$PvCO_2$, mmHg	**45**		
HCO_3v, mEq/L	**20-22**		

❍ What are the normal compensatory responses to alkalosis and acidosis?

The goal of homeostasis is to maintain constancy of the blood pH by maintaining a constant ratio between PCO_2 and HCO_3^-, which is accomplished as follows:

PRIMARY ACID/BASE DISORDER	COMPENSATORY RESPONSE
Increased PCO_2 (respiratory acidosis)	Increased HCO_3^- (metabolic alkalosis)
Decreased PCO_2 (respiratory alkalosis)	Decreased HCO_3^- (metabolic acidosis)
Increased HCO_3^- (metabolic alkalosis)	Increased PCO_2 (respiratory acidosis)
Decreased HCO_3^- (metabolic acidosis)	Decreased PCO_2 (respiratory alkalosis)

❍ How does alteration of arterial CO_2 correspond to changes in arterial pH?

DISORDER	PRIMARY	SECONDARY COMPENSATION

	DISORDER	
Metabolic Acidosis	Decreased $HCO3^-$	Expected $PCO_2 = 1.5 * HCO3^- + 8 (\pm 2)$ PCO_2 = last 2 digits of pH * 100
Metabolic Alkalosis	Increased $HCO3^-$	Expected $PCO_2 = 0.7 * HCO3^- + 20 (\pm 1.5)$
Respiratory Acidosis Acute (1-2 hr) Chronic (<12-24 hr) Respiratory Alkalosis Acute (1-2 hr) Chronic (<12-24 hr)	 Increased CO_2 Increased CO_2 Decrease CO_2 Decrease CO_2	 pH = 0.005 to 0.008 * PCO_2 and HCO3 = 0.1 * PCO_2 pH = 0.003 * PCO_2 and HCO3 = 0.35 * PCO_2 pH = 0.008 to 0.01 *PCO_2 and HCO3 = 0.2 * PCO_2 pH = 0.002 * PCO_2 and HCO3 = 0.5 * PCO_2

❍ **What is a better index of tissue CO_2, arterial or venous CO_2?**

Venous CO_2.

❍ **Is it possible to have the identical PCO_2 in arterial and mixed venous blood?**

During respiratory arrest, pulmonary arterial blood and systemic arterial blood have the same PCO_2. However, at the tissue level, the arteriolar PCO_2 is less than that of the tissue venous PCO_2.

❍ **What is the normal arterial-venous PCO_2 gradient and how would this gradient be affected by decreased cardiac output?**

The normal arterial-venous PCO_2 gradient is 4 to 6 mmHg. The arterial-venous PCO_2 gradient is increased by low cardiac output.

❍ **What is the affect of decreased cardiac output on the arterial PO_2?**

In most circumstances, cardiac output has no/minimal influence on arterial blood gas tensions.

Low cardiac output may decrease PaO_2 when there is a high pulmonary shunt fraction (Qs/Qt > 20%). In this case, the decreased cardiac output causes a sufficient reduction in mixed venous saturation such that the venous blood cannot be fully oxygenated during passage through the alveolar capillaries because of the presence of shunting.

❍ **What are the indications for $NaHCO_3$ administration?**

To replace gastroenteric bicarbonate losses, e.g., duodenal fistula.
To replace renal bicarbonate losses, e.g. renal tubular acidosis.
Treatment of acute hyperkalemia.
Treatment of tricyclic antidepressant overdose.
To correct severe metabolic acidosis only in the presence of adequate tissue perfusion and pulmonary ventilation (controversial).

❍ **For every ampule of $NaHCO_3$, how much CO_2 is generated?**

One 50 ml ampule of adult $NaHCO_3$ solution has the following properties, pH = 7.8, pK = 6.1, PCO_2 = 85, 1800 mOsm/L, Na = 892 mmol/L and it contains 44.6 mEq of bicarbonate.

Acutely about 10 to 15% of the administered $NaHCO_3$ is converted to CO_2 gas. Thus, a 44.6 mEq dose of bicarbonate generates 4.5 to 6.7 mEq of CO_2 that corresponds to about 100 to 150 mL of CO_2 gas. To prevent hypercapnia, the drug should be given slowly and necessitates a transient increase in the alveolar ventilation.

Eventually, most/all of the HCO_3^- is converted to CO_2 and 44.6 mEq of CO_2 corresponds to 1,000 ml of CO_2 gas.

❍ **How much sodium bicarbonate would you administer to correct a respiratory acidosis with the pH=7.21 and PCO_2 =90?**

None, its a (partially compensated) respiratory acidosis.

❍ **What are treatments for respiratory acidosis?**

Intubation
Increase minute ventilation
Decrease dead space ventilation
Correct auto-PEEP (air-trapping), e.g., bronchospasm, endotracheal tube obstruction.
Treat (prevent) pulmonary embolism
Reverse muscle weakness
Reverse sedatives and narcotics
Decrease CO_2 production (shivering, hyperthermia and excess glucose load due to hyperalimentation)
Nasal CPAP or BiPAP

❍ **What are the causes of high anion gap metabolic acidosis?**

The addition of strong acids to the ECF, with the exception of HCl, increases the number of unmeasured anions. Frequent causes can be remembered by the mnemonic:

M: methanol, congenital errors of metabolism
U: uremic acidosis
D: diabetic ketoacidosis
P: paraldehyde, phenformin
I: iron, isoniazid
L: lactic acidosis, D-lactic acidosis
E: ethanol, ethylene glycol
S: salicylate poisoning, solvents

❍ **What are the causes of normal anion gap metabolic acidosis?**

A normal anion gap acidosis is associated with a relatively high chloride, i.e. hyperchloremic metabolic acidosis.

<u>Gastrointestinal</u>
Diarrhea
Following bowel preparation
High output ileal fistula or external pancreatic fistula
Ingestion of substances that bind $NaHCO_3$: e.g., cholestyramine

<u>Renal</u>
Proximal (Type II) renal tubular acidosis: bicarbonate wasting due to impaired HCO_3^- reabsorption; distal acidification is intact; associated with hypokalemia
Distal (Type I) renal tubular acidosis: failure of distal nephron urinary acidification; associated with hypokalemia
Distal (Type IV) renal tubular acidosis: major problem is hyperkalemia

Other
Mineralocorticoid deficiency: i.e., hypoaldosteronism
Addition of HCl acid or one of its precursors: e.g., NH_4Cl
Post-hyperventilation metabolic acidosis
Dilutional acidosis: volume infusion with high chloride containing fluids (normal saline)

❍ **How are ketones detected?**

Ketones in urine can be assayed with the Acetest (employs the nitroprusside colorimetric reaction). This test, however, only detects acetoacetate (AcAc) and acetone. If beta-hydroxybutyrate is the predominate species the level of AcAc may be too low to be detected by the Acetest and the test result is falsely negative.

❍ **What is the treatment of alcoholic ketoacidosis?**

Saline infusion, glucose and thiamine.

❍ **What are the different kinds of metabolic alkalosis, how are they diagnosed and treated?**

Chloride responsive, urine chloride < 10 mmol/L
Volume contraction: e.g., diuretics
Loss of gastric acid: e.g., nasogastric suction
Post-hypercapnia

Chloride resistant, urine chloride > 20 mmol/L
High blood pressure: renovascular hypertension, renin producing tumor, hyperaldosteronism (tumor, licorice), Cushing syndrome and exogenous steroid use
Normal blood pressure: laxative abuse, Bartter's syndrome, severe hypokalemia and magnesium deficiency

❍ **What are the causes of respiratory alkalosis (hyperventilation)?**

Hypoxemia or tissue hypoxia
Pulmonary edema
Pulmonary embolism (air, fat, thromboembolism, amniotic fluid, etc).
Shock
Cyanide toxicity
Carboxyhemoglobin
Methemoglobin
Any pulmonary parenchymal disease
Any obstructive pulmonary process

Central
Agitation, anxiety, pain
CNS infection
Central hyperventilation associated with injury to midbrain and upper pons

Metabolic acidosis
DKA
Lactic acidosis
Ingestion of acids: aspirin and alcohol

Other
Sepsis
Pregnancy

Hepatic failure
Respiratory stimulants: progesterone

❍ **What is permissive hypercapnia?**

Permissive hypercapnia is the use of deliberate hypoventilation to prevent barotrauma and volutrauma. The tidal volume and often the respiratory rate are reduced to keep the ventilator pressures and volumes at a safer level. This strategy of ventilator management has gained acceptance in the management of patients with ARDS and severe asthma.

❍ **What would be the likely effect of continuous nasogastric drainage on blood pH?**

Metabolic alkalosis due to the removal of gastric HCl and other secretions. Gastric secretions may have pH as low as 2.0. Treatment is replacement of water, sodium and chloride deficits. During nasogastric suction, alkalemia can be prevented or reduced by administering gastric antacids, H_2-blockers or omeprazole.

❍ **What is the base excess (deficit) and how is it calculated?**

From examination of the equation:

$$CO_2 + H_2O \rightarrow H_2CO_3 \rightarrow H^+ + HCO_3^-$$

It is evident that changes in [CO_2] cause a similar direction change in [HCO_3^-]. The purpose of the base excess (BE) is to define the degree of elevation of [HCO_3^-] which is due only to a metabolic acid-base disorder. This is done mathematically by adjusting for any deviation in the CO_2 from a normal of 40 mm Hg. Base deficit (BD) is - BE. The normal base excess is 0 ± 2 mEq/L.

Base deficit can be determined from a Siggard-Andersen nomogram or it can be calculated according to one of several formulas. A two step method for calculating base deficit follows: During acute changes in respiration, assume that for every 10 mm Hg increase in PCO_2, the pH decreases 0.05 and for every 10 mm Hg decrease in PCO_2, the pH increases 0.1. (Editor's note: Observe the slightly different formuli used to estimate the pH change per PCO_2 change.)

First, determine the "corrected pH." For example, assume an uncorrected blood gas of pH = 7.10 and a PCO_2 of 80 mm Hg. The corrected pH is calculated as 7.40 - 0.005(80-40) = 7.20.

Next, from the predicted pH, calculate the base deficit according to the "2/3 formula":

$$\text{Base deficit} = 2/3 * 100 * (pH_{predicted} - pH_{measured})$$

From above, with pH = 7.10, PCO_2 =80, the predicted pH is 7.20.

$$BD = 2/3 * 100 * (7.20 - 7.10) = 2/3 * 100 * (0.10)$$
$$BD = 6.7 \text{ mEq/L}$$

❍ **What is the base deficit in a pure respiratory acidosis?**

By definition of base deficit, it should be 0. The formula, however, is an estimate, so it does not always exactly equal 0.

❍ **Other than acidosis, what are the causes of low anion gap?**

Hypoalbuminemia and IgG myeloma.

❍ **What is contraction alkalosis?**

Reduction in the circulating blood volume results in a hyperaldosterone state that stimulates sodium retention and loss of potassium and hydrogen ion.

❍ **What are the systemic effects of metabolic alkalosis?**

Respiratory depression
Systemic vasoconstriction
Coronary and cerebral vasoconstriction
Cardiac arrhythmias
Decreased cardiac output
Left shift of the oxyhemoglobin curve.
Glycolysis by disinhibition of phosphofructokinase
Decreased $[K^+]$
Decreased $[Ca^{2+}]$, possible tetany
Decreased renal acid secretion

❍ **What are the systemic effects of metabolic acidosis?**

Increased sympathetic tone leading to hypertension and tachycardia.
Increased release of stress hormones including epinephrine, norepinephrine, glucocorticoids, insulin, catecholamines and renin.
Ventricular dysrhythmias
Tachydysrhythmias with mild acidemia and bradydysrhythmias with severe acidemia
Decreased myocardial contractility
Increased $[K^+]$
Hyperventilation
Systemic arterial vasodilatation
Systemic venous constriction
Increased cerebral blood flow
Rightward shift of the oxyhemoglobin dissociation curve
Increased renal acid secretion

❍ **In a spontaneous ventilating patient, does metabolic alkalosis cause respiratory depression?**

Metabolic acidosis causes hyperventilation, but not all patients with metabolic alkalosis hypoventilate. It is possible to predict the PCO_2 for a given degree of metabolic alkalosis based on the empiric formula:

$$\text{Expected } PCO_2 = 20 + 0.7 * [HCO_3^-] \pm 1.5$$

❍ **What characteristic lab findings are associated with primary adrenal insufficiency?**

Hyperkalemia, hyponatremia, hypoglycemia, azotemia (if volume depletion is present) and a mild metabolic acidosis.

❍ **How should acute adrenal insufficiency be treated?**

Administration of hydrocortisone IV and crystalloid fluids containing dextrose.

❍ **What are the main causes of death during an adrenal crisis?**

Circulatory collapse and hyperkalemia induced arrhythmias.

❍ **What is thyrotoxicosis? What causes it?**

A hypermetabolic state occurring secondary to excess circulating thyroid hormone. Thyrotoxicosis is caused by thyroid hormone overdose, thyroid hyperfunction or thyroid inflammation.

❍ **What are the hallmark clinical features of myxedema coma?**

Hypothermia and coma.

❍ **What is the most important initial step in treating DKA?**

Volume replacement.

❍ **What are the neurologic signs and symptoms associated with hypoglycemia?**

Hypoglycemia may produce behaviorial and neurologic dysfunction. Neurologic manifestations include paresthesias, cranial nerve palsies, transient hemiplegia, diplopia, decerebrate posturing and clonus.

❍ **What laboratory finding occur in diabetic ketoacidosis?**

Elevated beta-hydroxybutyrate, acetoacetate, acetone and glucose. Ketonuria and glucosuria are present. Serum bicarbonate levels, PCO_2 and pH are decreased. Potassium levels may be elevated but will fall when the acidosis is corrected.

❍ **What is the basic treatment for DKA?**

Administer fluids. Start with normal saline, switch to 0.5 normal saline, include potassium (after the patient begins to urinate and if not hyperkalemic). Give insulin, 0.1 units/kg bolus followed by 5 to 10 units/hour. Add glucose to the IV fluid when the glucose level falls below 250 mg/dl and give the patient a phosphate supplement when the level drops below 1.0 mg/dl. Religiously monitor glucose, electrolytes (including anion gap), ketones, volume status and the patient's symptoms.

❍ **A 42 year-old female presents with a history of palpitations, sweating, diplopia, blurred vision and weakness. The husband states she has been confused, most notably before breakfast. What is the probable diagnosis?**

Islet cell tumor of the pancreas, which can result from fasting hypoglycemia.

❍ **What are the key features of non-ketotic hyperosmolar coma?**

Hyperosmolality, hyperglycemia and dehydration. Blood sugar levels are > 800 mg/dl, serum osmolality is > 350 mOsm/kg and serum ketones are negative.

❍ **What is the treatment for non-ketotic hyperosmolar coma?**

This is treated much like DKA with the caveat that the patient requires less insulin. It is important to initiate IV normal saline before giving insulin. Some suggest that an IV insulin bolus is not necessary in this condition.

❍ **Distinguish between lactic acidosis type A and B.**

Type A is associated with inadequate tissue perfusion, the resultant cellular anoxia and subsequent lactate and hydrogen ion accumulation. This condition usually occurs because of shock and is often seen in the ICU. Type B includes all forms of acidosis in which there is no evidence of tissue anoxia.

❍ **What pathognomonic findings and confirmatory lab tests are diagnostic of thyroid storm?**

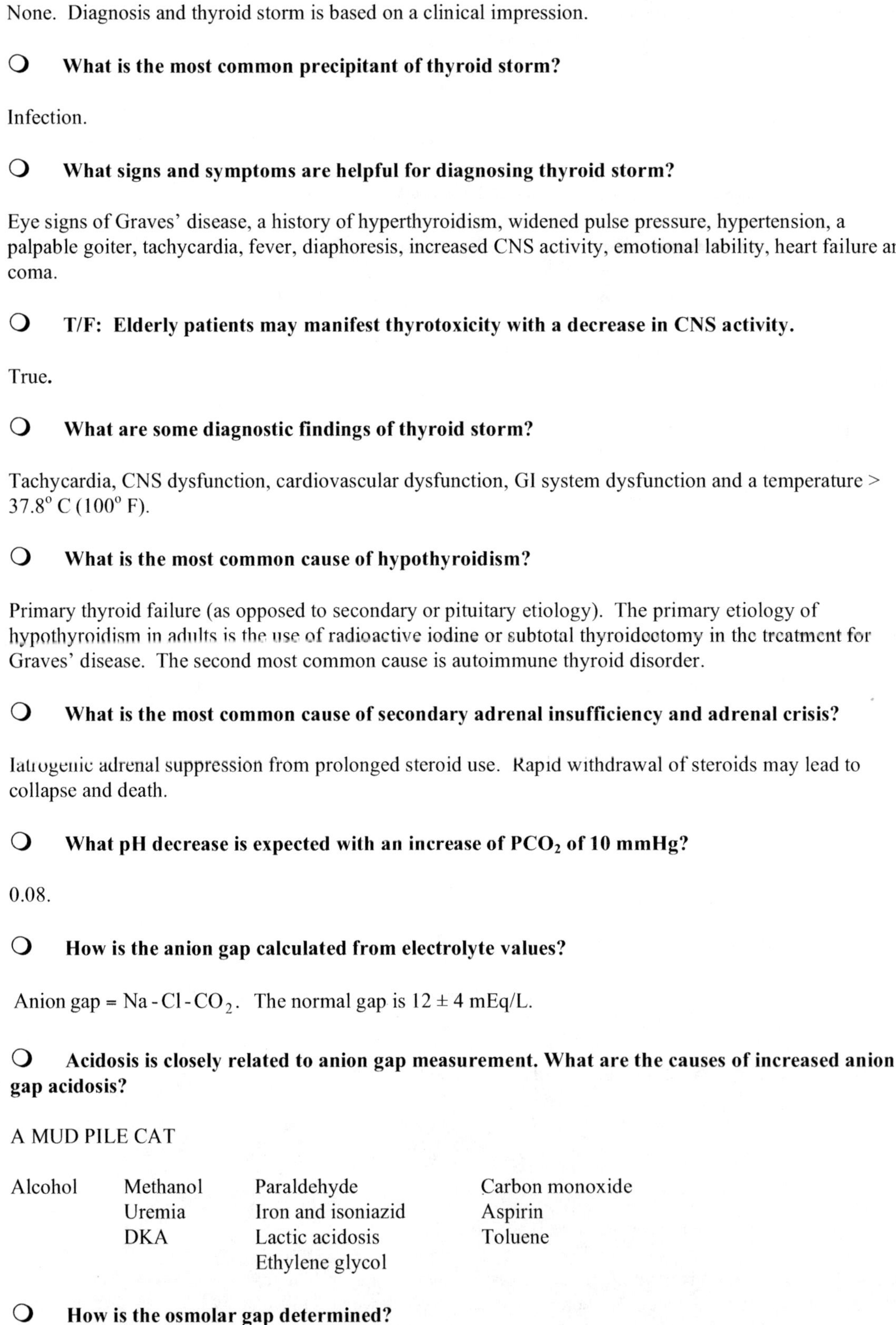

None. Diagnosis and thyroid storm is based on a clinical impression.

❍ **What is the most common precipitant of thyroid storm?**

Infection.

❍ **What signs and symptoms are helpful for diagnosing thyroid storm?**

Eye signs of Graves' disease, a history of hyperthyroidism, widened pulse pressure, hypertension, a palpable goiter, tachycardia, fever, diaphoresis, increased CNS activity, emotional lability, heart failure and coma.

❍ **T/F: Elderly patients may manifest thyrotoxicity with a decrease in CNS activity.**

True.

❍ **What are some diagnostic findings of thyroid storm?**

Tachycardia, CNS dysfunction, cardiovascular dysfunction, GI system dysfunction and a temperature > 37.8° C (100° F).

❍ **What is the most common cause of hypothyroidism?**

Primary thyroid failure (as opposed to secondary or pituitary etiology). The primary etiology of hypothyroidism in adults is the use of radioactive iodine or subtotal thyroidectomy in the treatment for Graves' disease. The second most common cause is autoimmune thyroid disorder.

❍ **What is the most common cause of secondary adrenal insufficiency and adrenal crisis?**

Iatrogenic adrenal suppression from prolonged steroid use. Rapid withdrawal of steroids may lead to collapse and death.

❍ **What pH decrease is expected with an increase of PCO_2 of 10 mmHg?**

0.08.

❍ **How is the anion gap calculated from electrolyte values?**

Anion gap = $Na - Cl - CO_2$. The normal gap is 12 ± 4 mEq/L.

❍ **Acidosis is closely related to anion gap measurement. What are the causes of increased anion gap acidosis?**

A MUD PILE CAT

Alcohol	Methanol	Paraldehyde	Carbon monoxide
	Uremia	Iron and isoniazid	Aspirin
	DKA	Lactic acidosis	Toluene
		Ethylene glycol	

❍ **How is the osmolar gap determined?**

Osmolar gap = measured osmolality - calculated osmolarity

$$\text{Calculated osmolality (mOsm/L)} = 2\ Na^{+} + \frac{\text{glu cos e}}{18} + \frac{BUN}{2.8}$$

(Normal osmolarity = 285 to 295 mOsm/L.)

❍ **How much do different substances contribute to the osmolar gap?**

	mg/dl to increase serum osmol 1 mOsm/L
Methanol	3.2
Ethanol	4.6
Ethylene glycol	6.2
Acetone	5.8
Isopropyl alcohol	6.0

Small amounts of methanol cause greater increases in osmolality. Note that the contribution to an osmolar gap due to ethanol may be calculated. This can be useful when mixed alcohol ingestion is suspected.

❍ **What else can narrow the differential of an anion gap acidosis?**

Methanol:	Visual disturbances and headache are common; can produce wide gaps
Uremia:	Must be advanced to contribute to gap
Diabetic ketoacidosis:	Usually occurs with both hyperglycemia and glucosuria
Alcoholic ketoacidosis:	Often has lower blood sugar and mild or absent glucosuria
Salicylates:	High levels required to contribute to gap
Lactic acidosis:	Can check serum level and has a broad differential
Ethylene glycol:	Causes calcium oxalate or hippurate crystals in urine

❍ **What causes an oxygen saturation curve to shift to the right?**

A shift to the right delivers more O_2 to the tissue. Remember:
CADET! Right face!
Hyper Carbia
Acidemia
2,3 DPG
Exercise
Incr'd Temperature
Release to tissues

❍ **What are the causes of normal anion gap metabolic acidosis?**

USED CRAP
Ureteroenterostomy
Small bowel fistula
Extra chloride (NH_4Cl or amino acid chlorides)
Diarrhea
Carbonic anhydrase inhibitors
Renal tubular acidosis
Adrenal insufficiency
Pancreatic fistula

❍ **What are the two primary causes of metabolic alkalosis?**

Loss of hydrogen and chloride from the stomach and overzealous diuresis with loss of hydrogen, potassium and chloride.

❍ **What are the key predisposing factors to hypoglycemia in diabetic patients on insulin?**

Exercise, poor oral intake, worsening renal function and medications.

❍ **What are the key therapies used to treat nonketotic hyperosmolar coma?**

Intravenous fluids and insulin.

❍ **What precipitants are likely to lead to DKA in an otherwise controlled diabetic?**

Infection, cardiac ischemia, medications, lack of compliance with insulin and diet.

❍ **Which medications are likely to worsen glucose control in a diabetic patient?**

The list is long but includes thiazide diuretics, beta-blockers, steroids, estrogens, phenytoin, cyclosporine and diazoxide.

❍ **What are the key factors leading to hypernatremia in a patient with non-ketogenic hyperosmolar coma?**

Profound dehydration with greater losses of water than salt as well as impaired thirst.

❍ **What are some complications of hypophosphatemia seen in DKA?**

Rhabdomyolysis, cardiac dysfunction, arrhythmias, hemolysis, poor neutrophil function.

❍ **What are the key factors predisposing to diabetic soft tissue infections?**

Microvascular disease, poor wound healing and trauma often masked by neuropathy.

❍ **What are usual glucose levels seen in patients with non-ketogenic coma?**

Often between 800 to 1000 mg/dl.

❍ **What are some agents used to treat severe diabetic gastroparesis?**

Cisapride and metoclopramide. Erythromycin has also been tried in very severe cases.

❍ **What dangerous abdominal infections occur in diabetic patients?**

Emphysematous cholecystitis, ischemic bowel, diverticular abscess, emphysematous pyelonephritis or pyonephrosis.

❍ **What antibiotic regimen is used to treat an elderly diabetic patient admitted to the hospital with a bilobar pneumonia?**

A third generation cephalosporin with erythromycin.

❍ **Diffuse abdominal pain with bloody stools and a high serum lactate in a diabetic might suggest what gastrointestinal disease?**

Ischemic or necrotic bowel.

❍ **What is the most common thyroid abnormality in hospitalized patients with non-thyroidal illness?**

Low T3 concentrations.

❍ **What is the major thyroid hormone binding protein?**

Thyronine binding globulin (TBG).

❍ **What are the components of the widespread changes that can occur in thyroid hormone status during critical illness?**

Alternations in the peripheral metabolism of thyroid hormone, TSH regulation and binding of thyroid hormone to TBG.

❍ **What is the major cause of a decreased T3 concentration in critical illness?**

Impaired peripheral conversion of T4 to T3 by inhibition of the deiodination process.

❍ **What single test of thyroid function would substantiate the diagnosis of euthyroid sick?**

An elevated reverse T3 (rT3).

❍ **What factors decrease TSH secretion?**

Major decreases occur with acute and chronic illness, adrenergic agonists, calorie restriction, dopamine and dopamine agonists, surgical stress and thyroid hormone metabolites. Minor decreases occur with carbamazepine, clofibrate, opiates, phenytoin and somatostatin.

❍ **What effect can pressor doses of dopamine have on TSH regulation?**

It decreases TSH levels to normal in patients with pre-existing hypothyroidism.

❍ **What factors increase T4 binding to TBG?**

Systemic factors such as liver disease, porphyria, HIV infection and the drugs including estrogens, methadone, clofibrate, heroin and tamoxifen.

❍ **What factors decrease T4 binding to TBG?**

Glucocorticoids, androgens, salicylates, phenytoin, tegretol and furosemide.

❍ **What accounts for the low T4 state seen in the critically ill patient?**

A decrease in the binding of T4 to serum protein carriers, decreased TSH level, decreased production of T4 and an increase in the nondeiodinative pathways of T4 metabolism.

❍ **What is the utility of TSH measurements for the evaluation of thyroid disease in critically ill patients?**

A normal test has a high predictive value for normal thyroid function, but an abnormal value of TSH alone is not useful.

❍ **What is the free T4 index (FTI)?**

FTI = Total T4 x T3 resin uptake.

❍ **What does the T3 resin uptake test measure?**

It quantitates the degree of saturation of the binding sites of TBG in the serum by T4 and T3.

❍ **What are the signs/symptoms of hypothyroidism?**

Decreased mental acuity, hoarseness, somnolence, cold intolerance, dry skin, brittle hair and weight gain. Physical exam reveals hypothermia, generalized edema, hypoventilation, sinus bradycardia and possibly hypertension.

❍ **T/F: Cardiac output (CO) is decreased in hypothyroidism.**

True.

❍ **What are the causes of alveolar hypoventilation in myxedematous hypothyroid patients?**

Respiratory center depression with decreased CO_2 sensitivity, defective respiratory muscle strength and airway obstruction due to tongue enlargement.

❍ **What associated laboratory abnormalities are expected in hypothyroidism?**

Hyponatremia, hypoglycemia, hypercholesterolemia and anemia

❍ **What hormone should uniformly be given with thyroid replacement in the hypothyroid myxedematous patient?**

Hydrocortisone.

❍ **What are the hemodynamic changes seen with thyroid storm?**

Tachycardia, increased cardiac output and decreased systemic vascular resistance (SVR).

❍ **What are the ophthalmologic signs in hyperthyroidism?**

Exophthalmos, lid lag, lid retraction and periorbital swelling.

❍ **What are the associated laboratory findings in hyperthyroidism?**

Hypercalcemia, hypokalemia, hyperglycemia, anemia, leukocytosis with a left shift, hyperbilirubinemia and increased alkaline phosphatase.

❍ **What is the initial treatment of thyroid storm?**

Intravenous fluids, acetaminophen, propranolol, propylthiouracil (PTU) and iodine.

❍ **What are the CNS manifestations of myxedema?**

Depression, memory loss, ataxia, frank psychosis and coma.

❍ **What are the common causes of hypothyroidism?**

Cessation of thyroid medication, autoimmune thyroid disease, decreased TSH, radioactive and surgical ablation and iodine deficiency/excess.

❍ **What is the first thyroid function test abnormality seen in hypothyroidism?**

TSH elevation (usually associated with a low T4).

❍ **A 45 year old female presents with a two year history of diffuse, tender thyroid enlargement, lethargy and a 20 pound weight gain. What is the most likely diagnosis?**

Hashimoto's thyroiditis.

❍ **What is the appropriate treatment for the above patient?**

Thyroid replacement therapy.

❍ **In a patient with hypothyroidism, what test would distinguish a hypothalamic defect from a pituitary defect?**

The TRH stimulation test.

❍ **What is the mechanism of action of propylthiouracil (PTU)?**

PTU interferes with the incorporation of iodine into the tyrosine residues of thyroglobulin. It also inhibits the peripheral conversion of T4 to T3.

❍ **What is the preferred definitive non-surgical treatment for Grave's disease?**

131-I radioablation.

❍ **What are the indications for surgical treatment of Grave's disease?**

Extremely large glands, presence of nodules, women in childbearing years and those opposed to radioiodine.

❍ **What is the preferred treatment for toxic multinodular goiter?**

Thyroid resection (lobectomy to total thyroidectomy) because 131-I treatment often needs repeated doses, does not reduce goiter size and may even cause acute enlargement.

❍ **How does PTH effect intestinal absorption of calcium?**

Indirectly through stimulation of vitamin D hydroxylation in the kidney.

❍ **A patient has serum calcium of 13 mg/dl and serum PTH of 400 mEq/ml. What is the most likely diagnosis?**

Primary hyperparathyroidism.

❍ **A 35 year old female has serum calcium of 8.5 mg/dl, serum PTH of 400 mEq/ml and serum creatinine of 5.6 mg/dl. What is the most likely diagnosis?**

Secondary hyperparathyroidism.

❍ **What is the first line therapy for patients with marked hypercalcemia or severe symptoms?**

Intravenous hydration followed furosemide (after achieving euvolemia).

❍ **What are the indications for calcium supplementation after thyroid parathyroid surgery?**

Circumoral paresthesias, anxiety, positive Chvostek's or Trousseau's sign, tetany, ECG changes or serum calcium less than 7.1 ml/dl.

❍ **What is the function of rT3?**

It is biologically inactive.

❍ **What are the signs/symptoms of hyperthyroidism?**

Anxiety, weight loss, heat intolerance, gastrointestinal disturbances, fever, arrhythmias, muscle weakness and tremors.

❍ **What is the differential diagnosis of thyrotoxicosis?**

Sepsis, pheochromocytoma, cocaine/amphetamine overdose, neuroleptic malignant syndrome and malignant hyperthermia.

❍ **What lab values would suggest a central cause of hypothyroidism?**

A low serum T4 in the presence of an inappropriately low TSH level.

❍ **What test is diagnostic for Grave's disease?**

Diffuse, increased uptake of 131I within a symmetrically enlarged gland.

❍ **Which organs are directly affected by PTH?**

Bone and kidney.

❍ **Which organs are affected by vitamin D?**

Intestines and bone.

❍ **What is the differential diagnosis for hypercalcemia?**

Hyperparathyroidism, malignancy, vitamin A or D intoxication, thiazide, diuretics, hyperthyroidism, milk-alkali syndrome, sarcoidosis, immobilization, Paget's disease, lithium, Addisonian crisis and idiopathic hypercalcemia of infancy.

❍ **What are the clinical characteristics associated with primary hyperparathyroidism?**

Urolithiasis, hypercalciuria, emotional disorder, osteoporosis, diminished renal function, hyperparathyroid bone disease and peptic ulcer disease.

❍ **What percentage of primary hyperparathyroidism is caused by a single adenoma?**

Approximately 80%.

❍ **What is the most common cause of hypoparathyroidism?**

Thyroid surgery.

❍ **What is the treatment for acute symptomatic hypocalcemia?**

Intravenous calcium gluconate.

❍ **What is the most common cause of chronic primary adrenal insufficiency (Addison's Disease)?**

Autoimmune disease.

❍ **What are the most common (non-medication) causes of acute secondary adrenal insufficiency?**

Sheehan's Syndrome (postpartum pituitary necrosis), bleeding into a pituitary macroadenoma and head trauma.

❍ **What diseases produce a slow insidious progression to primary adrenal insufficiency?**

Autoimmune diseases, tuberculosis, systemic fungal infections, CMV, Kaposi's sarcoma, metastatic carcinoma and lymphoma.

❍ **In a critical care setting, refractoriness to what type of medication suggests adrenal insufficiency?**

Catecholamines/vasopressors.

❍ **T/F: Orthostatic hypotension and electrolyte abnormalities are more common in primary adrenal insufficiency than secondary.**

True.

❍ **What are the most specific signs of primary adrenal insufficiency?**

Hyperpigmentation of the skin and mucosal membranes.

❍ **What therapy should be instituted in the interval until the results of an ACTH stimulation test is known in a critically ill patient?**

Empiric stress dose steroids should be given to treat a critically ill patient with adrenal insufficiency. Therapy can begin before the ACTH stimulation test using dexamethasone, as this will not interfere with cortisol assays.

❍ **What is the basis of the insulin induced hypoglycemia test for secondary adrenal insufficiency?**

Hypoglycemia induced by insulin stimulates the entire hypothalamus-pituitary-adrenal axis and the sympathetic nervous system. Plasma cortisol levels should exceed 20 g/dl.

❍ **What is the emergent steroid replacement in adrenal insufficiency?**

Hydrocortisone 100 mg intravenously every 8 hours.

❍ **What patients should receive fluorocortisone?**

Those with primary adrenal insufficiency.

❍ **What is the characteristic hemodynamic pattern of adrenal insufficiency?**

Decreased systemic vascular resistance and to a lessor degree, decreased cardiac contractility.

❍ **What drugs can impair cortisol synthesis in the critically ill patient?**

Ketoconazole, etomidate and aminoglutethimide.

❍ **T/F: Corticosteroids are effective in the treatment of septic shock.**

False.

❍ **A 45 year old male develops hypotension, lethargy, a hemoglobin of 12 gm/dl and a blood glucose of 34 mg/dl 24 hours after colectomy. His history is significant for a renal transplant 3 years ago. What is the most likely diagnosis?**

Addisonian crisis.

❍ **Where does aldosterone exert its primary effect?**

On the distal tubules and collecting ducts of the kidney, leading to an increase in the absorption of sodium from the urine in exchange for potassium, thereby aiding in water retention and restoring intravascular volume.

❍ **What are the metabolic effects of catecholamines seen during periods of stress?**

Increased glycogenolysis, gluconeogenesis, lipolysis and ketogenesis and inhibition of insulin use in peripheral tissues.

❍ **What stimuli cause release of ADH (vasopressin)?**

Plasma osmolality greater than 285 mOsm/L, decreased circulating blood volume, catecholamines, the renin-angiotensin system and opiates.

❍ **What are the characteristics of pituitary apoplexy due to hemorrhage?**

Severe headache, sudden visual loss, meningismus, decreased sensorium, bloody CSF and ocular palsy.

❍ **What condition is caused by an insufficient secretion of vasopressin from the posterior pituitary?**

Diabetes insipidus (DI).

❍ **How is the diagnosis of central DI established?**

By the water deprivation test.

❍ **What is the treatment of choice for central DI?**

Administration of exogenous vasopressin.

❍ **T/F: Vasopressin aids in the treatment of renal DI.**

False.

❍ **What is the etiology of Cushing's disease?**

Hypersecretion of ACTH by the pituitary.

❍ **What is the most likely diagnosis in a patient with Cushing's syndrome and low plasma ACTH levels?**

An adrenal tumor.

❍ **T/F: Most patients with Cushing's disease harbor microadenomas that lend themselves to complete surgical resection.**

True.

❍ **What is the most likely diagnosis of a patient who presents with palpitations, headaches, emesis, pounding pulse and retinitis?**

Pheochromocytoma.

❍ **What is the most likely diagnosis of a patient with elevated free cortisol levels, elevated plasma ACTH and persistent elevation of free cortisol after low dose and high dose dexamethasone administration?**

An ectopic source of ACTH production.

❍ **What tests are useful in differentiating hypercortisolism due to pituitary sources of ACTH from those due to ectopic sources of ACTH?**

The dexamethasone suppression test and the metyrapone test.

❍ **What is the most common cause of acute adrenocortical insufficiency?**

Withdrawal of chronic steroid therapy.

❍ **What is the most useful test to evaluate a patient suspected of having adrenocortical insufficiency?**

The rapid ACTH stimulation test.

❍ **What is the test of choice to confirm the clinical suspicion of a pheochromocytoma?**

Measurement of free epinephrine, norepinephrine or their metabolites.

❍ **When should a patient who is undergoing resection of a pheochromocytoma be given pre-operative α-blockers?**

Those patients with severe hypertension.

❍ **What are the classic electrolyte findings of hyperaldosteronism?**

Hypernatremia and hypokalemia.

❍ **What are the clinical manifestations of adrenal insufficiency?**

Fatigue, lethargy, anorexia, weight loss, depression, dizziness, orthostatic hypotension, nausea, vomiting, diarrhea, hyponatremia, hyperkalemia, hypoglycemia, normochromic/normocytic anemia, lymphocytosis and eosinophilia.

❍ **What symptoms should increase the suspicion of adrenal insufficiency in critically ill patients?**

Unexplained circulatory instability, fever without cause, hypoglycemia, hyponatremia, hyperkalemia, eosinophilia, unexplained mental status changes and disparity between the anticipated severity of disease and the actual state of the patient.

❍ **What is the action of ADH (antidiuretic hormone or vasopressin)?**

It causes increased rates of water reabsorption by enhancing hydrosmotic flow within the collecting ducts of the renal medulla.

❍ **What is renal diabetes insipidus (DI)?**

Failure of the kidneys to respond to an appropriate elevation of serum vasopressin.

❍ **What is the syndrome of inappropriate antidiuretic hormone (SIADH)?**

Hypersecretion of vasopressin.

❍ **What tumor most commonly causes ectopic ACTH secretion?**

Small cell carcinoma of the lung.

❍ **What is Waterhouse-Friderichsen syndrome?**

Acute adrenal hemorrhage secondary to sepsis.

❍ **What syndromes are associated with pheochromocytomas?**

MEN-IIa, MEN-IIb, von Recklinghausen's disease, tuberous sclerosis and Sturge-Weber disease.

❍ **What are some causes of factitious hyponatremia?**

Hyperglycemia, hyperlipidemia and hyperproteinemia.

❍ **What medications are likely to lead to acute hyperkalemia in a diabetic patient?**

NSAIDs, ACE inhibitors, beta-blockers, potassium sparing diuretics and salt substitutes (these are usually potassium salts).

❍ **What key complication is seen in diabetic patients on peritoneal dialysis?**

Peritonitis.

❍ **What are the major causes of sudden mortality in diabetic patients on dialysis?**

Vascular events including cardiac ischemia and stroke.

❍ **What are common causes of abdominal pain, nausea and vomiting in a diabetic patient?**

Diabetic gastroparesis, gallbladder disease, pancreatitis and ischemic bowel.

❍ **What usually causes hyperkalemia in a diabetic patient?**

Type IV renal tubular acidosis.

❍ **What refeeding phenomenon is seen in DKA patients undergoing treatment?**

Shifting of potassium, magnesium and phosphorus into cells.

❍ **Atypical chest pain in elderly diabetic individual should always suggest what syndrome?**

Diabetic patients have high a high risk of cardiac ischemia and this must always be strongly considered even if the pain is somewhat atypical.

❍ **What is a necrotizing perineal infection in a diabetic male?**

Fournier's gangrene which can spread very rapidly.

❍ **What necrotizing ear infection is seen in patient with DKA?**

Malignant otitis externa.

❍ **What is the strategy to treat hyperglycemia in pregnancy?**

These patients must have tight control achieved by multiple injections of insulin.

❍ **What adverse effect usually does not occur in a metformin overdose?**

Metformin does not cause hypoglycemia.

❍ **What causes an increase in acetone during treatment of DKA?**

The conversion of beta-hydroxybutyrate into acetone.

❍ **What does profound polyuria and dehydration in DKA reflect?**

Severe osmotic diuresis caused by glycosuria.

❍ **What are the usual causes of metabolic acidosis on patients with diabetes?**

In addition to ketoacidosis, diabetic patients are at risk for renal tubular acidosis as well as lactic acidosis.

❍ **What is the possible adverse effect seen during very rapid correction of severe hyperglycemia?**

Cerebral edema.

❍ **Primary adrenal insufficiency refers to destruction of which component of the hypothalamic-pituitary-adrenal axis?**

Adrenal gland.

❍ **Is orthostatic hypotension and electrolyte abnormalities more common in primary or secondary adrenal insufficiency?**

Primary because of aldosterone deficiency.

❍ **How is a corticotropin (ACTH) stimulation test performed to rule out adrenal insufficiency?**

After a baseline cortisol level is obtained (time 0), 250 ug of cosyntropin is given IV and cortisol levels are obtained at 30 and 60 minutes post-injection. Adrenal function is thought to be normal if the cortisol level drawn 30 or 60 minutes is $\geq$ 20 ug/dl.

❍ **Which patients should receive fludrocortisone?**

Patients with primary adrenal insufficiency should receive fludrocortisone as a substitute for aldosterone, guided by measurements of blood pressure, potassium and plasma renin activity.

❍ **What is the Somogyi phenomenon?**

A hyperglycemic event that results from an over zealous response by counter regulatory hormones during a period of hypoglycemia.

❍ **What is Schmidt's syndrome?**

A type II polyglandular autoimmune disease involving Addison's disease and IDDM, with or without lymphocytic thyroiditis.

❍ **Does the clinical presentation of adrenal insufficiency differ between primary and secondary causes?**

Yes. Primary causes involve the adrenals directly, while secondary causes involve the hypothalamic-pituitary axis. Also, primary insufficiency involves both glucocorticoids and mineral corticoids, while secondary insufficiency will only involve glucocorticoids.

❍ **Is Cushing's disease different than Cushing's syndrome?**

Cushing's disease results from pituitary adenomas, while Cushing's syndrome is elevated cortisol level from various causes, including paraneoplastic syndromes, primary adrenal tumors and exogenous use of cortisol.

❍ **What clinical manifestations are common to all patients with Cushing's syndrome?**

Moon faces, buffalo hump, obesity, hypertrichosis, hypertension, growth retardation, easy bruising, purple striae on the hips and abdomen and amenorrhea in girls.

❍ **How is Cushing's syndrome diagnosed?**

Using the dexamethasone suppression test. Patients with an ACTH dependent condition demonstrate suppression with the larger doses of dexamethasone while those with ectopic tumors cannot be suppressed at any level.

❍ **What type of RTA usually presents as an isolated condition?**

Type I - distal RTA.

❍ **What are the characteristic acid-base/electrolyte abnormalities associated with type I and type II RTA?**

Hypokalemic, hyperchloremic metabolic acidosis.

❍ **What are the characteristic acid-base/electrolyte abnormalities associated with type IV RTA?**

Hyperkalemic, hyperchloremic metabolic acidosis.

❍ **What is the underlying cause of type IV RTA?**

Decreased sodium reabsorption secondary to lack of aldosterone effect.

❍ **What are the sodium concentrations of the most common commercially available IV fluids?**

0.9 normal saline = 154 mEq/l
0.45 normal saline = 77 mEq/l
0.3 normal saline = 54 mEq/l
0.2 normal saline = 33 mEq/l

❍ **What disorder manifests with an autosomal dominant inheritance and is associated with episodic weakness or paralysis along with transient alterations in serum potassium?**

Periodic paralysis, most commonly associated with episodes of hypokalemia, but may occur with hyperkalemia as well. Patients are normal between attacks. The condition becomes progressively worse in adulthood.

❍ **How do you distinguish between endogenously produced and exogenously administered insulin?**

Endogenous - Insulin and C peptide levels correspond.
Exogenously - Insulin level elevated, C peptide level low.

❍ **What is the free T_4 index?**

The free T_4 index = T_4 total x T_3 resin uptake. Use of the free T_4 index allows for integration of binding abnormalities in assessment of thyroid hormone concentrations. In true thyroidal illness, the T_4 total and resin uptake move in parallel giving rise to an increased free T_4 index in hyperthyroidism and a decreased T_4 index in hypothyroidism. In non-thyroidal illness with abnormalities of TBG, the total T_4 and T_3 resin uptake move in reciprocal direction giving a normal free T_4 index.

Hyperthyroidism →	Increased free T_4 Index	=	↑ T_4 x ↑ T_3 Resin
Hypothyroidism →	Decreased free T_4 Index	=	↓ T_4 x ↓ T_3 Resin
Increased TBG →	Normal free T_4 Index	=	↑ T_4 x ↓ T_3 Resin
Decreased TBG →	Normal free T_4 Index	=	↓ T_4 x ↑ T_3 Resin

❍ **Should documented euthyroid sick syndrome be treated with supplemental thyroid hormone?**

No. Treatment has no effect on outcome and may be detrimental.

❍ **Are thyroid function tests necessary prior to the initiation of treatment for thyroid storm?**

No, this is a life threatening process and therapy should be initiated based upon the clinical findings and not waiting for results of thyroid testing.

❍ **Differentiate between non-ketotic hyperosmolar coma and DKA.**

In non-ketotic hyperosmolar coma, glucose is very high, often > 800. The serum osmolality is also very high, with average about 380. Nitroprusside test is negative.
In DKA, glucose is more often in the range of 600. The serum osmolality is approximately 350. Nitroprusside test is positive.

❍ **What focal signs may be present in a patient with non-ketotic hyperosmolar coma?**

These patients may have hemisensory deficits or hemiparesis. 10 to 15% of these patients have a seizure.

❍ **What ECG finding would you expect in myxedema coma?**

Bradycardia.

❍ **What is the major mineralocorticoid?**

Aldosterone. Aldosterone is regulated by the renin angiotensin system. Aldosterone increases sodium reabsorption and increased potassium excretion.

❍ **What key lab findings are expected in SIADH?**

Serum sodium is low and urine sodium is high.

❍ **What are the symptoms of thyrotoxicosis?**

Symptoms include weight loss, palpitations, dyspnea, edema, chest pain, nervousness, weakness, tremor, psychosis, diarrhea, abdominal pain, myalgias and disorientation.

Signs include fever, tachycardia, wide pulse pressure, CHF, shock, thyromegaly, tremor, weakness, liver tenderness, jaundice, stare and hyperkinesis. Mental status changes include somnolence, obtundation, coma or psychosis. Pretibial myxedema may be found.

❍ **What are the common causes of hypercalcemia?**

PAM P SCHMIDT.

P = Parathormone
A = Addison's
M = Multiple myeloma

P = Paget's

S = Sarcoidosis
C = Cancer
H = Hyperthyroidism
M = Milk - alkali syndrome
I = Immobilization
D = Vitamin D excess

T = Thiazides

❍ **When does alcoholic ketoacidosis commonly occur?**

It usually occurs in chronic alcoholics after an interval of binge drinking followed by one to three days of protracted vomiting, abstinence and decreased food intake.

❍ **What type of alcohol ingestion is associated with hypocalcemia?**

Ethylene glycol.

❍ **What type of alcohol ingestion is associated with hemorrhagic pancreatitis?**

Methanol.

❍ **What interstitial lung diseases are associated with diabetes insipidus?**

Eosinophilic granuloma or histiocytosis X.

❍ **What is the common mechanism of hyponatremia in pulmonary tumors and infections?**

Syndrome of inappropriate anti-diuretic hormone production (SIADH).

❍ **What type of lung cancer is commonly associated with hypercalcemia?**

Squamous cell carcinoma. The production of parathormone related peptide could produce hypercalcemia even without bony metastases.

❍ **What non-neoplastic pulmonary disease is often associated with hypercalcemia and hypercalciuria?**

Sarcoidosis.

❍ **What type of lung tumors can cause excessive ACTH production and Cushing's syndrome?**

Small cell carcinoma and carcinoid tumor.

TOXICOLOGY PEARLS

The young physician starts life with twenty drugs for each disease.
The old physician ends life with one drug for twenty diseases.
William Osler

❍ **What is the difference between carbamates and organophosphates?**

Carbamates produce similar symptoms as organophosphates. The bonds in carbamate toxicity are reversible.

❍ **A patient presents with miotic pupils, muscle fasciculations, diaphoresis and diffuse oral and bronchial secretions. The patient has an odor of garlic on his breath. What is the most likely diagnosis?**

Organophosphate poisoning.

❍ **What ECG changes may be associated with organophosphate poisoning?**

Prolongation of the QT interval and ST and T wave abnormalities.

❍ **What is the key laboratory finding in the diagnosis of organophosphate poisoning?**

Decreased red blood cell cholinesterase activity. The serum cholinesterase level (pseudocholinesterase) is more sensitive but less specific. RBC cholinesterase is regenerated slowly and can take months to approach normal levels.

❍ **Treatment of organophosphate poisoning?**

Decontamination, charcoal, atropine and pralidoxime.

❍ **Describe the features of each of the three stages of PCP intoxication.**

Stage I: patient is agitated or violent with normal vital signs.
Stage II: patient is tachycardic, hypertensive and unresponsive to pain.
Stage III: patient is unresponsive, has depressed respirations and seizures.

❍ **Explain how methylene blue functions as an antidote for methemoglobinemia.**

Methylene blue enhances NADPH dependent hemoglobin reduction by acting as a cofactor.

❍ **A patient presents with belladonna alkaloid poisoning resulting in anticholinergic effects. Explain the dangers of treating this patient with physostigmine.**

Physostigmine acts to increase acetylcholine levels. It can precipitate a cholinergic crisis resulting in heart block and asystole.

❍ **Does cyanide cause cyanosis?**

No, except secondarily when bradycardia and apnea precede asystolic arrest. Consider cyanide in an acidotic comatose patient without cyanosis and no hypoxia on ABG.

❍ **For what substances is activated charcoal is not effective?**

Alcohols, ions and acids and bases.

❍ **What is the appropriate treatment for QRS widening in tricyclic antidepressant (TCA) poisoning?**

$NaHCO_3$ is administered intravenously for patients with a QRS > 100 ms $NaHCO_3$ is bolused IV and repeated until the blood pH is between 7.50 and 7.55. An infusion of $NaHCO_3$ is then continued. Potassium levels must be closely monitored.

❍ **What is the appropriate treatment for TCA induced seizures?**

Benzodiazepines and barbiturates are the agents of choice. Phenytoin is not generally effective.

❍ **What is the treatment for TCA induced hypotension if a patient is resistant to fluid boluses and alkalinization?**

A directly acting α-agonist, such as norepinephrine, should be started. Dopamine acts in part by releasing norepinephrine. This agent may be depleted by the reuptake inhibition effect of the TCA.

❍ **What is the clinical presentation of anticholinergic poisoning?**

Mydriasis, tachycardia, hypoactive bowel sounds, urinary retention, dry axilla, hyperthermia and mental status changes. Remember:
Dry as a bone,
Red as a beet,
Mad as a hatter,
Hot as hades,
Blind as a bat.

❍ **What period of observation is required prior to medically clearing a TCA overdose?**

6 hours.

❍ **A 32 year-old female is prescribed meperidine for an open fracture. The patient is chronically on fluoxetine (Prozac). What is a potential complication?**

The serotonin syndrome.

❍ **What signs and symptoms are typical of the serotonin syndrome?**

Agitation, anxiety, sinus tachycardia, hyperthermia, shivering, tremor, hyperreflexia, myoclonus, muscular rigidity and diarrhea.

❍ **What are potential pharmacological treatments for the serotonin syndrome?**

Serotonin antagonists, such as methysergide and cyproheptadine. Benzodiazepines and propranolol have also been successfully employed.

❍ **A patient chronically on Nardil, an MAO inhibitor, drinks a glass of red wine. What potential toxicity may result?**

The tyramine reaction.

❍ **A patient, who ingests a toxic quantity of an MAO inhibitor, is in a hyperadrenergic state with a blood pressure of 240/160. What is the appropriate treatment?**

Short acting antihypertensives, such as phentolamine and nitroprusside, should be employed because the patient may develop refractory hypotension.

❍ **What are the major pharmacological effects of neuroleptics?**

Blockade of dopamine, α-adrenergic, muscarinic and histamine receptors.

❍ **What clinical findings occur with the neuroleptic malignant syndrome?**

Altered mental status, muscular rigidity, autonomic instability, hyperthermia and rhabdomyolysis.

❍ **Will charcoal bind lithium?**

No.

❍ **What are the signs and symptoms of lithium toxicity?**

Neurological signs and symptoms include tremor, hyperreflexia, clonus, fasciculations, seizures and coma. GI signs and symptoms consist of nausea, vomiting and diarrhea. Cardiovascular findings include ST-T wave changes, bradycardia, conduction defects and arrhythmias.

❍ **What is the treatment for lithium toxicity?**

Supportive care, normal saline diuresis, hemodialysis for patients with clinical signs of severe poisoning, renal failure or decreasing urine output.

❍ **What is the pharmacological effect of barbiturates and benzodiazepines?**

Both enhance chloride influx through the GABA receptor associated chloride channel. Benzodiazepines increase the frequency of channel opening, whereas barbiturates increase the duration of channel opening.

❍ **Alkalinization of the urine is beneficial in the management of what barbiturates?**

Long acting barbiturates, such as phenobarbital.

❍ **At what rate is alcohol metabolized in an acutely intoxicated person?**

About 20 mg/dl/hour.

❍ **What is the pharmacological treatment for alcohol withdrawal?**

Benzodiazepines.

❍ **Isopropanol is metabolized by what enzyme to what metabolite?**

Isopropanol is metabolized by alcohol dehydrogenase to acetone in the liver.

❍ **What is a normal osmolar gap?**

< 10 mOsm.

❍ **What is the toxic metabolic end product in methanol poisoning?**

Formic acid.

❍ **What methanol level mandates dialysis?**

25 mg/dL.

❍ **What cofactors are administered to a patient with ethylene glycol poisoning?**

Thiamine and pyridoxine. These cofactors will aid in transforming glyoxylic acid to nontoxic metabolites.

❍ **What are the three clinical phases of ethylene glycol poisoning?**

Stage I: Neurological symptomatology (inebriation)
Stage II: Metabolic acidosis and cardiovascular instability
Stage III: Renal failure

❍ **When should dialysis be initiated for ethylene glycol poisoning?**

For a serum level > 25 mg/dl, renal insufficiency or severe metabolic acidosis.

❍ **What may occur with too large a dose of naloxone in a chronic heroin user?**

Narcan may precipitate acute withdrawal.

❍ **What is the etiology of non-cardiogenic pulmonary edema after heroin injection?**

Unknown. May be delayed 24 to 48 hours after injection, although most patients present soon after injection. Treatment is the same as with any patient with ARDS.

❍ **What acid-base disturbance is typical for salicylate poisoning?**

Mixed respiratory alkalosis and metabolic acidosis.

❍ **T/F: A patient who ingests a large amount of enteric coated aspirin, and is asymptomatic for six hours in the emergency department, may be safely discharged home.**

False. The enteric coating delays absorption.

❍ **What is the treatment for a prolonged prothrombin time in salicylate poisoning?**

Parenteral vitamin K administration. Salicylates inhibit vitamin K epoxide reductase.

❍ **What are the indications for dialysis in salicylate poisoning?**

Persistent CNS involvement, ARDS, renal failure, severe acid-base disturbance, acute salicylate level > 100 mg/dl.

❍ **Can a patient present with salicylate poisoning and a therapeutic level?**

Yes. Patients with chronic salicylate poisoning have a large Vd and thus may present with mental status changes and a therapeutic level.

❍ **What are the 4 stages of acetaminophen (APAP) poisoning?**

Stage I: 30 minutes to 24 hours, nausea and vomiting
Stage II: 24 to 48 hours, abdominal pain and elevated LFTs
Stage III: 72 to 96 hours, LFTs peak, nausea and vomiting
Stage IV: 4 days to 2 weeks, resolution or fulminant hepatic failure

❍ **APAP poisoning produces what type of hepatic necrosis?**

Centrilobular necrosis.

❍ **What is the toxic metabolite of APAP?**

NAPQI. When the glucuronidation and sulfation pathways are saturated, APAP is metabolized by the P-450 system to the toxic metabolite N-acetyl-para-benzoquinoneimine (NAPQI).

❍ **According to the Rumack-Matthew nomogram, at what four hour APAP level should treatment be initiated?**

150 mg/ml.

❍ **How is the nomogram utilized in a patient who ingests an extended relief formulation of APAP?**

4 hour and 8 hour levels are obtained (at least).

❍ **What is the appropriate initial treatment of theophylline induced seizures?**

Benzodiazepines and barbiturates initially. Theophylline induced seizures warrant hemodialysis or hemoperfusion.

❍ **Why is multidose activated charcoal administration advocated for theophylline poisoning?**

Theophylline undergoes enterohepatic circulation.

❍ **What are the indications for Digibind administration in digoxin poisoning?**

Ventricular arrhythmias, hemodynamically significant bradyarrythmias that are unresponsive to standard therapy and potassium level greater than 5.0 mEq/L.

❍ **Why is calcium chloride administration contraindicated in digoxin poisoning?**

Digoxin inhibits the Na^+-K^+-ATPase. This mechanism increases the intracellular concentration of sodium. The sodium-calcium exchange pump is then activated, which leads to high intracellular concentrations of calcium. Calcium chloride administration would further increase intracellular calcium, which worsens myocardial irritability.

❍ **Can the digoxin level be followed after the administration of Digibind?**

No. Extremely elevated digoxin levels are measured after Digibind administration. The assay to measure digoxin does not discriminate between bound and unbound drug.

❍ **A patient on digoxin is bradycardic and hypotensive with significantly peaked T waves. What is the initial line of treatment?**

Administer 10 vials of Digibind intravenously while simultaneously treating the presumed hyperkalemia with insulin, glucose and sodium bicarbonate. Kayexalate is another therapeutic option.

❍ **What is the antidote for beta-blocker poisoning?**

Glucagon.

❍ **What is the biochemical rational for treatment with glucagon?**

Glucagon receptors, located on myocardial cells, are G protein coupled receptors that activate adenylate cyclase, leading to increased levels of intracellular c-AMP.

❍ **A 25 year old female presents status post ingestion of a sustained release calcium channel blocker. What is the disposition?**

Hospital admission to a monitored setting. Sustained release preparations have the capability of producing delayed toxicity.

❍ **What is the treatment for calcium channel blocker poisoning?**

IV calcium, isoproterenol, glucagon, transvenous pacer, atropine and vasopressors, such as norepinephrine, epinephrine or dopamine.

❍ **What is the mechanism and treatment for clonidine induced hypotension?**

Mechanism: Decreased cardiac output secondary to a decreased sympathetic outflow from the CNS.
Treatment: IV fluid administration and dopamine.

❍ **What typical eye response is related to clonidine poisoning?**

Pinpoint pupils.

❍ **Why does IV phenytoin administration lead to cardiovascular toxicity?**

The propylene glycol diluent is a myocardial depressant and vasodilator.

❍ **What are the four stages of iron poisoning?**

Stage I: Initial hour: gastrointestinal symptomatology, including abdominal pain, vomiting and diarrhea
Stage II: 6 to 24 hours: quiescent period during which time iron is absorbed
Stage III: > 12 hours: shock, metabolic acidosis, hepatic dysfunction, heart failure, cerebral dysfunction and renal failure
Stage IV: 1 day to 1 week: gastric outlet or small bowel obstruction secondary to scarring

❍ **What is the antidote to iron poisoning?**

Deferoxamine.

❍ **Carbon tetrachloride poisoning produces what type of liver damage?**

Centrilobular necrosis.

❍ **Methylene chloride is metabolized to which toxin?**

Carbon monoxide.

❍ **Oral hydrofluoric acid exposure may result in what life threatening electrolyte abnormalities?**

Hyperkalemia and hypocalcemia.

❍ **What is the antidote for cutaneous hydrofluoric acid exposures?**

Intradermal injection or intra-arterial infusion of calcium gluconate.

❍ **What enzyme is inhibited by organophosphates?**

Cholinesterase.

❍ **What are the two principal antidotes used for organophosphate poisoning?**

Atropine and pralidoxime.

❍ **What is the mechanism of cyanide toxicity?**

Electron transport inhibition. Cyanide binds to the ferric ion in cytochrome oxidase.

❍ **What items are contained within the Lilly Cyanide Antidote Kit?**

Amyl nitrite for inhalation, sodium nitrite and sodium thiosulfate for infusion. The nitrites induce methemoglobinemia. Thiosulfate enhances rhodanese activity and accelerates the degradation of cyanomethemoglobin.

❍ **What antihypertensive agent may induce cyanide poisoning?**

Nitroprusside.

❍ **What is "arterialization" of venous blood?**

High partial pressure of oxygen in venous blood. In cyanide poisoning, electron transport is inhibited leading to an inability to utilize oxygen as an electron acceptor. Consequently, venous blood contains a high partial pressure of oxygen.

❍ **A patient who is chronically on an oral hypoglycemic agent presents with a depressed mental status. Glucose level is 20 mg/dl. After an amp of D50 is administered, the patient returns to a normal mental status rapidly. What is the disposition of this patient?**

Hospital admission with serial glucose level determination. Oral hypoglycemic agents are long acting.

❍ **What is the antidote for isoniazid induced seizures?**

Pyridoxine.

❍ **A patient is administered a topical Cetacaine spray prior to endoscopy. The patient then complains of dyspnea and is noted to be cyanotic. What is the antidote?**

Methylene blue. Methemoglobinemia developed secondary to the local anesthetic.

❍ **A 32 year old female complains of vomiting and diarrhea which developed eight hours after ingesting an unknown type of mushroom. Is the mushroom potentially a hepatotoxin?**

Yes. Hepatotoxic cyclopeptide containing mushrooms induce a delayed onset of gastrointestinal symptomatology, generally occurring 6 hours after ingestion.

❍ **Under what circumstance is the use of Done's nomogram appropriate?**

Only when the patient has an acute single ingestion of a non-enteric coated ASA without recent prior use.

❍ **How does N-acetylcysteine (NAC, Mucomyst) work?**

NAC enters cells and is metabolized to cysteine, which serves as a glutathione precursor. Glutathione is a free radical scavenger.

❍ **Which measure of hepatic function is a better prognostic indicator in APAP overdose: liver enzyme levels or bilirubin level and prothrombin time?**

Bilirubin level and prothrombin time.

❍ **Clonidine is a centrally acting presynaptic α-2 adrenergic agonist that decreases the central sympathetic outflow. Although its primary use is to treat hypertension, clonidine has additional value in blunting withdrawal symptoms from opiates. A clonidine overdose closely resembles an overdose with which class of drugs?**

Opiates.

❍ **Which agent is a useful antidote for clonidine overdose?**

Naloxone.

❍ **What are a few substances that have anticholinergic properties?**

Antihistamines, cyclic antidepressants, phenothiazine, atropine, amanita mushrooms and Jimson weed.

❍ **What ECG abnormality is most common in patients who suffer from anticholinergic toxicity?**

Sinus tachycardia. Other dangerous arrhythmias include conduction defects and ventricular tachycardia.

❍ **Intermediate chain aliphatic hydrocarbons are responsible for most exposures to hydrocarbons. What is the most common complication of these liquids?**

Chemical pneumonitis caused by direct injury to the pulmonary parenchyma after aspiration.

❍ **Aromatic hydrocarbons, such as toluene present in glue, can be sniffed. Resulting effects most closely resemble those of what other class of compounds?**

Inhalational anesthetic agents. Initial excitatory response gives way to CNS depression.

❍ **Can solvent abusers be "scared to death"?**

Yes. Halogenated hydrocarbons can "sensitize" myocardium to catecholamines. Exertion or fright can lead to fatal arrhythmias.

❍ **Is charcoal useful for hydrocarbon ingestion?**

No.

❍ **T/F: Serum potassium tends to increase with digitalis intoxication.**

True.

❍ **T/F: A patient with acute digitalis overdose presents with frequent multifocal PVCs, peaked T waves and a K^+ of 6.2 mEq/L. The correct treatment is to first administer $CaCl_2$ as this is the fastest acting agent for reducing hyperkalemia.**

False. Although $CaCl_2$ is the fastest acting agent for treating hyperkalemia, administering Ca^+ to a patient with digitalis induced cardiac toxicity may cause serious arrhythmias.

❍ **What are the signs and symptoms of phenytoin toxicity?**

Seizure, heart blocks, bradyarrhythmias, hypotension and coma.

❍ **What is the treatment for a phenytoin overdose?**

Systemic support, charcoal, atropine for bradyarrhythmias and phenobarbital for seizures.

❍ **Nystagmus, ataxia and lethargy generally occur at what serum level of phenytoin?**

Nystagmus: 20 mg/ml
Ataxia: 30 mg/ml
Lethargy: 40 mg/ml

❍ **Beta-adrenergic antagonists have what three main effects on the heart?**

Negative chronotropy and inotropy and decreased AV nodal conduction velocity.

❍ **T/F: Beta-adrenergic antagonists can cause mental status changes and seizures.**

True.

❍ **A patient with a history of cyclic antidepressant overdose is found awake and alert by paramedics. What is the prognosis?**

Not enough information to assess. 25 to 50% of patients who die from cyclic overdose are awake and alert at the scene.

❍ **In cyclic antidepressant overdose, is the degree of toxicity closely related to QRS duration?**

QRS > 100 ms has a specificity of 75% and a sensitivity of 60% for serious complications. A normal ECG will not rule out a serious overdose. Of those with QRS > 100 ms, 30% will seize. Of those with QRS > 160 ms, 50% will develop arrhythmias.

❍ **T/F: Naloxone will move intra-alveolar fluid into the capillaries in a patient with heroin-induced pulmonary edema.**

False.

❍ **What is the treatment for narcotic overdose?**

Naloxone. Naloxone's duration of action is about 1 hour. Continuous infusion may be required.

❍ **What type of nystagmus is seen with PCP overdose?**

Vertical, horizontal and rotary. Vertical nystagmus is not common with other conditions/ingestions. The most common findings of a PCP overdose are hypertension, tachycardia and nystagmus.

❍ **What are the two most common complications of PCP intoxication?**

Hyperpyrexia and rhabdomyolysis.

❍ **What is the most common cause of chronic heavy metal poisoning?**

Lead.

❍ **Organophosphates are found in what kinds of compounds?**

Pesticides, flame retardants and plasticizers.

❍ **What is the mechanism of toxicity of organophosphate compounds?**

Inactivation of acetylcholinesterase at synapses of the central and peripheral nervous system.

❍ **What is the clinical presentation of acute organophosphate poisoning?**

Evidence of cholinergic excess, which includes:

Salivation, Lacrimation, Urination, Defecation, Gastrointestinal distress and Emesis (SLUDGE)
Pupil constriction, Bradycardia, Bronchoconstriction
Muscle weakness, Fasciculation
CNS effects: lethargy, confusion, agitation, coma and seizure

❍ **What is the usual cause of death in patients poisoned with organophosphates?**

Respiratory failure due to paralysis of respiratory muscles, diminished respiratory drive, copious pulmonary secretions and bronchoconstriction.

❍ **Skeletal muscle manifestation of organophosphate poisoning includes what symptoms?**

Fasciculation, weakness, involuntary twitching and hyperreflexia.

❍ **What is the drug of choice for counteracting the muscarinic effects of organophosphate poisoning?**

Atropine. Adequate atropinization is evidenced by the elimination of the muscarinic (SLUDGE) and CNS symptoms. High doses may be required.

❍ **What is the role of pralidoxime (2-PAM) in the management of the organophosphate poisoned patients?**

Reactivates acetylcholinesterase by uncoupling the organophosphate from the enzyme's binding site.

❍ **Cyanide's most important physiologic effect is a result of its inhibition of what mitochondrial enzyme?**

Cytochrome oxidase (cytochrome A_3), which catalyzes the final step in the electron transport chain, converting molecular oxygen to water.

❍ **What signs and symptoms are characteristic of cyanide poisoning?**

Odor of bitter almonds
CNS dysfunction - coma, obtundation, lethargy, stupor, agitation, anxiety and seizure
Gastrointestinal - abdominal pain and vomiting
Cardiovascular - hypotension and bradycardia

❍ **What metabolic disorder attends cyanide poisoning?**

Metabolic acidosis (lactic acidosis) secondary to anaerobic respiration.

❍ **On what basis is the diagnosis of cyanide poisoning made when patients present to the emergency department?**

Clinical grounds.

❍ **Does hyperbaric oxygen have a proven role in the management of cyanide poisoned patients?**

No.

❍ **What are the most important diagnostic studies to obtain in patients who have sustained smoke inhalation injury?**

Arterial blood gas, carboxyhemoglobin level, methemoglobin level and CXR. Hydrogen cyanide poisoning should be suspected in patients with profound metabolic acidosis.

❍ **What are the indications for emergent hyperbaric oxygen therapy?**

1) Loss of consciousness
2) Focal neurologic findings
3) Carboxyhemoglobin level greater that 25%
4) Myocardial ischemia
5) Pregnancy

❍ **What is the treatment for patients with asymptomatic CO level (< 25%)?**

100% oxygen by mask followed by observation.

❍ **What symptoms are typical of mild to moderate carbon monoxide (CO) poisoning?**

Headache, nausea, dizziness, weakness and difficulty concentrating.

❍ **What illnesses may be mimicked by carbon monoxide poisoning?**

Influenza, gastroenteritis and food poisoning.

❍ **How does carbon monoxide cause toxicity?**

Carbon monoxide has an affinity for hemoglobin 200 to 250 times greater than oxygen and displaces oxygen from its binding sites. It also causes a leftward shift of the oxyhemoglobin dissociation curve. These effects decrease oxygen delivery to the tissues.

❍ **What is the initial recommended treatment for carbon monoxide poisoning?**

100% oxygen by facemask or endotracheal tube.

❍ **What is the half life of COHb at 2.5 atm (in the hyperbaric chamber)?**

Approximately 20 minutes.

❍ **T/F: In a lethargic or unresponsive ethanol intoxicated patient, there is little need to search for further pathology.**

False. Before attributing a change in mental status simply to alcohol intoxication other etiologies such as hypoglycemia, subdural hematoma, hypothermia, subarachnoid bleed or ingestion of other drugs must be considered.

❍ **What is the most common arrhythmia induced by a heavy ethanol binge?**

Atrial fibrillation.

❍ **In chronic alcohol users, alcohol withdrawal seizures occur approximately how many hours after cessation of heavy alcohol consumption?**

6 to 48 hours from the time of the last drink.

❍ **Delirium tremens occurs how long after the cessation of alcohol consumption?**

On average 3 to 5 days.

❍ **What is the only proven means to enhance ethanol elimination?**

Hemodialysis.

❍ **What class of drugs is best to treat delirium tremens?**

Benzodiazepines.

❍ **Chronic alcohol abusers who are poorly nourished may develop Wernicke's encephalopathy as a result of what deficiency?**

Thiamine.

❍ **What is the classic triad of Wernicke's encephalopathy?**

Global confusion, oculomotor disturbances and ataxia.

❍ **What is the likely diagnosis in a chronic heavy alcohol abuser with the following history: little or no alcohol ingested for the past 1 to 2 days, abdominal pain, recurrent nausea and vomiting, decreased food intake, dehydration, a high anion gap acidosis and positive serum and urine ketones?**

Alcoholic ketoacidosis.

❍ **Which of the following alcohol ingestions is likely to cause ketosis but not a metabolic acidosis: methanol, isopropyl alcohol or ethylene glycol?**

Isopropyl alcohol.

❍ **T/F: A given blood level of isopropanol is more toxic than the same blood ethanol level.**

True.

❍ **What is the major metabolite of isopropyl alcohol?**

Acetone.

❍ **Which of the following alcohol intoxications is most likely to present with blurred vision or blindness: methanol, isopropyl alcohol or ethylene glycol?**

Methanol.

❍ **Which of the following alcohol intoxications may present with calcium oxalate crystals in the urine: methanol, isopropyl alcohol or ethylene glycol?**

Ethylene glycol.

❍ **T/F: Ethylene glycol is found most commonly in antifreeze/coolant fluids.**

True.

❍ **What constellation of findings should prompt consideration of ethylene glycol toxicity?**

Ethanol like intoxication (with no odor), large anion gap acidosis, increased osmolar gap, altered mental status leading to coma and calcium oxalate crystals in the urine.

❍ **What is the accepted antidote for methanol poisoning?**

Ethanol administration. Patients with high serum levels or who are very ill may also require hemodialysis.

❍ **A patient presents with complaints of headache, increasing lethargy, nausea and vomiting and decreased visual acuity. The patient is noted to have a significant metabolic acidosis and an increased osmolar gap. What is the likely etiology?**

Methanol poisoning.

❍ **How many hours after pure methanol ingestion before symptoms are noted?**

6 to 24 hr.

❍ **Hypocalcemia is most common in which alcohol ingestion: ethylene glycol, methanol, ethanol or isopropyl alcohol?**

Ethylene glycol.

❍ **In which type of alcohol ingestion may the urine appear to fluoresce under a Woods lamp?**

Ethylene glycol.

❍ **T/F: In a patient with a significant theophylline poisoning and recurrent vomiting, activated charcoal should be discontinued.**

False. For a patient with recurrent vomiting metoclopramide or ondansetron can be given to decrease vomiting and a slow continuous infusion through a nasogastric tube may be tried.

❍ **In life threatening theophylline overdose, what is definitive management?**

Charcoal hemoperfusion.

❍ **What are the indicators for charcoal hemoperfusion in theophylline overdose?**

Theophylline level > 90 mcg/ml at any time or a level > 40mcg/ml and any of the following: protracted vomiting (unable to tolerate charcoal), seizures, hypotension and ventricular arrhythmias.

❍ **Which of the following is not a common manifestations of significant theophylline toxicity: seizures, dysrhythmias, hypotension or visual disturbances?**

Visual disturbances.

❍ **T/F: Chronic exposure to theophylline leads to toxicity at lower levels than acute exposures.**

True.

❍ **When will sustained released theophylline tablets produce peak plasma concentrations?**

12 to 24 hours after ingestion.

❍ **What are the typical CNS findings in mild lithium toxicity?**

Rigidity, tremor and hyperreflexia.

❍ **What are the typical CNS findings in severe lithium toxicity?**

Seizures, coma and myoclonic jerking.

❍ **What is the primary system affected by lithium toxicity?**

Central nervous system.

❍ **T/F: Hydration status has little effect on lithium toxicity.**

False. Patients with lithium toxicity and dehydration require aggressive rehydration to establish euvolemia and normal urine output, while avoiding fluid overload.

❍ **What constitutes definitive therapy for moderate to severe lithium toxicity?**

Hemodialysis.

❍ **What are the indications for hemodialysis in lithium toxicity?**

Serum lithium level above 4.0 mEq/l, renal failure and severe clinical symptoms.

❍ **A 23 year old female arrives in the ED at 1:00 a.m. stating that she took three quarters of a bottle of Tylenol 1 hour ago. At what time should the acetaminophen level be drawn?**

The first acetaminophen level should be drawn at 5:00 a.m., 4 hours after ingestion. Waiting four hours after ingestion allows for complete absorption.

❍ **What is the primary organ system for acetaminophen metabolism?**

Acetaminophen is primarily metabolized in the liver. In adults, the primary mechanism for hepatic metabolism is glucuronidation.

❍ **What is the antidote for acetaminophen poisoning?**

N-acetylcysteine (NAC).

❍ **Is NAC effective after a dose of activated charcoal?**

There is no clinical evidence that the administration of activated charcoal inhibits the efficacy of oral N-acetylcysteine.

❍ **Within what period of time will NAC treatment provide maximum protection against hepatotoxicity?**

When given within 8 hours of an acetaminophen overdose. The efficacy of NAC decreases after this period.

❍ **What are the side effects of NAC?**

Nausea and vomiting are frequent side effects since NAC has an unpleasant smell and tastes like rotten eggs. Metoclopramide can be given to decrease vomiting.

❍ **Should acetaminophen levels be drawn on all patients who may have had an ingestion?**

Yes. Signs and symptoms of acetaminophen toxicity may be minimal in the first 8 hours. This is the time period that NAC is maximally effective. Many nonprescription medicines and pain medications contain acetaminophen.

❍ **A 32 year old man arrives in the ED after ingesting an unknown substance. What simple test can be done at the bedside to test for the presence of salicylates?**

The ferric chloride test is a qualitative, colorimetric test that can be done on urine. 10% ferric chloride is added drop by drop to 1 ml of urine obtained at least 2 hours after ingestion. A purple or purple-brown color indicates the presence of salicylate.

❍ **What mechanisms are used to enhance the elimination of a salicylate ingestion?**

Salicylate elimination can be enhanced by the use of multi-dose activated charcoal, by alkalinization of the urine to a pH between 7.5 to 8.0 and by hemodialysis.

❍ **What are the indications for hemodialysis of aspirin ingestion?**

Severe neurologic dysfunction, pulmonary edema, clinical deterioration despite decontamination and urine alkalinization, inability to alkalinize the urine or renal failure.

❍ **What methods can be used to decrease absorption of aspirin ingestion?**

Gastric lavage, multi-dose activated charcoal and whole bowel irrigation may be used to decrease absorption of salicylates.

❍ **What electrolyte deficiency must be corrected to maintain an alkaline pH of the urine?**

Hypokalemia.

❍ **What are the signs and symptoms of chronic salicylate intoxication?**

Hyperventilation, fever, dehydration, tremor, papilledema, agitation, paranoia, bizarre behavior, memory deficits, confusion and stupor. Neurologic abnormalities are more common in chronic ingestions.

❍ **A 70 year old women with a history of arthritis is brought to the ED by her son. He states that she is confused and hallucinating. The last time he saw her, she was "as sharp as a tack". She is not taking any medication according to her doctor. What ingestion should be considered?**

Chronic salicylate ingestion may present with delirium or dementia. Salicylates are contained in many over the counter preparations and may not be considered medication by patients.

❍ **What are the central anticholinergic toxic effects of cyclic antidepressants?**

Respiratory depression, agitation, lethargy, hallucinations, hyperthermia, ataxia, choreoathetoid movements, seizures and coma.

❍ **What are the peripheral anticholinergic toxic effects of cyclic antidepressants?**

Hypotension, decreased GI motility, dry flushed skin, urinary retention, sinus tachycardia and AV block.

❍ **What are the ECG findings in cyclic antidepressant overdoses?**

Sinus tachycardia, QRS prolongation and rightward terminal 40 msec of the frontal plane QRS complex (an R wave in lead aVR).

❍ **What level correlates with toxicity in cyclic antidepressant overdoses?**

There is no correlation between serum levels and symptoms of serious toxicity.

❍ **What classes of antidysrhythmic agents are contraindicated in cyclic antidepressant overdoses?**

Type 1A and 1C antidysrhythmic agents. They have quinidine like effects on the sodium channels and will enhance the cardiotoxicity of the cyclic antidepressants.

❍ **What are the acute manifestations of MAO inhibitor toxicity?**

Tachycardia, hypertension, neurologic and neuromuscular symptoms. Neurologic symptoms include irritability, confusion lethargy and hallucinations. Neuromuscular findings include hyperreflexia, tremors, fasciculations, myoclonus, rigidity and seizures.

❍ **A 30 year old man with a history of depression, on Nardil, presents to the ED with severe headache, nausea and vomiting after going to a wine and cheese party. His blood pressure is 190/130. What is the likely cause of his symptoms?**

Cheese has high concentrations of tyramine. MAOIs block the deamination of tyramine. This leads to an increase in pressor amines, which results in severe hypertension.

❍ **What over the counter cold medications should not be used by people taking MAOIs?**

Decongestants, antihistamines and products containing dextromethorphan

❍ **What is the most important first step in managing a patient with suspected poisoning?**

Not to forget your ABC's. Securing a patient's airway, allowing for adequate respiration (breathing) and supporting the circulation take precedence over other considerations.

❍ **What are the components of a "coma cocktail?"**

Dextrose, thiamine and naloxone.

❍ **What are the contraindications to the use of activated charcoal?**

Activated charcoal is useful in the absorption of a wide variety of compounds. However, it is not recommended in the ingestion of nonabsorbable corrosives such as strong acids or alkali and its presence obscures evaluation of injury by endoscopy. In hydrocarbon toxicity, where GI absorption is low, any provocation of vomiting might increase the chance of pulmonary aspiration.

❍ **A 20 year old man ingests potassium supplements and a large quantity of other medications, including amitryptyline, carbamazepine and acetaminophen. Should he receive activated charcoal?**

Like acids and alkali, ionized electrolytes such as potassium and the salts of bromide, cyanide, arsenic, fluoride, lithium and iron are not appreciably absorbed by charcoal. However, the other agents ingested here have significant GI absorption by activated charcoal. Although there is not enough information here to make definitive treatment priorities, it should be emphasized that in the setting of an unclear history of ingestion the benefits of charcoal are likely to outweigh its risks.

❍ **What is the osmolar gap?**

A discrepancy between calculated and measured serum osmolarity that occurs with certain low molecular weight toxins. Serum osmolarity normally ranges between 285 and 295 mOsm and equals $2(Na^+)$ + (BUN)/2.8 + (glucose)/18 + (ethanol)/4.6. A normal osmolar gap is less than 10.

❍ **What two agents produce severe metabolic acidosis and widen both the anion and osmolar gaps?**

Methanol and ethylene glycol.

❍ **The triad of depressed mental status, respiratory depressions and "pinpoint pupils" suggest what overdose?**

Opioid overdose.

❍ **Seizures are a manifestation of toxicity for which opioids in particular?**

Propoxyphene and meperidine. Even within a therapeutic dosing range, normeperidine, a meperidine metabolite, may lower the seizure threshold, especially in the setting of renal insufficiency.

❍ **You admit a pleasant elderly man with previously stable coronary artery disease for symptoms of unstable angina, four times in two weeks. A careful history elicits only a predeliction for eating barbecue grilled hot dogs. It is February. What laboratory test should you order?**

Carboxyhemoglobin level. The most common cause of death by poisoning in the United States is carbon monoxide poisoning and the presentation of toxicity with this agent can be as unlikely as new onset or worsening angina during the winter months in a patient with a charcoal or gas heater.

❍ **All suspected overdoses should be screened for what toxicity?**

Acetaminophen. It is ubiquitous, frequently a part of multi-drug poisonings and, in overdose, has deadly delayed consequences.

❍ **A 50 year old woman with a past history significant only for G6PD deficiency is being treated in the CCU for post-MI angina and VT. She complains to you of feeling very weak and having a terrible headache. You note dyspnea on exam, although the lung fields are clear and saturation on pulse oximetry is 100%. Her medications include IV nitroglycerin and lidocaine. After you draw blood for chemistry analysis, you note that it looks like chocolate. What toxicity should you consider?**

Methemoglobinemia. G6PD deficiency and the administered lidocaine and nitroglycerin would all predispose this patient. Oxygen saturation on pulse oximetry is typically (and falsely) elevated. Another classic finding is “chocolate colored” venous blood that retains this shade on exposure to air.

❍ **What antidote is available to treat the above toxicity?**

Methylene blue.

❍ **You are treating a 25 year old South American man who was resuscitated in an international airport terminal. His initial rhythm was ventricular fibrillation. Presently he is tachycardic and hypotensive. What drug toxicity and specific treatment modality should be strongly considered?**

Cocaine smugglers may swallow packets of cocaine (“body packers”) and develop significant toxicity if the packets rupture, including arrhythmias, hyperthermia and intractable seizures. Whole bowel irrigation eliminates drug packets from the GI tract.

❍ **What major pathophysiologic mechanisms underlie cocaine’s toxic effects on the cardiovascular system?**

1) Potentiates the actions of the sympathetic nervous system by blocking presynaptic reuptake of dopamine and norepinephrine. This results in increased inotropy, tachycardia and hypertension.
2) Induces coronary artery spasm, with possible increased focal effects in atherosclerotic areas.
3) Induces platelet activation and aggregation, which may help to induce thrombus formation.

❍ **What arrhythmia is pathognomonic for digoxin toxicity?**

Bidirectional ventricular tachycardia. It is characterized by a regular (beat-to-beat) alteration of two QRS complexes. The site of origin may be junctional or ventricular.

❍ **What happens to the digoxin level immediately after the administration of digoxin Fab fragments?**

Total serum digoxin levels rise, sometimes more than tenfold, secondary to displacement of drug from tissue and extracellular compartments into plasma where it binds to the Fab fragments. When there is concern of a possible rebound phenomenon (Fab-digoxin complex dissociation in patients with renal failure and delayed drug excretion) free plasma levels should be measured.

❍ **A 13 year old boy is brought into the emergency department with what you believe to be a cholinesterase inhibitor poisoning. After initial stabilization what study can you obtain to definitively establish the diagnosis?**

Plasma and red blood cell cholinesterase levels.

❍ **What drugs should be avoided in G-6-PD deficiency?**

ASA, phenacetin, primaquine, quinine, quinacrine, nitrofurantoin, sulfamethoxazole, sulfacetamide and methylene blue. These are all oxidants.

❍ **Antidote for lead?**

Dimercaptosuccinic acid (DMSA) or calcium EDTA.

❍ **Name five drugs or conditions that cause hypertension or tachycardia.**

Sympathomimetics
Withdrawal
Anticholinergics
MAO Inhibitors
Phencyclidine (PCP). Mnemonic for this is SWAMP.

❍ **Name six common drugs that can cause hyperthermia.**

Salicylates
Anticholinergics
Neuroleptics
Dinitrophenols
Sympathomimetics and PCP.

❍ **What is a mnemonic for remembering drugs that are radiopaque?**

BAT CHIPS!

B = barium
A = antihistamines
T = tricyclic antidepressants

C = chloral hydrate, calcium, cocaine condoms
H = heavy metals
I = iodine
P = phenothiazines, potassium
S = slow-release (enteric coated) bezoars of aspirin

❍ **Match the poison with the antidote.**

1) Acetaminophen	**a) Deferoxamine**
2) Anticholinergics	**b) Digoxin antibody**
3) Arsenic	**c) Dimercaptosuccinic acid or penicillamine**
4) Carbon monoxide	**d) Acetylcysteine (Mucomyst)**
5) Digoxin	**e) Oxygen**
6) Iron	**f) Atropine and 2-PAM**
7) Lead	**g) Physostigmine (rarely; may cause cholinergic toxicity)**
8) Mercury	**h) Calcium EDTA or penicillamine**
9) Methanol or ethylene glycol	**i) Naloxone**
10) Narcotics	**j) Ethanol**
11) Organophosphates	**k) Penicillamine**

Answers: (1) d, (2) g, (3) k, (4) e, (5) b, (6) a, (7) h, (8) c, (9) j, (10) i and (11) f.

❍ **Describe the clinical characteristics of carboxyhemoglobin concentrations for the ranges of 10 to 70%.**

10%: Frontal headache
20%: Headache and dyspnea
30%: Nausea, dizziness, visual disturbance, fatigue and impaired judgment
40%: Syncope and confusion
50%: Coma and seizures
60%: Respiratory failure and hypotension
70%: May be lethal

❍ **What is the appropriate treatment for cyanide poisoning?**

Amyl nitrite and sodium nitrite IV, followed by sodium thiosulfate IV.

ENVIRONMENTAL PEARLS

It is your work in life that is the ultimate seduction.
Pablo Picasso

❍ **How is frostnip treated?**

Frostnip is the only form of frostbite that can be treated at the scene. It is treated by warming the affected area(s) by hand, by breathing on the skin or by placing the exposed extremities in the armpit. The affected part should not be rubbed because this action does not thaw the tissues completely.

❍ **What is appropriate treatment for frostbite?**

The exposed extremity should be rewarmed rapidly by immersing the affected area in 42°C circulating water for 20 minutes or until flushing is observed. Do not use dry heat. Refreezing thawed tissue greatly increases damage. Remember to provide tetanus prophylaxis. Débride white or clear blisters because toxic mediators (prostaglandin and thromboxanes) may be present. However, leave hemorrhagic blisters intact. Topical antibiotics, such as silver sulfadiazine, may be used.

❍ **What are some common complications of frostbite?**

Rhabdomyolysis, permanent depigmentation of the extremity and an increased probability of a subsequent injury caused by cold conditions. Extremity frostbite may result in later x-ray findings of irregular, fine, punched-out lytic lesions on the MTP, PIP and DIP joints.

❍ **What are the four degrees of frostbite?**

First degree: Erythema and edema.
Second degree: Blister formation.
Third degree: Necrosis.
Fourth degree: Gangrene.

❍ **What complications are associated with hypothermia?**

Coagulopathy, confusion, disorientation, decreased immune response, platelet dysfunction, reduced cardiac function, decreased cardiac output, vasoconstriction and hypotension.

❍ **What measures can be instituted to treat hypothermia?**

Increasing the room temperature, using intravenous fluid and blood warmers, heating ventilator gases and using warming blankets.

❍ **As the patient re-warms, what problems can arise?**

Development of metabolic acidosis, shivering, hypotension and tachycardia.

❍ **A patient's temperature is 30° Celsius. During cardiac arrest defibrillation was unsuccessful. What treatment is recommended?**

Active warming should precede further defibrillation attempts and medication administration.

❍ **At what altitude does acute mountain sickness typically develop?**

8000 feet.

❍ **What organ is most commonly affected in a radiation accident?**

The skin. Burns may take up to 2 weeks to become clinically apparent.

❍ **What is the LD_{50} for a radiation victim?**

Within 60 days: 450 rads. LD_{90}: 700 rads.

❍ **A patient presents with two small puncture wounds and a halo lesion with a circular area of pallor surrounded by a ring of erythema. What is the diagnosis?**

Black widow spider envenomation.

❍ **Describe the presentation of black widow spider envenomation versus scorpion envenomation.**

Black widow victims typically stay in one position for a few seconds to a few minutes before moving. They also have a halo lesion. Scorpion victims present with a constant writhing and abnormal eye movements.

❍ **What are the indications for administering antivenin in a black widow spider envenomation?**

Severe pain, dangerous hypertension and pregnant women with moderate to severe envenomations.

❍ **Can a scratch from a rattlesnake result in a serious envenomation?**

Yes. However, up to 25% of rattlesnake bites do not result in envenomation.

❍ **What patients who have been bitten by a rattlesnake will develop serum sickness following antivenom administration?**

Most patients who receive more than 5 vials will develop serum sickness. Symptoms may range from mildly viral-like to severe urticarial rash and arthralgias. Treatment includes antihistamines, corticosteroids and analgesics.

❍ **A patient presents with a human bite wound that was inflicted while he was in a mental ward. What bacterium is likely?**

Eikenella corrodens, anerobic streptococci and staphylococcus.

❍ **What is the frequency of eye injury in lightning strike victims?**

Fifty percent develop structural eye lesions. Cataracts are the most common and develop within days to years. Unreactive dilated pupils may not equal death because transient autonomic instability may occur.

❍ **What is the most common otologic injury in lightning strike victims?**

Tympanic membrane rupture (50%). Hemotympanum, basilar skull fracture, acoustic and vestibular deficits may also occur.

❍ **What is the most common arrhythmia found in patients with hypothermia?**

Atrial fibrillation. Other ECG findings include PAT, prolongation of the PR, QRS or QT waves, decreased P wave amplitude, T wave changes, PVCs or humped ST wave segment adjacent to the QRS complex (Osborn waves).

❍ **A 24 year old baseball player presents with a history of light-headedness, headache, nausea and vomiting. Upon examination, the patient has a HR of 110, RR of 22, BP of 90/60 and is afebrile. Profuse sweating is noted. What is the diagnosis?**

Heat exhaustion.

❍ **A 27 year-old marathon runner presents confused and combative. Her temperature is 105° F. Why must renal function be monitored?**

This patient has heat stroke. Rhabdomyolysis may occur 2 to 3 days after injury.

❍ **How should a honeybee's stinger be removed?**

Scrape it out. Squeezing with a tweezers or finger may increase envenomation.

❍ **Should burn victims have their blisters debrided?**

Yes. They contain vasospastic agents and should be drained.

❍ **An Osborn (J) wave seen on ECG is associated with what disorder?**

Hypothermia.

❍ **Hypothermia is defined as a core temperature below what level?**

35° C.

❍ **How is a sodium metal wound debrided?**

Cover with mineral oil and excise retained metal fragments.

❍ **Is lightning AC or DC?**

DC. It may cause asystole and respiratory arrest.

❍ **What type of arrhythmia is expected with AC shock?**

Ventricular fibrillation.

❍ **How long should an asymptomatic lightning strike victim be monitored?**

Several hours, as CHF may be delayed.

❍ **What is the most common cause of death in CO poisoning?**

Cardiac arrhythmias.

❍ Are the elderly more prone to become hypothermic?

Yes. Several factors make the elderly more susceptible to hypothermia. These include loss of muscle mass, increased surface area to body mass ratio, decreased cutaneous vasoconstrictor response and decreased heat production.

❍ List the four mechanisms of heat loss from the body.

The four mechanisms of heat loss are:

1) Radiation: Transfer of heat from a warm to a cold body via electromagnetic radiation.
2) Convection: Air abutting the body is heated by way of its direct contact to the patient. Since warm air is less dense it rises and is replaced by cooler air.
3) Evaporation: Water on the body's surface evaporates, the latent heat of vaporization comes from the patient whose temperature consequently falls.
4) Conduction: This is the direct transfer of heat energy through a substance.

❍ Which are the sites that contribute to evaporative heat loss?

Evaporation accounts for heat loss from the skin and respiratory tract.

❍ What is the typical pattern of body temperature decline in the operating room?

Typically there is an initial precipitous fall in the first hour. This is followed by a second phase lasting 2 to 3 hours characterized by a gradual decrease in temperature. Finally there is a plateau phase.

❍ What is the mechanism underlying this fall in body temperature?

These changes are not seen in unanesthetized volunteers in the operating room. This must be due to factors intrinsic to anesthesia and not the environment that accounts for this decline. Anesthesia results in peripheral vasodilatation allowing warm blood from the core to mix with cold blood from the shell. This mixing results in a fall in body temperature.

❍ What is the effect of general anesthesia on metabolic rate?

General anesthesia causes a reduction of metabolic rate of approximately 15%.

❍ What are the effects of hypothermia on the central nervous system?

Mild hypothermia (32 to 35°C) will decrease cerebral metabolic rate by 15 to 20%, which combined with general anesthesia will provide some degree of protection against hypoxia and ischemia. The MAC of volatile agents is reduced by approximately 5% for every degree centigrade reduction in body temperature. Hypothermia is associated with delayed emergence from general anesthesia. Body temperatures of less than 30°C can produce narcosis.

❍ What are the cardiovascular side effects of hypothermia?

When temperature falls below 35°C there is significant vasoconstriction, increasing central blood volume. Further falls in temperature to below 32°C are associated with a decrease in cardiac output and delays in electrical conduction. At temperatures less than 30°C increased ventricular irritability is encountered, with increased danger for ventricular fibrillation. Hypothermia below 28°C is associated with decreased contractility and further reductions to below 20°C results in cardiovascular collapse because of decreased peripheral resistance.

❍ Is respiratory function compromised by hypothermia?

There are a variety of pulmonary changes associated with hypothermia including a decrease in hypoxic ventilatory drive, attenuation of hypoxic pulmonary vasoconstriction, increased bronchiolar tone and respiratory depression. Hypothermia has been cited as one of the reasons for reintubation in the recovery room following anesthesia.

❍ How does hypothermia affect the metabolism of anesthetic drugs?

Hypothermia impairs both hepatic and renal functions. Any drug that is dependent on either of these organs for clearance will accumulate. The duration of action of vecuronium and pancuronium are prolonged by hypothermia.

❍ What are the hematologic consequences of hypothermia?

As body temperature falls, vasomotor tone increases resulting in a increase in plasma volume. This results in a diuresis, the loss of free water resulting in a increase in viscosity. Because of this there tends to be sludging with an increased risk of vascular occlusion. Additionally there is a reversible sequestration of platelets by the reticular endothelial system and decline in platelet function. These two factors together with an inhibition of the coagulation cascade, lead to an increased risk in bleeding.

❍ What are the metabolic consequences of hypothermia?

There is a temperature dependent decrease in metabolic rate. In addition hypothermia is associated with increased protein catabolism and decreased insulin secretion.

❍ How is renal function affected by hypothermia?

Renal blood flow is decreased to a greater extent than cardiac output. Initially, there is a cold induced diuresis because of a decreased secretion of anti-diuretic hormone and an impaired renal reabsorption of sodium. As temperatures fall further, both urine output and renal concentrating ability become impaired.

❍ What are the consequences of shivering?

Shivering is the rhythmical contraction and relaxation of small muscle groups. It results in a significant increase in oxygen consumption and CO_2 production. If this increase in metabolic activity is not met by increased minute ventilation, respiratory acidosis ensues. If cardiac output is not increased, to meet the increased O_2 demand, then mixed venous oxygen levels will decrease and the patient will possibly develop tissue hypoxia.

❍ Which modalities are available in order to treat shivering?

The most reliable method to prevent shivering is to prevent intraoperative hypothermia. Conservation of radiant heat loss can prevent shivering. Another method that can be used for skin warming is the forced air exchange blanket. There are pharmacological methods to treat shivering, the most popular being meperidine.

❍ Can warming fluids aid in the prevention of hypothermia?

Yes. Cold banked blood should always be warmed. Rapid and large volumes of crystalloid or colloid should be warmed. If a massive transfusion is anticipated then a rapid infusion system that can deliver blood at 37°C at rates of 250 to 500ml/min should be used.

❍ What are the consequences of post-operative rewarming?

If a patient is hypothermic in the immediate post-operative period and then rewarmed, there are two physiologic consequences: vasodilation and shivering. The vasodilation may unmask underlying hypovolemia resulting in hypotension and tachycardia.

❍ **Which test is most reliable in predicting the severity of radiation exposure 48 h post exposure?**

Absolute lymphocyte count. Presence or absence of GI symptoms following near lethal doses is a good indicator as well.

❍ **What distinguishes heat stroke from heat exhaustion?**

Heat exhaustion is progressive loss of electrolytes and body fluid depletion. Therapy is rehydration.

Heat stroke occurs when temperatures are above 42 °C and enzyme systems cease to function normally. As a result, there is necrosis, denaturing and organ failure. Heat stroke requires much more aggressive treatment than simple fluid rehydration.

Remember - in patients with an altered sensorium and a core temperature above 42 °C, always suspect heat stroke. Half of patients will be diaphoretic.

❍ **What lab abnormalities may be found with heat stroke?**

Elevations in SGOT, SGPT, LDH, BUN, creatinine, CPK and other indices of rhabdomyolysis.

❍ **How should a patient with heat stroke be treated?**

1) Cool the patient with cool water and fans.
2) Pack the axillae, neck and groin with ice.
3) Maintain euvolemia.
4) Treat shivering with chlorpromazine (Thorazine) IV.

❍ **What complications can result from heat stroke?**

Renal failure, rhabdomyolysis, DIC and seizures. Remember antipyretics will not help.

ANESTHESIOLOGY AND NUTRITION MANAGEMENT PEARLS

"Seeking the food he eats
And pleased with what he gets"
As You Like It,
Shakespeare

❍ **What is the functional residual capacity (FRC)?**

The FRC is the volume of gas in the lungs at the end of a normal expiration. It represents the balance between the elastic nature of the lungs to collapse in and of the chest wall to spring out. The expiratory reserve volume and the residual volume make up the FRC.

❍ **What is the closing capacity?**

The closing capacity is approximately the residual volume in normal individuals. It represents the lung at which the small airways close inhibiting the flow of gas.

❍ **What is the relationship between the FRC and the closing capacity forms the basis for post-operative ventilatory changes?**

The FRC is normally larger than the closing capacity. During a tidal breath the small airways stay open throughout inspiration and expiration. If the closing capacity becomes larger than the FRC, the tidal breath may only partially open the small airways or not at all. This results in areas of atelectasis and ventilation/perfusion mismatch.

❍ **What changes does general anesthesia confer that causes a restrictive ventilatory defect in the post-operative setting?**

Relaxation of the diaphragm, chest wall relaxation, loss of respiratory compliance and a shift of the blood volume from the chest into the abdomen. After thoracic or abdominal surgery, all lung volumes are reduced. The VC and FRC can be reduced as much as 50 to 70% in the first 24 hours post surgery. These changes start shortly after anesthesia induction and can last as long 7 to 14 days.

❍ **During induction of general anesthesia, what happens to the diaphragm?**

The diaphragm shifts cephalad in the supine patient. This accounts for a loss of 340 to 750 cc of lung volume.

❍ **How do intravenous anesthetics affect the respiratory muscles?**

Intravenous anesthetics depress the contractility of the diaphragm.

❍ **How do volatile anesthetics affect respiratory muscle function?**

Depresses it.

❍ **How does epidural anesthesia affect diaphragm function?**

Animal studies indicate that phrenic nerve activity is reduced through the transmission of inhibitory signals from somatic or visceral afferent nerves. Epidural anesthesia ablates these inhibitory signals. Phrenic nerve transmission increases and the diaphragm improves.

❍ **How do epidural narcotics affect diaphragm function?**

Epidural narcotics ameliorate pain, but do not affect diaphragm function. Intrathecal opioids will depress ventilatory function centrally in a dose dependent fashion.

❍ **How often is phrenic nerve paralysis found after cardiac surgery?**

Less than 10%.

❍ **After cardiac surgery, what variables are associated with severe atelectasis?**

The variables associated with severe atelectasis post-cardiac surgery include the number of saphenous vein grafts, the use of internal mammary artery grafts, the duration of cardiac bypass time and whether or not the pleural space was entered.

❍ **How long may hypoxemia last beyond upper abdominal or thoracic surgery?**

Hypoxemia may last days to weeks after thoracic or upper abdominal surgery. This correlates with a reduced FRC and an increased closing capacity.

❍ **How is induction of anesthesia associated with hypoxia?**

Induction of general anesthesia is associated with increased dead space ventilation, shunting of blood and inhibition of hypoxic vasoconstriction.

❍ **How much can dead space be increased with general anesthesia?**

The combined effect of the anesthesia circuit and redistribution of ventilation can result in dead space as much as 50% of the tidal volume. If total ventilation is not increased alveolar hypoventilation occurs resulting in hypercapnia and hypoxemia.

❍ **What is a shunt?**

Shunt is the phenomenon of perfusing areas of non-ventilated lung (atelectatic). We normally shunt about 2 to 5% of our cardiac output. During general anesthesia this can increase to 8%. The increase is greatest in patients who are obese or have pre-existing pulmonary conditions.

❍ **What is absorption atelectasis?**

Atelectasis that occurs when 100% oxygen is administered. Without the presence of slowly diffusing nitrogen, the oxygen is completely absorbed from the airspaces resulting in atelectasis.

❍ **What is hypoxic vasoconstriction (HPV)?**

HPV is the normal vasoconstriction that occurs in the pulmonary circulation in response to hypoxia. The lung attempts to shift blood flow from poorly ventilated to well ventilated areas in an effort to preserve normal ventilation -perfusion relationships.

❍ **How fast does the $PaCO_2$ rise in an apneic patient?**

Without ventilatory support the $PaCO_2$ will rise 2 to 3 mmHg/minute.

❍ **What are the most important defense mechanisms of the lung to environmental and infectious agents?**

The mucociliary transport and the cough reflex.

❍ **How is the cough reflex impaired past surgery?**

Pain and the use of narcotic analgesia inhibit cough. In addition respiratory muscle dysfunction reduces the expulsive force and the effectiveness of the cough.

❍ **How long past general anesthesia is the mucociliary clearance reduced?**

Mucociliary clearance is reduced for 2 to 6 days past general anesthesia. This is the result of ciliary damage from dry anesthetic gases, increased mucus viscosity and reduced clearance from areas of atelectasis.

❍ **How may phrenic nerve injury occur during cardiac surgery?**

The classic mechanism is that of "phrenic nerve frostbite" from cardioplegia solution. In addition the phrenic nerve can be mechanically injured during the dissection of the internal mammary artery because of its anatomic proximity.

❍ **What recommendations can be made to reduce the incidence of atelectasis post cardiac surgery?**

The use of careful technique in the mobilization of the internal mammary artery, use of a pericardial insulating pad, avoidance of entry into the pleural space and recovery of as much cardioplegia solution as possible before it enters the pulmonary circulation.

❍ **How long may changes in respiratory function last past a thoracotomy?**

Several weeks.

❍ **What is the effect of a thoracotomy on respiratory system compliance?**

Compliance may decrease by as much as 75%. This markedly increases the work of breathing.

❍ **Unique to lung surgery is the intraoperative collapsing of one lung to facilitate surgery. Why doesn't this technique result in profound intraoperative hypoxia?**

Hypoxic pulmonary vasoconstriction. The lung shifts most of its circulation to the well ventilated lung. The collapsed lung needs to be periodically reinflated to prevent prolonged post-operative hypoxia.

❍ **What are the effects of a sternotomy on post-operative pulmonary function?**

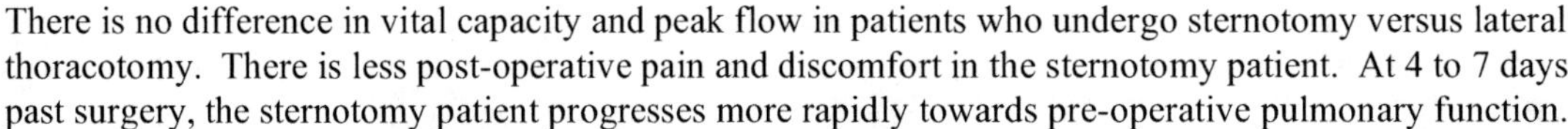

There is no difference in vital capacity and peak flow in patients who undergo sternotomy versus lateral thoracotomy. There is less post-operative pain and discomfort in the sternotomy patient. At 4 to 7 days past surgery, the sternotomy patient progresses more rapidly towards pre-operative pulmonary function.

❍ **What anatomic changes occur post-pneumonectomy?**

On the operated side the mediastinum shifts, the hemidiaphragm elevates and the rib interspaces become smaller. The remaining lung distends. There is no new lung growth.

❍ **What should be done to keep the mediastinum neutral post-pneumonectomy?**

Nothing. Attempts to limit mediastinal shift with thoracoplasty and plombage result in scoliosis to the operated side and worsened pulmonary function. The pneumonectomized space will fill with fluid shortly post-pneumonectomy and then fibrose. Care should be taken not to drain this fluid. Many surgeons will leave only a small chest tube for 24 hours to assess for bleeding or air leak.

❍ **What are risk factors for post-operative pulmonary complications?**

The anatomic site for surgery, general debility, chronic obstructive lung disease, poor pre-operative PFTs, obesity, cigarette smoking and pre-operative hypercapnia.

❍ **What techniques can be used to lessen pulmonary complications?**

Lung expansion techniques. The goal is to promote alveolar ventilation and to normalize the FRC.

❍ **What is IPPB?**

Intermittent positive pressure breathing. Early studies showed its application reduced the incidence of complications over controls. However, it is no more effective than deep breathing exercises and incentive spirometry. IPPB is best reserved for those patients where active lung inflation is not possible even with patient cooperation (such as muscular dystrophy and kyphoscoliosis).

❍ **What is non-invasive mechanical ventilation?**

It is the application of positive pressure breathing via the use of a tight fitting mask. The mask can be uncomfortable. The advantage may be in that often obviates the need for intubation and the risks thereof.

❍ **What is CPAP?**

Continuous positive airway pressure.

❍ **What is BiPAP?**

Bilevel positive airway pressure. An expiratory pressure and an inspiratory pressure are dialed in per the needs of the patient. A tightly fitting nasal mask the interface to the patient.

❍ **What are mechanisms of post extubation airway closure?**

Laryngeal edema, laryngospasm and failure of vocal cord abduction due to trauma. These problems may be anticipated when no air leak is detected upon deflation of the endotracheal tube cuff, the intubation was traumatic or neck surgery was performed.

❍ **What medical therapies are available to treat laryngeal edema?**

Nebulized racemic epinephrine, corticosteroids and heliox.

❍ **What is heliox?**

Heliox is a commercially available mixture of helium and oxygen. Either 80% helium and 20% oxygen or 70% helium and 30% oxygen. It has a density one third that of air. The reduced density decreases airway resistance and flow resistive work. It can be used as a temporizing technique while managing upper airway obstruction.

❍ **What is the most common organism in wound infections?**

Staphylococcus.

❍ **T/F: Botulism never occurs in a post-operative wound.**

False.

❍ **A patient who develops a reddish-brown exudate within 6 hours of an appendectomy most likely has a wound with what type of infection?**

Clostridium. Necrotizing fasciitis, dehiscence and sepsis may result if not treated promptly.

❍ **What are the indications for surgical treatment of a chylothorax?**

Failure of non-operative therapy after 7 to 14 days, continued drainage of more that 1500 ml per day in adults, persistent electrolyte abnormalities or malnutrition.

❍ **What special anesthetic and surgical considerations are necessary before anesthetic induction in patients with large anterior or middle mediastinal masses?**

Airway compression from the mass could result in airway occlusion during the induction of anesthesia and vascular collapse from a compromised venous return to the heart.

❍ **What should be immediately available during the induction of anesthesia in patients with large mediastinal masses?**

Rigid bronchoscopy. It can be used to establish an airway and ventilate the patient if airway occlusion occurs.

❍ **The sudden onset of a continuous cough with copious serosanguinous sputum while a patient is recovering from a pneumonectomy is pathognomonic for what condition?**

Post-operative bronchopleural fistula.

❍ **What is the initial bedside therapy for an acute bronchopleural fistula following pneumonectomy?**

Turn the patient operated side down to prevent the aspiration of pleural fluid into the contralateral lung and perform a tube thoracostomy.

❍ **What are the risk factors for post-operative bronchopleural fistula following pulmonary resection?**

Diabetes mellitus, malnutrition, radiation therapy, infection, inflammation or devascularization of the bronchial stump and residual tumor at the site of bronchial closure.

❍ **In the surgical patient, circulatory failure and accumulation of lactic acid frequently cause metabolic acidosis. What is the appropriate treatment?**

Assuming adequate cardiac function, volume resuscitation with fluid or blood restores circulation and hepatic clearance of lactate.

❍ **What metabolic changes occur with acute illness?**

Catabolism, negative protein balance, hypermetabolic state and hyperglycemia.

❍ **Hypermetabolic states commonly occur in what patients?**

Patients with burns, neurological injury, sepsis and multiple trauma.

❍ **What are the nutritional parameters that can be followed in a critically ill patient?**

Indirect calorimetry, protein measurements (albumin, prealbumin, transferrin and retinol binding protein), 24-hour nitrogen balance study and daily weights.

❍ **When is indirect calorimetry inaccurate?**

If the patient is hyperactive, hyperventilating, when the inspired oxygen concentration is above 60% and in the presence of an air leak.

❍ **Using indirect calorimetry, how is resting energy expenditure calculated?**

Resting energy expenditure (kcal/day) = 3.94 x VO_2 (L/day) + 1.11 x VCO_2 (L/day)

❍ **What is the basal energy expenditure as predicted by the Harris-Benedict equation?**

Men: 66.473 + (13.75 x weight in kg) + (5.0 x height in cm) – (6.8 x age in years)
Women: 655.09 + (9.56 x weight in kg) + (1.84 x height in cm) – (4.67 x age in years)

❍ **In a 70 kg man in acute renal failure and unable to tolerate enteral feedings, what considerations should be accounted for in ordering total parenteral nutrition?**

Minimize fluids, avoid excess protein content (unless the patient is on hemodialysis) and closely monitor and adjust electrolytes and divalent cations.

❍ **What is in a nutritional formula designed for patients with hepatic failure?**

Higher levels of branched chain amino acids and lower concentrations of aromatic amino acids. This is to minimize the development of encephalopathy.

❍ **What are the goals of nutritional therapy?**

Maintain lean body mass, minimize catabolism, preserve organ function and promote immune function.

❍ **When should enteral nutrition be started?**

Most proponents believe enteral nutrition should be started as soon as possible, preferably in the first 24 hours after injury or surgery (assuming no ileus).

❍ **What proportion of critically ill and injured patients are catabolic or hypermetabolic?**

Nearly all.

❍ **Are immunocompetence and vital organ function dependent upon nutritional support?**

Yes. Both are secondary goals of nutritional support.

❍ **What is the predominant energy source used during starvation by a healthy subject?**

Lipids.

❍ **How long does the body's reserve of carbohydrates last during starvation?**

Glycogen stores are consumed within 24 hours.

❍ **Does the metabolic rate increase or decrease during starvation in a healthy subject?**

Decrease.

❍ **Are adaptation mechanisms seen with starvation similar to those seen in critically ill patients?**

No. There is impaired protein conservation and a persistent hypermetabolic response in the critically ill patient.

❍ **With the onset of critical illness, what factors are thought to raise resting energy expenditure and protein turnover?**

Catecholamines and cortisol.

❍ **How does the insulin resistance associated with critical illness affect substrate use?**

Insulin resistance decreases the peripheral use of glucose and increases proteolysis.

❍ **Is there any rationale for overfeeding or underfeeding critically ill patients?**

No. Both have been shown to be detrimental. The goal is to meet the metabolic needs of the patient.

❍ **What are the serum half-lives of albumin and prealbumin?**

18 days and 2 to 3 days, respectfully.

❍ **What two methods are frequently used to assess nutritional status in critically ill patients?**

Indirect calorimetry and nitrogen balance.

❍ **As a patient's FIO_2 requirements increase, is indirect calorimetry more or less accurate in measuring energy expenditure?**

Less.

❍ **What other factors are sources of errors with indirect calorimetry?**

Air leaks from endotracheal tubes and the need for extrapolation of measurements to 24 hours.

❍ **What is the equation for nitrogen balance?**

Nitrogen Balance = Nitrogen intake - Nitrogen loss
= (Protein (g) / 6.25) - ((Urine Urea Nitrogen / 0.8) + 3)

❍ **How much protein is required for balance in a healthy stable adult?**

Approximately 0.6 g/kg ideal body weight/day.

❍ **What is the goal of protein delivery?**

To achieve a positive nitrogen balance.

❍ **What is the optimal calorie-to-nitrogen ratio for critically ill patients?**

100 : 1 to 200 : 1.

❍ **What is the recommended starting point for non-protein calorie needs for hypermetabolic critically ill patients?**

25 kcal/kg ideal body weight/day.

❍ **What is the most common manifestation of excessive carbohydrate administration?**

Hyperglycemia.

❍ **Can lipid emulsions be useful in patients needing volume restriction or demonstrating carbohydrate intolerance?**

Yes. Lipids are calorie dense compared to dextrose solutions.

❍ **What minimum percentage of total calories should be supplied as lipid to prevent fatty acid deficiency?**

Five percent of total calories at minimum.

❍ **How long does it take non-stressed patients receiving lipid-free total parenteral nutrition (TPN) to demonstrate evidence of essential fatty acid deficiency?**

Within four weeks. Hypermetabolic patients within ten days.

❍ **Can lipids administered parenterally hurt cellular immunity?**

There is data to suggest lipids cause reticuloendothelial dysfunction and immune suppression.

❍ **What clinical symptoms are seen with hypophosphatemia brought on by refeeding a malnourished patient?**

Weakness and congestive heart failure.

❍ **What is the main energy source of enterocytes?**

Glutamine.

❍ **Besides an energy source, what role does glutamine play in the gut?**

It is thought to be important in maintaining intestinal structure and function.

❍ **How much glutamine has been included in standard amino acid solutions used with total parenteral nutrition (TPN)?**

None, due to its instability in parenteral solutions.

❍ **Is glutamine an essential amino acid?**

No. However, during times of metabolic stress, intracellular glutamine stores are markedly depleted, indicating supplementation may be beneficial.

❍ **Arginine, a semi-essential amino acid, is considered to be vital to what body system?**

The immune system.

❍ **Can branched-chain amino acids improve the outcome in critically ill patients?**

No. Some suggest it may be helpful in patients with hepatic encephalopathy.

❍ **Have immunoenriched diets, containing substrates such as omega-3 fish oils, arginine and RNA nucleotides, been found to improve outcome?**

Yes, a number of recent studies suggest improvement using enteral immunoenriched formulas.

❍ **What is the preferred route for the delivery of nutrition, enteral or parenteral?**

The enteral route.

❍ **When should nutritional support be started?**

As soon as a hypermetabolic state (e.g., trauma or sepsis), underlying malnutrition or an expected delay in resuming an oral diet of > 5-10 days is recognized.

❍ **What complications are associated with enteral nutrition?**

Complications involve routes of access to the GI tract (e.g., feeding tube displacement and obstruction), the GI tract itself (e.g., nausea, vomiting and diarrhea) or the metabolic system (e.g., hyperglycemia and hypophosphatemia).

❍ **T/F: Bowel sounds are a good index of small bowel motility.**

False.

❍ **Has pre-operative nutritional support for malnourished patients been shown to be reduce post-operative morbidity?**

Yes, for those with severe malnutrition.

❍ **In which patients is parenteral nutritional support indicated?**

When enteral access is unobtainable, enteral feeding contraindicated or when the level of enteral nutrition fails to meet requirements.

❍ **In which patients is intravenous nutritional support unlikely to be of benefit?**

Those expected to start oral intake in 5 to 7 days or with mild injuries.

❍ **Typically, what feeding route requires a greater length of time to reach full support?**

Enteral.

❍ **Can lipids be given through a peripheral vein?**

Yes. They are iso-osmotic, unlike the concentrated dextrose solutions that should be infused centrally.

❍ **Are omega-3 fatty acids (fish oil) or omega-6 fatty acids thought to be anti-inflammatory?**

Omega-3 fatty acids.

❍ **What are the complications of parenteral nutrition?**

Those associated with catheter insertion (e.g., pneumothorax), the indwelling line (e.g., line sepsis, thrombosis), lipid emulsions (e.g., pancreatitis, reticuloendothelial dysfunction) and GI tract complications (e.g., cholestasis, acalculous cholecystitis).

❍ **Can overfeeding result in difficulty weaning a patient from mechanical ventilation?**

Yes. This is related to increased energy expenditure, oxygen consumption and CO_2 production with a resultant increase in respiratory rate and minute ventilation.

❍ **Can underfeeding result in difficulty weaning a patient from mechanical ventilation?**

Yes. Malnutrition can cause respiratory muscle weakness and ventilator dependence.

❍ **Among protein, fat and carbohydrate, which can provide the most energy per molecule and which the least?**

Fat generates the most energy at 9 kcal/g while amino acids provide 4 kcal/g and glucose only 3.4 kcal/g.

❍ **During times of glycogen depletion what source of energy is utilized by tissues that are obligate glucose users?**

Protein is the only other source of glucose. Conversion of amino acids to alpha-keto analogues allows the proteins to be used in gluconeogenesis. Lipids are highly inefficient since only the glycerol portion of the triglyceride molecule can be used for glucose synthesis.

❍ **What are the major metabolic and physiologic effects of glucose, protein and fat during times of stress?**

Gluconeogenesis is increased by the liver while peripheral glucose use is reduced, resulting in hyperglycemia. Skeletal muscle undergoes increased proteolysis which can manifest as muscle wasting and increased excretion of uninary free nitrogen. Fat metabolism is also increased in an effort to decrease the amount of glucose being used.

❍ **Define the term respiratory quotient (RQ).**

The respiratory quotient is the ratio of carbon dioxide produced to oxygen consumed.

❍ **What is the mechanism behind the increase in body temperature seen during the stress response?**

The increase in body temperature is caused by pyrogens, namely IL-I, which is released from macrophages. The pyrogens subsequently stimulate PGE_2 which up-regulates the thermoregulatory center in the hypothalamus.

❍ **Why are alanine and glutamine so important during periods of stress?**

Alanine and glutamine are the major carriers of nitrogen for use in protein synthesis. In addition, glutamine serves as a major fuel for the gastrointestinal tract and inflammatory cells and provides ammonium groups to the kidney for help in acid excretion.

❍ **What is the initial response of circulating insulin and glucagon level after injury?**

Initially insulin levels are low and glucagon levels high. This is thought to be secondary to elevated levels of epinephrine which decreases insulin secretion.

❍ **What is the role of arginine in patients following severe injury or sepsis?**

Although arginine is considered a nonessential amino acid, during times of significant stress its stores can be rapidly depleted. Arginine has been shown to enhance certain immunologic functions, especially in macrophages and lymphocytes. It is thought that this may have some beneficial outcomes on wound healing.

❍ **What are cytokines and which ones play a primary role in the stress response?**

Cytokines are a group of protein mediators stimulated by cell injury, inflammation or infection, that include interleukins, interferons, tumor necrosis factor and colony stimulating factors. TNF, IL-1, IL-2 and IL-6 are thought to play a significant role in the stress response.

❍ **What happens to serum concentrations of ADH and aldosterone after surgery?**

The stress of anesthesia and surgery lead to an elevation in ADH and aldosterone as the body attempts to hold onto salt and fluid. This, in part, accounts for the decrease in urine output seen in patients post-operatively as well as some of the third spacing of fluid seen three to four days after surgery.

❍ **Where is aldosterone produced and what is its stimulus for secretion?**

Aldosterone is a mineralocorticoid secreted from the zona glomerulosa of the adrenal gland. Its secretion is stimulated by ACTH, angiotensin II, increased serum potassium concentration and decreased serum sodium.

❍ **Where does aldosterone exert its primary effect and what is this effect?**

Aldosterone works primarily on the distal tubules and collecting ducts of the kidney, leading to an increase in the absorption of sodium from the urine in exchange for potassium and thereby aiding in water retention.

❍ **What are the effects of catecholamines on alpha, beta-l and beta-2 receptors during times of stress?**

Catecholamines cause arteriolar vasoconstriction through alpha receptors, increased cardiac inotropy and chronotropy through beta-l receptors and arteriolar vasodilation in muscle through the beta-2 receptors. All of these actions are to aid in the fight or flight response that is seen during periods of stress.

❍ **What are the metabolic effects of catecholamines seen during periods of stress?**

Catecholamines increase glycogenolysis, gluconeogenesis, lipolysis, ketogenesis and antagonize insulin in peripheral tissues. All of these actions aid in providing more substrate for repair of injured tissue.

❍ **What is the net result of uncomplicated starvation on glucose, protein and lipid metabolism?**

The end result of uncomplicated starvation is to shift from glucose utilization to lipid utilization while minimizing protein metabolism.

❍ **T/F: During periods of sepsis administration of exogenous glucose suppresses protein catabolism, as seen in starvation.**

False. Administration of glucose does not suppress protein catabolism during sepsis.

❍ **T/F: Stress ulcers can be caused by burns, trauma, sepsis, hemorrhage, renal failure, ARDS and brain injury and commonly cause bleeding in these situations.**

True. Any injury that leads to a stress response can cause stress ulcers.

❍ **T/F: During an inflammatory response albumin, prealbumin and transferrin are among the acute phase proteins whose synthesis is increased.**

False. Albumin, prealbumin and transferrin are not considered acute phase proteins. Their synthesis is actually decreased during periods of stress.

❍ **Which of the following statements is incorrect?**
1) Hepatic gluconeogenesis is increased during periods of sepsis/stress.
2) Skeletal muscle proteolysis is increased during periods of sepsis/stress.
3) A shift from glucose to lipid as a fuel source occurs during periods of sepsis/stress.

All statements are true.

❍ **What happens to serum triglyceride, free fatty acid and glycerol levels during stress/sepsis?**

Elevated triglyceride levels and normal to elevated fatty acid and glycerol levels are seen during stress/sepsis. This is thought to be secondary to the increased lipolysis stimulated by cortisol, catecholamines and glucagon.

❍ **How does worsening liver failure seen in sepsis/trauma effect the clearance of aromatic amino acids as opposed to branched chain amino acids and what is the significance of this?**

Liver failure leads to a decreased ability to clear AAAs, a situation that does not occur with BCAs. The excess AAAs are thought to be metabolized to false neurotransmitters which may antagonize the effects of catecholamines or cross the blood brain barrier and cause encephalopathy.

❍ **What protein sparing event occurs early on in starvation?**

Early on in starvation the brain, which has the largest obligate requirements for glucose, begins to use ketones instead of glucose for energy. This reduction in the need for glucose minimizes the amount of proteolysis that is occurring.

❍ **A 30 year old woman is endotracheally intubated and needs nutrition. She has a functioning gastrointestinal tract. What are the advantages of enteral nutrition when compared to parenteral nutrition?**

Enteral nutrition is more physiologic, has a trophic effect on gastrointestinal cells, avoids the need for a central venous catheter and its complications and costs less.

❍ **What is total energy expenditure (TEE)?**

The amount of calories burned by an individual in a 24 hour period. It is the sum of basal metabolic rate, activity related energy expenditure, illness related energy expenditure and the thermogenic effect of feeding.

❍ **How does the change in resting energy expenditure (REE) differ in the critically ill patient versus the starving person?**

REE increases during acute illness and decreases during non-stressed starvation.

❍ **What is the respiratory quotient (RQ)?**

The ratio of carbon dioxide produced to oxygen consumed. When carbohydrate is the fuel it is 1.0, for protein it is 0.8 and for fat it is 0.7. An RQ of greater than 1.0 indicates fat synthesis and an RQ less than 0.7 is consistent with ketones as the source of fuel
.

❍ **What does indirect calorimetry measure?**

Gas exchange at steady-state. Measured values are inspired and expired oxygen fractions, inspired and expired carbon dioxide fractions and minute ventilation. Oxygen consumption and carbon dioxide production are calculated using these measurements.

❍ **During starvation, as in the pre-operative period, what are the main organs involved in glucose production?**

Liver and kidney.

❍ **By what mechanism does the body supply itself with glucose if there is no dietary carbohydrate?**

Gluconeogenesis (conversion of protein to glucose) from body protein.

❍ **A previously healthy 20 year old woman is injured in a motor vehicle accident. The day following admission her serum albumin is noted to be 2.8. Why is her serum albumin low?**

The decreased albumin in this patient is a marker of the injury response rather than of impaired nutrition.

❍ **What happens to nitrogen reserves after trauma?**

Nitrogen reserves are mobilized due to accelerated protein catabolism.

❍ **What is the maximum osmolarity of solutions that should be infused into a peripheral vein?**

Nine hundred mOsm. Parenteral nutrition solutions are commonly greater than 1500 mOsm and require central venous access for delivery.

❍ **A critically ill patient's intravenous access is via a peripherally inserted central catheter (PICC). Can solutions with an osmolarity of greater than 900 mOsm be infused through a PICC?**

Yes. Although the insertion site is peripheral, the catheter tip is in a central vein and thus there is no osmolarity restriction.

❍ **A 40 year old woman has had a small intestine resection. What minimum length of small bowel is required for enteral absorption of nutrients and below which parenteral nutrition must be considered?**

A minimum of 100 centimeters of small intestine is needed to sustain life.

❍ **A previously healthy, well nourished, non-stressed, 38 year old man requires parenteral nutrition. What is his protein requirement?**

Between 0.8 and 1.0 gram per kilogram of body weight.

❍ **A 55 year old man is scheduled for a distal splenorenal shunt for esophageal varices. His total parenteral nutrition (TPN) solution (Hepatamine) contains less aromatic amino acids and more branched-chain amino acids than standard solutions. What is the indication for this solution?**

Hepatic encephalopathy. In hepatic failure there is an elevation of phenylalanine and methionine (aromatic amino acids) and a decrease in leucine, isoleucine and valine (branched-chain amino acids). This formula is used in an attempt to normalize plasma amino acids, based on the theory that hepatic encephalopathy may be due to this plasma amino acid change and a resulting imbalance of neurotransmitters in the brain.

❍ **What maximum percent of daily caloric intake should be from fat?**

Thirty to 60 percent.

❍ **When fat emulsions are administered, which patients should have monitoring of serum triglyceride levels?**

Patients with hyperlipidemias, acute pancreatitis, pulmonary insufficiency, hepatic failure and sepsis.

❍ **At what level of serum triglycerides should the fat and glucose administration be decreased?**

If serum triglyceride level exceeds 500 mg/dl.

❍ **When ordering total parenteral nutrition (TPN) the concentrations of what two electrolytes must be monitored to prevent precipitation?**

Calcium and phosphate.

❍ **When total parenteral nutrition (TPN) is prescribed, what anions are generally used to form sodium and potassium salts?**

Chloride and acetate.

❍ **When is it indicated to prescribe acetate or increased acetate in total parenteral nutrition (TPN)?**

For metabolic acidosis, usually non-anion gap acidosis in which bicarbonate loss is the cause of the acidosis. It is not indicated for compensated respiratory alkalosis, in which hyperchloremia maintains electronegativity.

❍ **What nutritional deficiency should be considered if a patient has unexplained lactic acidosis?**

Thiamine deficiency.

❍ **How is lactate cleared from the blood?**

By the liver using gluconeogenic and oxidative pathways. A normal liver can remove up to 400 grams per day of lactate.

❍ **What metallic nutrient may require supplementation in patients on long term total parenteral nutrition (TPN) because it is not part of multi-trace elements (MTE)?**

Iron.

❍ **A patient on total parenteral nutrition (TPN) has severe diarrhea. What trace element may need to be supplemented?**

Zinc.

❍ **An order is placed for multi-trace elements as "MTE-5." What five trace elements are included?**

Zinc, copper, chromium, manganese and selenium.

❍ **An order is placed for multivitamins as "MVI-12." What vitamin is excluded and must be added separately to total parenteral nutrition (TPN) solutions?**

Vitamin K.

❍ **What vitamin deficiency can be caused by gastric or ileal resection?**

Vitamin B_{12}. There is loss of intrinsic factor with gastric resection and loss of the absorptive site with ileal resection.

❍ **The non-essential amino acid glutamine is not contained in commercial parenteral nutrition solutions. Why not?**

Because of stability and shelf-life limitations. Although the body is capable of making large quantities of glutamine, in stress states glutamine consumption exceeds production and glutamine depletion results. It is thought of as "conditionally essential" but whether or not administering glutamine improves patient outcome remains to be determined.

❍ **What is the goal for calculated nitrogen balance in a critically ill patient?**

Positive 2 to 6 grams of nitrogen per day.

❍ **Protein requirements are often stated in terms of nitrogen requirement. How do you determine the content of nitrogen in dietary protein?**

Grams of dietary protein divided by 6.25 approximates grams of nitrogen.

❍ **What are the three categories of complications related to total parenteral nutrition (TPN)?**

Mechanical complications related to insertion of the central venous access catheter, metabolic complications and infection.

❍ **A 50 year old trauma victim is started on total parenteral nutrition (TPN) and has new onset hyperglycemia. Why?**

The "diabetes of trauma" is due to a combination of inhibition of insulin secretion, increased glucagon release and reduced peripheral use of glucose.

❍ **Which factor contributes more to an increase in carbon dioxide production, a high carbohydrate to fat ratio in the feeding solution or a high caloric intake resulting in overfeeding?**

A high caloric intake resulting in overfeeding.

❍ **What are the untoward effects of overfeeding in a critically ill patient?**

Increased carbon dioxide production, increased oxygen consumption, fluid overload, hepatic steatosis and hyperglycemia. An increased carbon dioxide production may impede weaning from mechanical ventilation.

❍ **A 45 year old man has not had adequate nutrition due to nausea and emesis for many days before total parenteral nutrition (TPN) is started. What mineral may be severely decreased during re-feeding?**

Serum phosphate. Hypophosphatemia may be associated with severe muscle weakness and a need for mechanical ventilation.

❍ **What are three options for handling total parenteral nutrition (TPN) during the intra-operative period?**

Continue the TPN as ordered, discontinue the TPN by tapering over several hours during the pre-operative period or replace TPN with ten percent dextrose during surgery.

❍ **During prolonged surgery, what laboratory tests should be monitored because a patient is receiving total parenteral nutrition (TPN)?**

Plasma glucose and potassium.

ALLERGY, RHEUMATOLOGY AND TRANSPLANTATION PEARLS

I don't want to achieve immortality through my work.
I want to achieve it through not dying.
Woody Allen

❍ **What is an orthotopic graft?**

A graft placed in the anatomic position normally occupied by such tissue.

❍ **What chromosome contains the major histocompatibility complex (MHC)?**

Chromosome 6.

❍ **Which MHC antigens best trigger the proliferation of allogenic lymphocytes?**

Human leukocyte antigen (HLA) class II antigens (HLA-D, DR, DQ and DW/DR).

❍ **T/F: Grafts between HLA-identical siblings will reject if chronic immunosuppression is not utilized after transplantation.**

True.

❍ **What are the methods of determining the degree of histocompatibility between donor and recipient?**

MHC matching and mixed lymphocyte culture (MLC).

❍ **What is the most common use of the MLC?**

Related bone-marrow transplantation.

❍ **What triggers the rejection reaction after transplantation?**

The immune response to the HLA antigens on the cells of the transplanted organ/tissue.

❍ **What is the mechanism of action of azathioprine (AZ)?**

It is a purine analog (antimetabolite) that interferes with DNA synthesis.

❍ **What is the mechanism of action of FK 506?**

It inhibits T-cell activation and maturation.

❍ **What is the role of methotrexate in chronic immunosuppression?**

It is used clinically only for bone marrow transplantation as graft-versus-host (GVH) prophylaxis.

❍ **What are the clinical uses of cyclophosphamide?**

It is used in renal transplant patients when liver toxicity prohibits the use of azathioprine and for bone marrow recipients.

❍ **What side effects are specific to cyclophosphamide?**

Prompt fluid retention, severe hemorrhagic cystitis and cardiac toxicity.

❍ **What combination of drugs provides the most effective immunosuppression with the fewest side effects?**

Cyclosporine and prednisone and/or azathioprine.

❍ **What are the adverse effects of cyclosporine?**

Hirsutism, neurotoxicity, hyperkalemia, nephrotoxicity, hypertension and tremors.

❍ **T/F: The potency of FK 506 is much greater than that of cyclosporine.**

False.

❍ **What are the characteristics of chronic steroid administration?**

A cushingoid appearance, hypertension, weight gain, peptic ulcers, gastrointestinal bleeding, euphoric personality changes, cataract formation, hyperglycemia, diabetes, osteoporosis and avascular necrosis of bone.

❍ **What is the prototypic monoclonal antibody in clinical immunosuppression?**

OKT3.

❍ **What is the most common cause of death in transplant recipients?**

Infection.

❍ **What are the typical manifestations of CMV infection in transplant patients?**

A mild febrile illness followed by an antibody response and regression of viral symptoms.

❍ **What are the most frequent malignancies seen in transplant patients?**

Those that are common to immunosuppressed patients. Most are epithelial or lymphoid in origin (i.e., carcinoma in situ of the cervix, carcinoma of the lip, squamous or basal cell carcinoma of the skin and B cell lymphoma).

❍ **Which drugs are used most often to prevent lung rejection?**

Cyclosporine, azathioprine and corticosteroids.

❍ **What are the histopathological findings in acute lung rejection?**

Perivascular mononuclear cellular infiltrate and lymphocytic bronchitis or bronchiolitis.

❍ **What are the clinical findings in acute lung rejection?**

Dyspnea, fever, hypoxemia and infiltrates on CXR.

❍ **How is acute lung rejection diagnosed?**

Histologically, with transbronchial lung biopsy. BAL does not distinguish between infection and rejection.

❍ **What is the treatment for acute lung rejection?**

High dose steroids. If this fails, OKT3 or ATL is used.

❍ **What is the typical manifestation of chronic lung rejection?**

Progressive dyspnea with decline in FEV1 (at least 20% from baseline), usually after three months.

❍ **Is tissue necessary to make the diagnosis of chronic lung rejection?**

No, not in the correct clinical scenario. Biopsy is useful to rule out concurrent acute rejection and infection.

❍ **What is the histological hallmark of chronic lung rejection?**

Obliterative bronchiolitis and fibrointimal thickening of arteries and veins.

❍ **What is the treatment for chronic lung rejection?**

Augmented steroids, OKT3, ATL and FK506 have been used. The response is generally poor.

❍ **What is the most common cause of infectious complications associated with lung transplantation?**

Bacterial, which often occur early after the transplantation. Gram negative organisms are the most common.

❍ **What is the most common viral infection associated with lung transplantation?**

CMV, which occurs 1 to 3 months post-transplantation. Ganciclovir is the treatment and occasionally CMV hyperimmune globulin is added.

❍ **Who is at risk for CMV pneumonitis?**

The seronegative recipient with a seropositive donor is at risk for primary disease. The seropositive recipient may develop reactivation disease. Ganciclovir is often given to patients at high risk for CMV disease.

❍ **What other viral infections occur after lung transplantation?**

RSV and herpes simplex. The latter has been less common since the use of prophylactic regimens containing acyclovir or ganciclovir.

❍ Which fungal infections are the most common in lung transplant patients?

Candida and aspergillus.

❍ Which prophylactic drug has drastically reduced the incidence of PCP?

Bactrim.

❍ What is post-transplant lymphoproliferative disorder in a lung transplant recipient?

This is a proliferation of cells, either polyclonal or monoclonal, that usually occurs in the lung. The polyclonal variety is responsive to a reduction in immunosuppressive agents. The monoclonal variety is a lymphoma that requires chemotherapy. The response is poor, in general. These conditions are thought to be related to infection with EBV.

❍ What is the reimplantation response?

This is a capillary leak syndrome thought to be due to ischemia and reperfusion of the grafted lung. It usually occurs in the first few days. The treatment is supportive care.

❍ What are the indications for single, double or heart-lung transplantation?

Single: COPD, primary pulmonary hypertension, IPF or other interstitial lung diseases
Double: cystic fibrosis, primary pulmonary hypertension, COPD
Heart-lung: Eisenmenger's syndrome (in congenital heart disease), primary pulmonary hypertension

❍ EBV infection is linked with what late complication (years)?

Post transplant lymphoproliferative disorder.

❍ When is Pneumocystis carinii pneumonia most likely to be seen in a transplant patient?

2 to 6 months post transplantation.

❍ What immunosuppressive agents have the highest risk of reactivating CMV infection?

Azathioprine and OKT3/antilymphocyte globulin.

❍ What tests should be performed for rejection surveillance in a heart-lung transplant recipient?

Pulmonary function tests
Systemic arterial oxygen saturation
Chest roentgenogram
Transbronchial biopsy

❍ Fever, sternal tenderness, erythema and purulent drainage suggest what diagnosis 48 hours post-operative heart transplantation?

Mediastinitis caused by S. aureus, S. epidermidis or gram negative bacilli.

❍ What is the most common site of bacterial infection in all types of transplant patients?

Lung (35%).

❍ **What is graft versus host disease (GVHD)?**

Engraftment of immunocompetent donor cells into an immunocompromised host, resulting in cell-mediated cytotoxic destruction of host cells if an immunologic incompatibility exists.

❍ **When does acute GVHD present and what are the typical manifestations?**

Acute GVHD typically occurs around day 19 (median), just as the patient begins to engraft and is characterized by erythroderma, cholestatic hepatitis and enteritis.

❍ **A 30 year-old female is 21 days status-post bone marrow transplant (BMT) and presents with a fever, maculopapular rash over 30% of her body, >1,000 ml diarrhea/day and rising LFTs, with a total bilirubin of 4 mg/100ml. What is the clinical stage of GVHD?**

Stage 2.

❍ **The above patient, four days later, has evidence of generalized erythroderma with desquamation, severe abdominal pain with no bowel movements and a total bilirubin of 16mg/100ml. What is the clinical stage of GVHD?**

The patient has progressed to stage 4.

❍ **What is the clinical definition of chronic GVHD (cGVHD)?**

As early as 60 to 70 days status-post engraftment, the patient exhibits signs of a systemic autoimmune process, manifesting as Sjogren's syndrome, systemic lupus erythematosus, scleroderma, primary biliary cirrhosis and commonly experiences recurrent infection with encapsulated bacteria, fungi or viruses.

❍ **What agent may be a treatment alternative for patients with high risk GVHD or with refractory chronic GVHD?**

Thalidomide.

❍ **What drugs increase blood levels of cyclosporine?**

Ketoconazole
Erythromycin
Methylprednisolone
Warfarin
Verapamil
Ethanol
Imipenem-cilastatin
Metaclopropamide
Fluconazole

❍ **What drugs decrease blood levels of cyclosporine?**

Phenytoin
Phenobarbital
Carbamazepine
Valproate
Nafcillin
Rifampin

❍ **What are significant toxic side effects of cyclosporine therapy?**

Neurotoxic: tremors, paraesthesia, headache, confusion, somnolence, seizures and coma.
Hepatotoxic: cholestasis, cholelithiasis and hemorrhagic necrosis.
Endocrine: ketosis, hyperprolactinemia, hypertestosteronemia, gynecomastia and impaired spermatogenesis.
Metabolic: hypomagnesemia, hyperuricemia, hyperglycemia, hyperkalemia and hypocholesterolemia.
Vascular: hypertension, vasculitic hemolytic-uremic syndrome and atherogenesis.
Nephrotoxic: oliguria, acute tubular damage, fluid retention, interstitial fibrosis and tubular atrophy.

❍ **What drugs may exacerbate the nephrotoxicity of cyclosporine?**

Aminogylcosides, amphotericin B, acyclovir, digoxin, furosemide, indomethacin and trimethoprim.

❍ **What are the long term effects of corticosteroid treatment?**

Growth failure, cushingoid appearance, hypertension, cataracts, GI bleeding, pancreatitis, psychosis, hyperglycemia, osteoporosis, aseptic necrosis of the femoral head and suppression of the pituitary-adrenal axis.

❍ **What is the overall risk for developing a secondary malignancy, as compared to the general population?**

The risk is 6.7 times that of the general population.

❍ **What are some common immunosuppressive drugs?**

Cyclosporine, azathioprine, prednisone, OKT3 (monoclonal antilymphocyte antibody) and FK506.

❍ **Child's Class C chronic liver disease is associated with what clinical manifestations?**

Serum bilirubin > 3, serum albumin < 3, PT of INR > 2, comatose neurologic state, difficult to control ascites and a wasting neurologic condition.

❍ **What are some causes of encephalopathy in liver transplant candidates?**

Gastrointestinal bleeding or other protein loads, hepatic coma secondary to cerebral edema and elevated intracranial pressure.

❍ **What conditions predispose liver transplant patients to renal failure?**

1) Hypovolemia.
2) Ascites formation.
3) Hepatorenal syndrome.

❍ **On induction for lung transplantation, patients with severe chronic obstructive pulmonary disease (COPD) are often hemodynamically unstable. Why?**

COPD patients are frequently very volume depleted. On induction and commencement of positive pressure ventilation, they have a tendency to auto-peep secondary to air trapping and "breath stacking," severely reducing venous return and cardiac output. These patients should be preloaded with crystalloid and ventilated with shallow tidal volumes and a long expiratory time.

❍ **T/F: Permissive hypercapnia is never utilized in lung transplantation.**

False. Ventilation is often marginal in lung transplantation patients, particularly during one lung ventilation. An elevated PCO_2 is accepted so long as the pH is maintained above 7.20.

❍ **Describe some of the factors considered when making decisions for induction of the cardiac transplant patient.**

Recognition of the patient's limited cardiac reserve is paramount. Frequently the patient has a full stomach. Drug doses should be adjusted for a prolonged circulation time and reduced volume of distribution associated with the low cardiac output state. Beta-receptor down regulation and receptor uncoupling frequently results in an unpredictable response to sympathomimetic agents.

❍ **What are the primary indications for heart-lung transplantation (HLTx)?**

Congenital heart disease with or without Eisenmenger's complex and primary pulmonary hypertension are the two main indications for HLTx.

❍ **Describe some methods for controlling pulmonary vascular resistance (PVR) in the heart-lung transplantation patient during induction and the pre-bypass period.**

Pre-oxygenation is critical. Induction is generally accomplished with a high dose of an opiate and a small dose of a cardiostable induction agent such as etomidate or midazolam. Ketamine is contraindicated because of its deleterious effects on PVR. Vasoactive drugs are frequently required. Some useful combination therapies include prostaglandin E_1, amrinone/milrinone or nitroglycerin for PVR reduction combined with norepinephrine for increased systemic blood pressure and cardiac contractility.

❍ **Describe rate control for the heart transplanted patient.**

The transplanted heart frequently has two SA nodes. The native SA node is isolated from the myocardium by the suture line and does not influence the heart rate, although its P-wave may be visible on the EKG. The SA node from the donor heart controls the heart rate, but because of the resultant denervation it is isolated from sympathetic and parasympathetic modulation. Direct acting positive chronotropic agents are required to increase heart rate.

❍ **In a patient undergoing renal transplantation, is succinylcholine contraindicated?**

Succinylcholine is only contraindicated if the patient has an elevated serum potassium level, risk factor for malignant hyperthermia or some other pre-existing medical condition that could cause the potassium level to become elevated (such as paralysis, muscular dystrophy, etc.) due to succinycholine administration.

❍ **In a patient needing renal transplantation list some common pre-operative problems that are often encountered?**

These problems include inadequate or excessive intravascular volume, electrolyte abnormalities, hypertension, anemia, concurrent drug therapy or complications associated with DM (cardiac and vascular).

❍ **In a patient needing renal transplantation why is the hemoglobin level low?**

Chronic anemia with hemoglobin levels of 5 to 7 results from decreased production of erythropoietin and diminished red cell survival time. Iron absorption from the gastrointestinal tract may also be decreased in patients with ESRD leading to iron deficiency.

❍ **In a patient needing renal transplantation how are the serum cholinesterase levels affected?**

The serum cholinesterase levels should be normal in renal failure patients, whether or not they are undergoing dialysis.

❍ **In a patient who is to receive a cadaveric kidney transplant what pre-operative medications should be considered?**

Most cadaveric kidney transplants are performed on an emergency basis and, therefore, most of the patients are considered to have a full stomach. H_2-antagonists and a gastric motility drug as metoclopramide should be considered. The patient should also receive any chronic antihypertensive or cardiac medication that is scheduled.

❍ **In a patient with ESRD needing renal transplantation are platelets affected?**

The platelet count is often low but the primary affect is on platelet function. Prolonged bleeding time and decreased platelet adhesiveness occur.

❍ **In a patient with ESRD needing renal transplantation what coagulation problems other than platelet dysfunction can be present?**

The vitamin K dependent coagulation factors (II, VII, IX, X) and factor V tend to be low.

❍ **In a patient who has undergone renal transplantation what are some of the early post-operative complications?**

Renal artery occlusion, hyperacute rejection, acute renal failure, graft rupture, wound infection and urinary fistula.

❍ **In a patient who has undergone renal transplantation what are the signs of rejection?**

Decreased urine output, fever and increased serum creatinine. The kidney is often enlarged and tender to palpation. A renal biopsy is necessary to verify the diagnosis.

❍ **In a patient who has undergone renal transplantation what are some of the common immunosuppressive drugs used?**

Azathioprine, corticosteroids, cyclosporine, monoclonal antibiodies and antilymphocyte globulin (ALG).

❍ **What is the primary indication for pancreas transplantation?**

Transplantation of the pancreas is the best method by which to establish a constant glycemic state in diabetic patients with permanent normalization of glycosylated hemoglobin.

❍ **How does pancreatic islet transplantation differ from pancreas transplantation?**

Pancreatic islet transplantation is a form of selective transplantation since only the cells required by the recipient are transplanted. When only the islet cells are transplanted complications related to the exocrine portion of the pancreas are eliminated.

❍ **What type of anesthesia is required for pancreatic islet cell transplantation?**

The transplantation of islet cells is performed by injecting purified islet suspension into the portal vein. Sedation combined with local anesthesia is usually all that is needed. This form of transplantation is often performed in the intensive care unit, not the operating room.

❍ **What are the clinical manifestations of the acute GVH reaction?**

Skin rash, hepatic dysfunction, diarrhea, wasting and myelosuppression.

❍ **How is the diagnosis of acute GVH reaction confirmed?**

Skin biopsy.

❍ **What is the treatment for acute GVH reaction?**

FK 506 or cyclosporine plus steroids.

❍ **T/F: Transplantation of insulin-producing islet cells (beta cells) is sufficient to achieve glucose hemostasis.**

True.

❍ **What are the most common liver diseases for which liver transplantation is required?**

Chronic active hepatitis, cholestatic liver disease, biliary atresia and alcoholic cirrhosis.

❍ **How is rejection differentiated from ischemia, viral infection and cholangitis?**

Percutaneous liver biopsy.

❍ **What findings suggest cholangitis?**

PMNs within the portal tracts.

❍ **What are the most common causes of encephalopathy following liver transplantation?**

Gastrointestinal bleeding or other protein loads and hepatic coma secondary to cerebral edema and increased intracranial pressure.

❍ **Why is adequate venous access so critical in patients undergoing liver transplantation?**

Because liver transplantation is associated with major volume losses secondary to coagulopathies.

❍ **A 50 year old male, status-post liver transplant, has rapidly rising serum bilirubin and transaminases as well as hyperkalemia, hypoglycemia and coagulopathy. What is the most likely diagnosis?**

Thrombotic occlusion of the hepatic artery or portal vein.

❍ **What is the appropriate treatment for the above patient?**

Retransplantation.

❍ **T/F: The sinus node of the donor heart becomes the dominant pacemaker.**

True.

❍ **What is the most common regimen of immunosuppression following cardiac transplantation?**

Triple therapy with oral cyclosporine, azathioprine and prednisone.

❍ **What drugs are used in "rescue" therapy for cardiac rejection?**

Cytolytic agents (OKT3, ATG and ALG).

❍ **What biopsy findings suggest Grade 2 cardiac rejection?**

Focal infiltrates with myocyte necrosis.

❍ **What signs and symptoms are associated with cardiac rejection?**

Malaise, fatigue, dyspnea/orthopnea, tachycardia, a ventricular gallop, rales and edema.

❍ **What are the indications for double-lung transplantation?**

Cystic fibrosis, bronchiectasis, pulmonary hypertension, correctable congenital defects and emphysema.

❍ **How is CMV lung disease in a transplanted lung established?**

By finding inclusion bodies in lung tissue obtained by transbronchial biopsy.

❍ **What is the standard immunosuppressive management following renal transplantation?**

Cyclosporine, azathioprine and prednisone.

❍ **What is the differential diagnosis for early anuria following renal transplantation?**

Hypovolemia, thrombosis of the renal artery or vein, hyperacute rejection, compression of the kidney or obstruction to urine flow.

❍ **T/F: An allograft is a tissue or organ graft between two individuals of the same species.**

True.

❍ **What is a syngeneic graft?**

A graft between identical twins.

❍ **Which class of immunoglobulins is responsible for urticaria (hives) and angioedema?**

IgE.

❍ **Which class of drugs is commonly associated with angioedema?**

Angiotensin-converting-enzyme (ACE) inhibitors. A patient who has suffered angioedema from one ACE inhibitor should not be prescribed another one. ACE-triggered angioedema can occur at any time during the course of therapy.

❍ **What drug is the most common pharmaceutical cause of true allergic reactions?**

Penicillin

❍ **How long after exposure to an allergen does anaphylaxis occur?**

Seconds to 1 hour.

❍ **After penicillin, what is the most common cause of anaphylaxis-related deaths?**

Insect stings. Approximately 100 deaths occur in the US annually because of anaphylaxis induced by insect stings.

❍ **A patient on a beta-blocker who develops anaphylactic cardiovascular collapse may not respond to epinephrine or dopamine infusions. What drug can be used in this setting?**

Glucagon.

❍ **Cite an example for each of the four major types of allergic reactions: Type I (immediate hypersensitivity); type II (cytotoxic); type III (Arthus reaction); and type IV (delayed hypersensitivity).**

Type I:	Asthma, food allergies (IgE).
Type II:	Transfusion reaction (IgG and IgM).
Type III:	Serum sickness, post streptococcal glomerulonephritis (complex activates complement).
Type IV:	Skin testing (activated T-lymphocytes).

❍ **Which of the four types of allergic reactions can be caused by a drug allergy?**

All of them.

❍ **Myocardial infarction can occur with which two rheumatic diseases?**

Kawasaki disease and polyarteritis nodosa (PAN).

❍ **What diagnostic procedure is indicated for a patient with rheumatoid arthritis who presents with dysphagia, hoarseness and stridor?**

Urgent laryngoscopy to assess the paired cricoarytenoid joints. These joints can cause airway compromise if they become fixed in a closed position.

❍ **What is the treatment of choice for a patient in anaphylactic shock?**

Epinephrine intravenously.

❍ **How does relapsing polychondritis affect the airway?**

Approximately 50% of patients with relapsing polychondritis have airway involvement and may present with pain and tenderness over the cartilaginous structures of the larynx. Dyspnea, stridor, cough, hoarseness and erythema and edema of the oropharynx and nose may also be exhibited.

❍ **How should patients with airway involvement from relapsing polychondritis be managed?**

Admit these patients for high-dose steroids and for close observation. Repeated exacerbations may lead to severe airway compromise and asphyxiation.

❍ **A patient on chronic steroids presents with weakness, depression, fatigue and postural dizziness. What pathological process should be suspected? What is the treatment?**

Adrenal insufficiency. The treatment is to administer large "stress doses" of steroids.

❍ **What cardiac complication commonly occurs with SLE, juvenile rheumatoid arthritis and rheumatoid arthritis?**

Pericarditis.

❍ **What causes fatality in hereditary angioedema?**

Edema of the larynx.

❍ **What neurologic disorders, if present, serve as diagnostic criteria for SLE?**

Seizures and psychosis.

❍ **What pharmacologic agents are most commonly associated with drug-induced lupus?**

Anticonvulsants, hydralazine and isoniazid.

❍ **What are the major causes of SLE mortality?**

Nephritis, with resultant renal failure
Central nervous system complications
Infection
Pulmonary lupus
Myocardial infarction

❍ **Which form of vasculitis may be seen after infection with Hepatitis B?**

Polyarteritis nodosa.

❍ **What side effects might one rarely see with administration of IV gamma globulin?**

Anaphylaxis, chills, fever, headache and myalgia.

❍ **What rare vasculitis should be considered in an 18 year-old African-American girl with obscure hypertension, increased ESR and fever?**

Takayasu's arteritis.

❍ **A patient with a slowly progressive course of dermatomyositis is most susceptible to what disease complication?**

Calcinosis, which is deposition of calcium in subcutaneous tissue.

❍ **An 18 year-old female presents with complains of fever and malaise one week prior to the development of 1 to 3 cm painful, red, ovoid nodules on her shins bilaterally. Bilateral hilar lymphadenopathy is demonstrated on chest x-ray. What is the diagnosis?**

Erythema nodosum associated with sarcoidosis.

❍ **Behcet syndrome is characterized by recurrent oral and genital ulcers and ocular inflammation. What additional symptoms are associated with a particularly poor prognosis?**

CNS abnormalities, such as cranial nerve palsies and psychosis.

❍ **What is the clinical scenario of Familial Mediterranean Fever and what is the attributed cause?**

Amyloid deposition is the cause of this condition, which manifests with proteinuria that progresses to nephrotic syndrome and renal failure.

❍ **What is the treatment?**

Colchicine.

❍ **What inflammatory conditions might one expect in secondary amyloidosis?**

JRA, cystic fibrosis, inflammatory bowel disease and chronic infections, such as tuberculosis.

❍ **Anti dsDNA antibodies are most indicative for what disease?**

Systemic lupus erythematosus.

❍ **The presence of antineutrophil cytoplasmic antibodies (c-ANCA) with a diffuse staining pattern in serum immunofluorescence is most commonly associated with what disease?**

Wegener's Granulomatosus.

❍ **What is the best screening test for SLE?**

ANA should be demonstrable in all patients with active SLE.

❍ **What hematologic conditions are seen with patients who have SLE?**

Anemia, thrombocytopenia and leukopenia.

❍ **What class of anesthetic drugs is most likely to be responsible for an allergic reaction in the operating room?**

Muscle relaxants especially succinylcholine. An allergy to one muscle relaxant means that the patient may be sensitive to another relaxant even if there has not been exposure to it previously because these agents share quaternary ammonium groups that are able to bind antibodies.

❍ **Is there really cross-reactivity between penicillins and cephalosporins?**

Yes. Anaphylaxis to a cephalosporin can occur in a penicillin allergic patient.

❍ **Do you need to give both H1 and H2 receptor antagonists for an anaphylactic episode?**

Yes. Many studies have confirmed that to maximally block the histamine receptors with both H1 and H2 receptor antagonists decreases the severity of reactions involving histamine release more effectively than H1 receptor blockade alone.

❍ **Matching transplants:**

1. Autograft **a. Donor and recipient are genetically the same.**
2. Heterotrophic **b. Donor and recipient are the same person.**

3. Isograft	**c. Donor and recipient are of the same species.**
4. Orthotopic	**d. Donor and recipient belong to different species.**
5. Allograft	**e. Transplantation to a normal anatomical position.**
6. Xenograft	**f. Transplantation to a different anatomical position.**

Answers: (1) b, (2) f, (3) a, (4) e, (5) c and (6) d.

❍ **What transplant organ can be preserved the longest?**

The kidney. Kidneys can be preserved in cold storage for up to 48 hours, the pancreas and liver for 8 hours and the heart for 4 hours. Viability can be extended by using cold storage solutions, such as Collins solution and UW-Belzer solution.

DERMATOLOGY PEARLS

He: "You have beautiful skin!"
She: "Yes and it covers my whole body."
Woody Allen

❍ **Rank these skin conditions in order of decreasing risk for mortality: erythema multiforme minor, toxic epidermal necrolysis and erythema multiforme major (Stevens-Johnson Syndrome).**

Toxic epidermal necrolysis > erythema multiforme major (Stevens-Johnson syndrome) > erythema multiforme minor.

❍ **What is the mortality in erythema multiforme minor?**

0%.

❍ **T/F: Oral lesions are very common in erythema multiforme minor.**

False.

❍ **T/F: Oral lesions are very common in erythema multiforme major.**

True.

❍ **What disease produces erythematous plaques with dusky centers and red borders resembling bull's eye targets?**

Erythema multiforme. This disease can also produce non-pruritic urticarial lesions, petechiae, vesicles and bullae.

❍ **What is the appropriate management for toxic epidermal necrolysis (TEN)?**

Admit the patient for management similar to that required for extensive second-degree burns. The mortality rate of TEN can be as high as 50% because of fluid loss and secondary infections.

❍ **What drugs are most commonly implicated in toxic epidermal necrolysis?**

Sulfa and other antibiotics, phenylbutazone, barbiturates and other antiepileptic drugs.

❍ **What can cause erythema multiforme?**

Viral or bacterial infections, drugs of nearly all classes and malignancy.

❍ **What are Beau lines?**

Transverse grooves in the nailbed that are caused by the disruption of the nailbed matrix secondary to systemic illness. Illness can actually be dated by these lines as nails grow 1 mm per month.

❍ **What are the most common causes of allergic contact dermatitis?**

Poison ivy, poison sumac, poison oak, ragweed, topical medications, nickel, chromium, rubber, glue, cosmetics and hair dyes.

❍ **A mother brings her 17 year-old boy to you a week after you prescribed ampicillin for his pharyngitis. Mom says he developed a rash over his torso, arms, legs and even the palms of his hands. Upon examination, the patient has an erythematous, maculopapular rash. What might the child have other than pharyngitis?**

Infectious mononucleosis. In almost 95% of patients with Epstein-Barr viruses that are treated with ampicillin, a rash will develop. The rash and subsequent desquamation will last about a week.

❍ **Ecthyma most commonly presents on what body parts?**

The lower legs. Ecthyma is similar to impetigo but can also be associated with a fever and lymphadenopathy. The most common infecting agent is Staphylococcus aureus. This infection is most prevalent in moist, warm climates.

❍ **What is the most common bullous disease?**

Erythema multiforme. The typical erythema multiforme lesion is the iris lesion (a gray center with a red rim). These lesions are symmetrical and most frequently found on the distal extremities spreading proximally. Patients may also have plaques, papules and bullous lesions. The disease most commonly occurs in children and young adults.

❍ **What type of reaction is erythema multiforme?**

Hypersensitivity. Bullae are subepidermal, the dermis is edematous and a lymphatic infiltrate may be present around the capillaries and venules. In children, infections are the most important cause. In adults, drugs and malignancies are more common causes. EM is often seen during epidemics of adenovirus, atypical pneumonia and histoplasmosis.

❍ **What are the features of Staphylococcal scalded skin syndrome (SSSS)?**

This condition begins with the appearance of patches of tender erythema followed by loosening of the skin and denuding to glistening bases. SSSS is commonly found in children younger than 5 and is due to a toxin that induces cleavage within the epidermis under the stratum granulosum.

❍ **What area does Staphylococcal scalded skin syndrome (SSSS) usually affect?**

The face around nose and mouth, neck, axillae and groin. The disease commonly occurs after upper respiratory tract infections or purulent conjunctivitis. Nikolsky's sign is present when lateral pressure on the skin results in epidermal separation from the dermis.

❍ **How can SSSS be distinguished from scalded skin syndrome caused by drugs or chemicals?**

In drug or chemical etiologies, the skin separates at the dermoepidermal junction. In staphylococcal induced SSSS, the skin separates more superficially within the epidermis. This drug-induced TEN carries up to 50% mortality as a result of fluid loss and secondary infection. On microscopic exam of SSSS, intraepidermal cleavage occurs and a few acantholytic keratinocytes can be seen. In the non-staphylococcal type, cellular debris, inflammatory cells and basal cell keratinocytes are present.

❍ **What is the treatment of SSSS?**

Anti-staphylococcal antibiotic, local wound care and IV fluids. Corticosteroids are contraindicated.

❍ **A patient presents with fever, myalgias, malaise and arthralgias. On exam, findings include bullous lesions of the lips, eyes and nose. The patient indicates eating is very painful. What should the family be told about the patient's prognosis?**

Stevens-Johnson syndrome has a mortality of 5 to 10% and may have significant complications including corneal ulceration, panophthalmitis, corneal opacities, anterior uveitis, blindness, hematuria, renal tubular necrosis and progressive renal failure. Scarring of the foreskin and stenosis of the vagina can occur. Supportive care treatment is best managed in a burn unit.

❍ **What is the treatment of a tetanus prone wound?**

Surgical debridement, human tetanus immune globulin (TIG) IM (do not inject into wound) and penicillin G or metronidazole.

❍ **How can the development of decubitus ulcers be prevented?**

Change the patient's position every 2 hours, keep the skin clean and dry, use protective padding at potential sites of ulceration, (e.g., heel pads or ankle pads) and keep patients on egg crate mattresses or the equivalent. Daily foot examination is important in diabetic patients.

❍ **What organism is the most common cause of bullous impetigo?**

Coagulase positive Staphylococcus aureus.

❍ **What is another name for erythema multiforme major?**

Stevens-Johnson syndrome.

❍ **What antibiotics are most likely to cause a photoallergic drug reaction?**

Tetracycline and sulfonamides.

OBSTETRICS AND GYNECOLOGY PEARLS

To my embarrassment I was born in bed with a lady.
Wilson Mizner

❍ **What anticoagulant is safe in pregnancy?**

Heparin. Warfarin is contraindicated.

❍ **What is the pulmonary complication of tocolytic therapy?**

Pulmonary edema.

❍ **Which agents are associated with this syndrome?**

Terbutaline, ritadrine and magnesium sulfate.

❍ **What are the major consequences of amniotic fluid embolism?**

Cardiopulmonary arrest and DIC.

❍ **What are the potential mechanisms of cardiopulmonary arrest?**

Mechanical obstruction of pulmonary vasculature, alveolar capillary leak, pulmonary edema from LV failure and anaphylaxis.

❍ **How is amniotic fluid embolism diagnosed?**

By demonstrating fetal squames in the buffy coat preparations of blood and by pulmonary microvascular cytology of blood drawn from the distal lumen of a PA catheter.

❍ **What is the treatment for amniotic fluid embolism?**

Supportive.

❍ **What is the normal PCO_2 in pregnancy?**

30 to 34 mmHg. This is due to chronic mild hyperventilation secondary to elevated progesterone.

❍ **What is the predominant change in lung volumes in pregnancy?**

Decrease in functional residual capacity by as much as 15 to 25%.

❍ **T/F: In pregnancy the elevated diaphragm decreases tidal volume.**

False. The tidal volume actually increases and accounts for much of the increased minute ventilation and mild respiratory alkalosis.

❍ **T/F: The decreased functional residual capacity results in early airway closure in pregnancy.**

False.

❍ **Why is the incidence of thromboembolism increased in pregnancy?**

Venous stasis from uterine pressure on the inferior vena cava, increase in clotting factors, increased fibrinogen and decreased fibrinolysis.

❍ **What special considerations exist when cardiac arrest occurs in a pregnant patient?**

During chest compression, a wedge under the right hip should be used to minimize aortocaval compression. For the pregnant patient who is unconscious due to airway obstruction, chest thrusts are performed rather than abdominal thrusts.

❍ **What is the effect of pregnancy on acid-base considerations?**

Pregnancy is characterized by a chronic, compensated respiratory alkalosis. The pH is typically 7.40 to 7.45, $PaCO_2$ 28 to 32 mmHg and serum HCO_3^- 18 to 21 mEq/L.

❍ **What is the effect of pregnancy on the A-a O_2 gradient?**

In the upright position, pregnancy is associated with a normal A-a O_2 gradient. However, in the supine position, the A-a gradient increases secondary to increased ventilation-perfusion inequality because of the enlarged uterus impinging upon the lungs.

❍ **What is the most common non-gynecologic condition presenting with lower abdominal pain?**

Appendicitis.

❍ **How long after the removal of Norplant capsules must patients wait to become pregnant?**

Ovulation usually occurs within 3 months.

❍ **What is the most common heart problem in pregnant women?**

Congenital heart disease.

❍ **What is Meigs' syndrome?**

Ascites and hydrothorax in the presence of an ovarian tumor.

❍ **What are the most common sites for metastasis of ovarian carcinoma?**

The peritoneum and omentum.

❍ **T/F: A woman with pelvic inflammatory disease (PID) is likely to have an exacerbation of symptoms when she menstruates.**

True. The breakdown of the cervical mucus antibacterial barrier allows bacteria to ascend from the lower tract to the upper tract. Pelvic examination, intercourse and exercise can all exacerbate symptoms.

❍ **What two organisms cause most cases of PID?**

Neisseria gonorrhea and Chlamydia trachomatis.

❍ **Which patients with PID should be admitted?**

Patients who are pregnant, have a temperature > 38° C (100.4° F), are nauseated or vomiting (which prohibits oral antibiotics), have a pyosalpinx or tubo-ovarian abscess, peritoneal signs, have an IUCD, show no response to oral antibiotics or for whom the diagnosis is uncertain.

❍ **What are the criteria for diagnosis of PID?**

All of the following must be present: (1) adnexal tenderness, (2) cervical and uterine tenderness and (3) abdominal tenderness. In addition, one of the following must be present: (1) temperature > 38° C, (2) endocervix Gram's stain positive for gram-negative intracellular diplococci, (3) leukocytosis > 10,000/mm^3, (4) inflammatory mass on ultrasound or pelvic examination or (5) WBCs and bacteria in the peritoneal fluid.

❍ **What changes occur in the cardiovascular system of a pregnant patient?**

Plasma volume increases 50%, pulse increases 12 to 18 beats per minute, stroke volume increases 25% and hematocrit drops, due to hemodilution.

❍ **What causes dependent and non-dependent edema in pregnant women?**

Compression of veins by the growing uterus causes dependent edema, whereas hypoalbuminemia can cause non-dependent edema.

❍ **What is pregnancy-induced hypertension?**

An increase in the systolic pressure > 30 mm Hg or an increase in diastolic pressure > 15 mm Hg over baseline, measured on 2 separate occasions, at least 6 hours apart.

❍ **What is Sheehan's syndrome?**

Anterior pituitary necrosis following postpartum hemorrhage and hypotension. It results in amenorrhea, decreased breast size and decreased pubic hair.

❍ **What are some common teratogens?**

Alcohol, anticonvulsants, coumadin, DES, isotretinoin, lithium, methimazole and propylthiouracil.

❍ **Describe the effect pregnancy has on (1) cardiac output, (2) BP, (3) heart rate, (4) coagulation, (5) sedimentation rate, (6) leukocytes, (7) blood volume, (8) tidal volume, (9) bladder, (10) BUN/Cr and (11) GI system.**

1) Cardiac output:	Increases
2) BP:	Falls in second trimester; returns to normal in third
3) Heart rate:	Increases
4) Coagulation:	Factors 7, 8, 9 and 10 and fibrinogen increase; others remain unchanged
5) Sed rate:	Elevates
6) Leukocytes:	Increase (up to 18,000)
7) Blood volume:	Increases; no change in RBC; dilutional "anemia" is physiologic

8) Tidal volume:	Increases 40%
9) Bladder:	Displaced superiorly and anteriorly
10) BUN/Cr:	Decreases because of increased GFR and renal blood flow
11) GI:	Gastric emptying and GI motility decrease; alkaline phosphatase increases; peritoneal signs such as rigidity and rebound are diminished or absent

❍ **What is the most common surgical complication during pregnancy?**

Appendicitis. Cholecystitis is the second most common.

❍ **How is the appendix displaced during pregnancy?**

Superiorly and laterally. Diagnosis of appendicitis in pregnant patients may be further complicated by the fact that a normal pregnancy can itself cause an increased WBC. Prompt diagnosis is important because the incidence of perforation increases from 10% in the first trimester to 40% in the third.

❍ **What viral or protozoal infections require extensive work-up during pregnancy?**

TORCH
Toxoplasma gondii
Rubella
Cytomegalovirus
Herpes genitalis

❍ **Can iodinated radiodiagnostic agents be used in pregnant patients?**

No. They should be avoided because concentration in the fetal thyroid can cause permanent loss of thyroid function.

❍ **What percentage of pregnancies are ectopic?**

1.5%. Ectopic pregnancies are the leading cause of death in the first trimester.

❍ **What is the most common presentation of ectopic pregnancy?**

Amenorrhea followed by pain.

❍ **What is the most common finding on pelvic exam in a patient with an ectopic pregnancy?**

Unilateral adnexal tenderness.

❍ **Define preeclampsia.**

HTN after 20 weeks of gestational age with generalized edema or proteinuria.

❍ **Define eclampsia.**

Preeclampsia plus grand mal seizures or coma.

❍ **Should BP be lowered acutely in a preeclampsia patient?**

Dangerous HTN (>170/110) should be gradually lowered with hydralazine IV. Definitive treatment for preeclampsia and eclampsia is delivery.

❍ **3 days post-partum a patient presents with fever. On exam, a foul lochia and tender boggy uterus is present. What is the most likely diagnosis?**

Endometritis, which typically occurs 1 to 3 days post-partum.

❍ **Why is Rh status important in a pregnant patient?**

Rh negative with Rh positive fetus can result in fetal anemia, hydrops and fetal loss. Rh immunoglobulin should be given to all Rh negative patients. The usual amount of RhoGAM may be inadequate in the setting of trauma. A Kleihauer-Betke assay can quantitate fetomaternal hemorrhage.

❍ **An 8 month pregnant patient presents to the ED with profuse bleeding. What must be ruled out with ultrasound before a pelvic exam is performed?**

Placenta previa.

❍ **Risk factors for placenta previa?**

Previous cesarean section, previous placenta previa, multiparity, multiple induced abortions and multiple gestations.

❍ **Risk factors for abruptio placentae?**

Smoking, hypertension, multiparity, trauma and previous abruptio placenta.

❍ **What are the clinical features of abruptio placentae?**

Placental separation before delivery is associated with vaginal bleeding (78%), abdominal pain (66%), as well as tetanic uterine contractions, uterine irritability and fetal death.

❍ **What is the normal fetal heart rate?**

120 to 160 beats per minute. If bradycardia is detected, position the mother on her left side and give oxygen.

❍ **How should a diagnostic peritoneal lavage be performed for a pregnant patient?**

Use an open supraumbilical approach. Always make sure a nasogastric tube and Foley catheter are in place.

❍ **When can one auscultate the fetal heart?**

Ultrasound: 6 weeks.

Doppler: 10 to 12 weeks.

Stethoscope: 18 to 20 weeks.

ETHICS, PAIN MANAGEMENT AND PSYCHIATRIC PEARLS

"It is difficult to say what is impossible, for the dream of yesterday is the hope of today and the reality of tomorrow."
Robert H. Goddard, at his high school graduation, 1904.

❍ **What are some principles of medical ethics?**

Beneficence, nonmaleficence and autonomy.

❍ **What is an ethical dilemma?**

When two or more ethical principles conflict. An example of this is a patient who wishes to have a treatment that is not indicated. This is a conflict of autonomy and nonmalfeasance.

❍ **What is a health care proxy?**

This is an individual who acts as a surrogate in making decisions regarding another individual's health care should the person become unable to do so. This is usually the spouse of the patient.

❍ **What is power of attorney?**

This document declares an individual who has the legal right to make decisions regarding the health care of an individual who is unable to do so.

❍ **What is a living will?**

A living will specifies that certain medical procedures (CPR, etc) not be performed in the event that the patient lacks the capacity to decline the procedures.

❍ **What is an advance directive?**

This document is a living will or a durable power of attorney for health care.

❍ **T/F: A patient who is fully coherent and is a Jehovah's Witness is having a massive lower GI hemorrhage. The patient is an adult and refuses blood products. The physician is legally bound to coerce the patient to receive blood because withholding it may result in the patient's death.**

False. The principle of autonomy dictates that this patient may refuse blood products even if it results in his/her death.

❍ **What must be present to decide that a patient has the capacity to make health care decisions?**

The patient must have knowledge of the options and their consequences and an understanding of the costs and benefits of the options relative to a set of stable values.

❍ **T/F: A patient who refuses a recommendation by their physician is incapacitated to make health care decisions.**

False.

❍ **T/F: It is unethical to withdraw a patient from a ventilator who has end stage COPD and inoperable lung cancer, is of sound mind and requests such a maneuver.**

False.

❍ **T/F: A patient with stage I bronchogenic carcinoma has pulmonary edema requiring mechanical ventilation. You explain this to the patient and he agrees with proceeding with intubation and mechanical ventilation. His wife refuses. The physician should not intubate the patient.**

False. The principle of autonomy declares that each individual is the ultimate arbiter of his or her own health care.

❍ **In the above patient, what should the physician do next?**

Speak to the wife. It could be that she is unaware that the tumor is potentially curable and that the pulmonary edema can be remedied by medications.

❍ **May a physician disclose the content of a medical record to someone other than a patient (or, in the case of a minor or ward, to the patient's parent or guardian)?**

No.

❍ **May a physician disclose the content of a medical record to another health care professional in the regular course of treatment?**

Yes.

❍ **May a physician disclose the content of a medical record under a court order?**

Yes.

❍ **May a physician disclose the content of a child's medical record to school officials who request it?**

No.

❍ **In artificial insemination by donor, where the mother is married, who is considered the legal father?**

The mother's husband.

❍ **May a physician be found liable for a child's reaction to a vaccine she/he administers?**

Only if a typical reasonable competent physician would not have acted as the physician did.

❍ **Is there an ethical difference between withholding and withdrawing life-support measures in patients with acute respiratory failure?**

Ethical principles underlying the decision to withhold intubation and mechanical ventilation apply equally when patients or proxies request discontinuance of care for patients who have no hope for an acceptable and meaningful recovery.

❍ **Are physicians required to honor properly established advance directives by a patient with severe COPD to forego intubation and mechanical ventilation?**

Respect for patient autonomy requires a physician to honor such requests or transfer the patient's care to another physician who can honor the patient's directives.

❍ **When can respiratory depression be seen with spinal opioids?**

Early (30 min.) respiratory depression can be seen with lipophilic opioids, while delayed (3-10 hours) respiratory depression is more commonly seen with hydrophilic opioids such as morphine. Early depression is thought to be due to rapid brain penetration by lipophilic compounds.

❍ **What are the mechanisms of opioid-induced hypotension?**

Histamine release, bradycardia, vasodilation and decreased sympathetic tone.

❍ **T/F: Certain opioids may cause myocardial depression and tachycardia.**

True.

❍ **What are the effects of fentanyl on the cardiac conduction system?**

Fentanyl slows AV node conduction, prolongs the duration of the action potential, the R-R interval, the QT interval and the AV node refractory period.

❍ **Are opioids arrhythmogenic?**

No. Opioids are safe to use in patients with WPW syndrome.

❍ **What is the time to maximal respiratory depression after an IV dose of fentanyl or morphine?**

Fentanyl 5 to 10 min. and morphine 30 min.

❍ **How should opioid-induced seizures be treated?**

With benzodiazepines and barbiturates. Naloxone will generally not reverse seizure activity, especially when induced by normeperidine.

❍ **Which opioid is effective in treating shivering?**

Meperidine. It is effective in treating post-operative, transfusion-related or epidural anesthesia related shivering.

❍ **What is the impact of hepatic disease on opioid pharmacokinetics?**

Decrease clearance, longer elimination half-life. If jaundice and decreased albumin accompany liver disease, patients are more sensitive to opioids.

❍ **What are the effects of renal disease on opioid effects?**

Morphine may show a longer duration of action due to reduced volume of distribution and decreased elimination of active metabolites. Normeperidine accumulation and toxicity can occur. Fentanyl is not significantly altered by renal failure.

❍ **How do opioids affect the respiratory pattern?**

Decrease in rate, tidal volume and minute ventilation. The pattern may also be irregular.

❍ **Which anesthetics when combined with opioids can lead to cardiovascular depression?**

Nitrous oxide, volatile anesthetics, propofol and barbiturates.

❍ **What are the relative potency differences between the opioids?**

Drug	IM	oral
Morphine	10	30
Hydromorphone	1.5	7.5
Meperidine	75	300
Methadone	10	12.5
Codeine	120	200

❍ **What are the most hydrophilic opioids?**

Morphine>meperidine>methadone>alfentanil>fentanyl>sufentanil

❍ **What is the appropriate conversion ratio from IV to epidural opioids?**

IV to epidural = 10:1

❍ **What are the advantages of patient controlled epidural analgesia?**

The ability to titrate analgesic doses in proportion to individual levels of pain intensity, lower total dose requirements compared to other systems, decreased sedation and increased patient satisfaction.

❍ **What are some of the common side effects of opiates and their treatments?**

Side effect	Treatment
Nausea	Phenothiazines, metoclopramide
Sedation	Naloxone
Constipation	Laxatives, stool softeners
Urinary retention	Reduction of dosage, catheterization
Pruritis	Diphenhydramine, naloxone
Respiratory depression	Naloxone

❍ **What are the advantages and disadvantages of methadone administration?**

Advantages include long half-life, can be administered in a liquid form, high bioavailability and no active metabolites.
Disadvantages include accumulation and longer time to reach steady state than other opioids.

❍ **What are the differences between epidural fentanyl and morphine?**

Agent	Onset	Peak	Duration
Morphine	20 min.	30-60 min.	12-24 hr.

Fentanyl	5-10 min.	20 min.	3-6 hr.

❍ **Which epidurally administered opioid has the fewest side effects?**

Fentanyl.

❍ **Why are IM injections of opioids a poor choice for post-operative analgesia?**

Variable blood levels, unpredictable absorption, delayed onset, lag to peak analgesic effect and pain. PCA administration eliminates these problems.

❍ **What are the major advantages of epidural opioid administration?**

Improved pain relief, steady pain relief, decreased post-operative morbidity, improved pulmonary function and shortened hospital stays.

❍ **What are the signs of impending epidural opioid toxicity?**

Altered mental status, decreased level of consciousness, oxygen desaturation, decreased respiratory rate, miosis, increased CO_2 levels.

❍ **What is the mechanism of action of the nonsteroidal anti-inflammatory drugs?**

Inhibition of the cyclooxygenase and lipoxygenase pathways of prostaglandin synthesis.

❍ **What are the major contraindications to the use of NSAIDs in the post-operative period?**

Recent history of GI bleed and ulcers, severe insensitivity to the NSAIDs, impaired renal function and any significant hematologic abnormality that might predispose to bleeding.

❍ **What is the estimated potency of ketorolac compared to narcotic medications?**

Ketorolac 30 mg has potency similar to about 5-10 mg of parenteral morphine.

❍ **What agent has been shown to prevent NSAID gastropathy?**

Misoprostol has been shown to reduce the incidence of gastric lesions when taken four times each day. Because of its cost and side effect profile of diarrhea, it is reserved clinically for those who absolutely require it.

❍ **What are the effects of NSAIDs and aspirin on platelet function?**

All NSAIDs produce reversible inhibition of platelets. Aspirin produces irreversible platelet function. The effects of the NSAIDs persist until the drug is mostly eliminated. Those with longer half-lives have an increased incidence of complications as well.

❍ **When might it be advantageous to use epidural over IV PCA medication in the post-operative period?**

Upper abdominal, vascular and thoracic surgeries benefit from epidural analgesics.

❍ **A patient complains of back pain after an epidural. What information is important to know to determine the actual etiology of this patient's pain?**

Back pain can be caused by catheter pressure on the skin, infection, hematoma or even pre-existing back pain. Assess for neurological deficits. An abscess usually appears at least 5 days post-placement. Hematoma can occur spontaneously and can cause paralysis rapidly. Always assess complaints of back pain in epidural patients completely.

❍ **How much time do you have from the onset of an epidural hematoma to decompress it before permanent neurological damage occurs?**

6 to 8 hours is the generally accepted rule.

❍ **What are the disadvantages of using opioid agonist/antagonists or partial agonists in post-operative pain?**

These agents have a ceiling effect on analgesia above which there is no benefit to analgesia with increased dose. Above this ceiling effect these agents have adverse psychomimetic effects and other adverse effects. These agents are not as potent analgesics as conventional opioid agonists.

❍ **What is the appropriate breakthrough dose of oral opioid medication in a patient taking controlled-release opioid for post-operative pain?**

Patients should be given 1/4 to 1/3 the dose of the scheduled controlled-release preparation every 3 to 4 hours for breakthrough pain. Therefore if a patient is taking 30 mg of controlled-release morphine sulfate every 12 hours, a dose of 10 mg immediate release morphine is adequate when pain is particularly severe.

❍ **What are the important terms associated with patient-controlled analgesia?**

Dose: the amount of medication (based upon patient age, renal function, body habitus) prescribed which the patient may self-administer.
Bolus: the initial amount of medication (loading dose) given when the patient first begins PCA. Generally 2 to 3 times the dose.
Lockout: the time interval between which a patient may not receive additional doses of the agent prescribed. Generally 6 to 10 minutes.
Basal: the continuous background infusion prescribed in addition to the dose made available to the patient.

❍ **What is the purpose of naloxone infusion in patients receiving epidural opioids?**

In very small amounts administered by continuous IV infusion naloxone reverses sedation, nausea, vomiting, pruritis and urinary retention which may be caused by epidural opioids. At low doses naloxone does not reverse analgesia.

❍ **When is a caudal catheter better than an epidural catheter?**

In very small children and infants the placement of the caudal catheter is technically very easy and the space is better defined than the epidural space. This is an option in adults with multiple vertebral fractures in whom epidural analgesics are desired.

❍ **What are non-surgical (post-operative) reasons to consider epidural analgesia?**

Patients with multiple rib or sternal fractures are very good candidates for the analgesic benefits of epidural opioid/local anesthetic mixtures.

❍ **With what procedures has epidural analgesia been shown to be particularly beneficial?**

Procedure	Benefit

Thoracotomy	Pulmonary function
Joint replacement	Decreased DVT, earlier ambulation
Vascular procedures	Improved blood flow, patency
Pediatric cardiac	Decreased ventilator time and hospital stay
Abdominal surgery	Earlier return of bowel recovery

❍ **What is the best way to manage post-operative pain in the patient with a current problem of illegal opioid abuse and addiction?**

"PRN" injections are to be avoided. After a thorough and frank discussion about the pain and expectations about pain relief the patient should receive adequate doses of either scheduled oral or IV opioids or preferably, IV PCA with a background infusion. Consideration must be made for the patient's tolerance to "usual" doses of opioids. Larger bolus doses should be anticipated. Adjunct analgesics such as NSAIDs may be appropriate.

❍ **What are commonly encountered side effects of epidurally administered local anesthetic infusions?**

In large quantities a partial sympathetic block may precipitate hypotension, particularly orthostatic hypotension. With more dilute concentrations this is avoided. Mild motor or sensory loss may occur. Urinary retention, particularly in the very young or the elderly male patient, may occur.

❍ **What are the signs and symptoms of an epidural hematoma?**

Severe back pain and radiating lower extremity pain followed quickly by weakness, paralysis and sensory losses are ominous signs. Loss of bowel and bladder function is a later sign. These findings all require immediate and emergent evaluation.

❍ **What is the work-up for a suspected epidural hematoma?**

1) Immediate history and thorough neurological evaluation.
2) The catheter should be left in place.
3) Neurosurgical consultation.
4) MRI evaluation of the epidural space.
5) Surgical evacuation may be required.

❍ **What are non-pharmacological approaches to managing post-operative pain?**

T.E.N.S. (transcutaneous electrical nerve stimulation) has been studied and shown to be effective in some post-op pain states. Hypnosis and biofeedback as well as heat/cold therapy and massage are also advocated and efficacious.

❍ **What are the major physiologic adverse effects of uncontrolled post-operative pain?**

System	Adverse Effect
Gastrointestinal	Ileus
Cardiovascular	Increased sympathetic effect (BP, Pulse) and angina
Pulmonary	Atelectasis, hypoxia, shunting and CO_2 retention
CNS	Altered mental status and stress
Immunologic	Impaired wound healing

❍ **What is the prevalence of alcoholism in the US?**

Ten to fifteen percent is the lifetime prevalence. Ten percent of men and 3.5 % of women are alcoholic.

❍ **What laboratory changes are suggestive of alcoholism?**

Look for an increase in ALT, AST, alkaline phosphatase, amylase, bilirubin, cholesterol, GGT, LDH, MCV, prothrombin time, triglycerides and uric acid. Look for a decrease in BUN, calcium, hematocrit, magnesium, phosphorus, platelet count and protein.

❍ **Describe the symptoms of alcohol withdrawal and their temporal relations.**

Hallucinations:	Auditory, visual and tactile occur 24 hours after the patient's last drink.
Autonomic hyperactivity:	Tachycardia, hypertension, tremors, anxiety and agitation occur 6 to 8 hours after the patient's last drink.
Global confusion:	Occurs 1 to 3 days after the patient's last drink.

❍ **What is the most common mental illness in large cities?**

Substance abuse. Substance abuse is prevalent in rural communities as well but the addiction percentages are lower. Incidentally, opiates are predominantly a city drug, while marijuana, alcohol and amphetamines are found in both rural and urban settings.

❍ **A patient presents with tearing eyes, a runny nose, tachycardia, piloerection, abdominal pains, nausea, vomiting, diarrhea, insomnia, pupillary dilation and leukocytosis. What is the diagnosis?**

Opiate withdrawal.

❍ **What is the difference between methadone and heroin?**

Methadone causes analgesia, but does not cause euphoria. Habituation occurs with both drugs. The withdrawal symptoms of methadone are less severe but last longer.

❍ **What are a few substances that might mimic generalized anxiety when ingested?**

Nicotine, caffeine, amphetamine, cocaine and anticholinergic agents. Alcohol and sedative withdrawal can also mimic this disorder.

❍ **Bereavement generally lasts how long?**

6 months. Full melancholic syndrome, hallucinations and suicidal ideation are not common in bereavement.

❍ **Why can a patient taking lithium experience polyuria?**

Long term lithium ingestion can cause nephrogenic diabetes.

❍ **What are some common laboratory findings associated with eating disorders?**

Hyponatremia, hypokalemia, hypocalcemia, hypophosphatemia, anemia, hypoglycemia, starvation ketoacidosis, abnormal glucose tolerance, hypothyroidism due to low T3 levels, persistently elevated cortisol due to starvation, low FSH, LH and estrogens and elevated growth hormone.

❍ **What is dementia?**

Disturbed cognitive function that results in impaired memory, personality, judgment or language. Dementia has an insidious onset, but it may present as acute worsened mental state when the patient is facing other physical or environmental stresses.

❍ **What is delirium?**

"Clouding of consciousness" that results in disorientation, decreased alertness and impaired cognitive function. Acute onset, visual hallucinosis and fluctuating psychomotor activity are all commonly seen. These symptoms are variable and may change within hours.

❍ **What are two major causes of dementia?**

Alzheimer's disease and multi-infarction.

❍ **Name some over-the-counter and "street" drugs that may produce delirium or acute psychosis.**

Salicylates, antihistamines, anticholinergics, alcohols, phencyclidine, LSD, mescaline, cocaine and amphetamines.

❍ **What is a dystonic reaction?**

A very common side effect of neuroleptics. It involves muscle spasms of the tongue, face, neck and back. Severe laryngospasm and extraocular muscle spasms may also occur. Patients may bite their tongue leading to an inability to open the mouth, tongue edema or hemorrhage.

❍ **How do you treat a dystonic reaction?**

Diphenhydramine or benztropine.

❍ **What are the five Kubler-Ross stages of dying?**

1) Denial
2) Anger
3) Bargaining
4) Depression
5) Acceptance
Patients may undergo all or only a few of these stages.

❍ **A 24 year-old male presents complaining of pleuritic pain, palpitations, dyspnea, dizziness and tingling in his arms and legs. What is your diagnosis?**

Hyperventilation syndrome. This is frequently associated with anxiety.

❍ **What is an extreme case of fictitious disorder?**

Munchausen's syndrome. These patients may actually try to cause harm to themselves (e.g., by injecting feces into their veins) and are very accepting or seeking of invasive procedures. Munchausen by proxy is another example. In this disease the patient seeks medical care for another, usually a child.

❍ **What is the difference between low potency and high potency neuroleptics?**

Low potency neuroleptics have greater sedative, postural hypotensive and anticholinergic effects. High potency neuroleptics have greater extrapyramidal effects.

❍ **Neuroleptic medications are formulated in low, medium and high potency. What are some of these medicines and their categories?**

Low potency:	Chlorpromazine (Thorazine)
Medium potency:	Perphenazine (Trilafon)
High potency:	Haloperidol, droperidol (Inapsine), thiothixene (Navane), fluphenazine (Prolixin) and trifluoperazine (Stelazine)

❍ **Why is haloperidol one of the preferred neuroleptics?**

It can be used IM in emergencies plus it has few side effects. It does, however, have a high frequency of extrapyramidal effects.

❍ **You are considering chemical restraint. What are your options?**

Benzodiazepines:
1) Lorazepam (Ativan)
2) Midazolam (Versed)
3) Diazepam (Valium)

Sedative hypnotics:
1) Haloperidol (Haldol)
2) Droperidol (Inapsine)

Benzodiazepines may be given in combination with the sedative hypnotics above to both hasten and potentiate their effect. Titrate to effect and monitor appropriately.

❍ **A patient has ingested a phenothiazine and is hypotensive. What is the preferred pressor?**

Norepinephrine.

❍ **What may happen when ethanol is combined with an anxiolytic (benzodiazepine)?**

Death due to their combined respiratory depressive effects.

❍ **What should be used to treat a hypertensive crisis caused by the combination of an MAO inhibitor and a sympathomimetic agent?**

An alpha-adrenergic antagonist agent as IV phentolamine or a potent intravenous vasodilator as nitroprusside.

❍ **Name some drugs contraindicated in a patient who is taking MAO inhibitors.**

Meperidine (Demerol) and dextromethorphan can cause a sympathomimetic crisis. Other agents to avoid include ephedrine, sympathomimetic amines in cold remedies, amphetamines, cocaine and methylphenidate (Ritalin).

❍ **Name the three common MAO inhibitors (chemical and brand name).**

1) Phenelzine (Nardil).
2) Isocarboxazid (Marplan).
3) Tranylcypromine (Parnate).

❍ **Can a person acquire post-traumatic stress disorder (PTSD) if he/she did not actually witness a disturbing event?**

Yes. According to the DSM-IV, one can ex`perience PTSD if an event, such as a violent personal assault, a serious accident or the serious injury of a close friend or family member, is learned of indirectly. PTSD can also occur after a person hears of a life threatening disease affecting a friend or family member.

❍ **List some life threatening causes of acute psychosis.**

WHHHIMP
Wernicke's encephalopathy.
Hypoxia.
Hypoglycemia.
Hypertensive encephalopathy.
Intracerebral hemorrhage.
Meningitis/encephalitis.
Poisoning.

❍ **What signs and symptoms suggest an organic source for psychosis?**

Acute onset, disorientation, visual or tactile hallucinations, age under 10 or over 60 and any evidence suggesting overdose or acute ingestion, such as abnormal vital signs, pupil size and reactivity or nystagmus.

❍ **A 30 year-old female complains of calf pain, a headache, shooting pain when flexing her right wrist, random epigastric pain, bloating and irregular menses, all of which cannot be explained after medical examination. What is the diagnosis?**

Somatization disorder that is characterized by many unexplained medical symptoms involving multiple systems. In order to diagnose a patient with somatization disorder, one must have 4 or more unexplained pain symptoms. Symptoms generally begin in childhood and are fully developed by age 30. This is more common in women than men.

❍ **Who is more successful at suicide, men or women?**

Males (3:1). However, women attempt suicide three times as often as men.

❍ **Major depression and bipolar affective disorder account for what percentage of suicides?**

50%. Another 25% are due to substance abuse and another 10% are attributed to schizophrenia.

❍ **What psychiatric problems are associated with violence?**

Acute schizophrenia, paranoid ideation, catatonic excitation, mania, borderline and antisocial personality disorders, delusional depression, posttraumatic stress disorder and decompensating obsessive/compulsive disorder.

❍ **What are the prodromes of violent behavior?**

Anxiety, defensiveness, volatility and physical aggression.

❍ **What are the potential side effects of naloxone administration?**

Tachycardia, ventricular arrhythmias, cardiac arrest, hypertension, pulmonary edema, reversal of analgesia and precipitation of withdrawal syndrome.

❍ What are the characteristic withdrawal symptoms when opioids are discontinued?

Nausea, vomiting, mydriasis, diarrhea, anorexia, piloerection, yawning, abdominal pain, muscle spasms and leukocytosis.

❍ Explain the significant features of each "axis" in the DSM-III official diagnostic criteria and nomenclature for psychiatric illnesses.

Axis I Organic brain syndromes caused by intoxication or physical illness and major psychiatric disorders including psychosis, affective disorders and disorders of substance use.
Axis II Personality disorders including antisocial, schizoid and histrionic types.
Axis III Medical problems such as heart disease and infections.
Axis IV Life events that contribute to the patient's problems.
Axis V Patient's adaptation to these problems.

❍ According to Holmes and Rahe, what are life's top 10 most stressful events?

1) Death of spouse or child
2) Divorce
3) Separation
4) Institutional detention
5) Death of close family member
6) Major personal injury or illness
7) Marriage
8) Job loss
9) Marital reconciliation
10) Retirement

RANDOM MULTIPLE CHOICE AND TRUE/FALSE PEARLS

❍ **What is a satisfactory initial tidal volume and rate setting for a patient with emphysema?**

A: 12 mL/kg of patient's estimated body weight at 12 breaths per minute
B: 12 mL/kg of patient's ideal body weight at 18 breaths per minute
C: 18 mL/kg of patient's ideal body weight at 18 breaths per minute
D: 10 mL/kg of patient's ideal body weight at 10 breaths per minute
E: 15 mL/kg of patient's ideal body weight at 6-8 breaths per minute

The correct answer is D. In a patient with chronic obstructive pulmonary disease, the initial selected tidal volume and rate are slightly reduced to avoid hyperinflation and hyperventilation.

❍ **Which of the following is the proper amount of physiologic positive end-expiratory pressure (PEEP) to add on the initial ventilator setup when instituting mechanical ventilation?**

A: 2 cm water pressure
B: 7 cm water pressure
C: 4 cm water pressure
D: Difference between the peak and plateau pressure
E: 0 cm water pressure

The correct answer is E. Because PEEP is not a benign mode of therapy, most physicians believe that using the least amount of PEEP is better and that zero PEEP is best. Therefore, the initial ventilator setup involves the use of high fractions of inspired oxygen to oxygenate rather than immediately defaulting to PEEP. If the patient cannot be adequately oxygenated despite using a high fraction of inspired oxygen, then PEEP is appropriate.

❍ **(T/F): When considering mechanical ventilation, a patient who requires 8 cm water of positive end-expiratory pressure (PEEP) for oxygenation should have 8 sighs per hour at a volume of 1.5 times the tidal volume delivered as a single sigh.**

The correct answer is False. Sighs used in combination with PEEP increase the risk of barotrauma; therefore, the use of sighs is not recommended.

❍ **(T/F): The inspiratory-to-expiratory (I:E) ratio can be decreased by increasing the inspiratory flow rate.**

The correct answer is True. The I:E ratio can be adjusted by increasing the inspiratory flow rate, decreasing the tidal volume, and decreasing the ventilatory rate. Attention to the I:E ratio is important for avoiding barotrauma in patients with obstructive airway disease (eg, asthma, chronic obstructive pulmonary disease).

❍ **(T/F): When starting mechanical ventilation, the fraction of inspired oxygen (FIO_2) should initially be set at 40%.**

The correct answer is False. When initiating mechanical ventilation, the highest priority is to provide effective oxygenation. After intubation, a 100% FIO_2 should always be used until adequate oxygenation has been documented based on post-intubation and post-mechanical ventilation arterial blood gas values. A short period on FIO_2 of 100% is not dangerous for patients on mechanical ventilation and offers the clinician several advantages. An FIO_2 of 100% protects the patient against hypoxemia if unrecognized problems develop from the intubation procedure. If the PaO_2 is measured while the patient is on an FIO_2 of 100%, the clinician can easily calculate the next desired FIO_2 and can quickly estimate the shunt fraction. Simply stated, until the patient is stabilized on mechanical ventilation, the initial FIO_2 should be 100%. Then, the FIO_2 can be decreased as the clinical situation allows.

❍ **(T/F): Objective data have documented that the newer modes of mechanical ventilation are more successful for ventilating patients than conventional methods.**

The correct answer is False. No strong evidence supports the use of non-conventional modes of mechanical ventilation. Most physicians use alternative methods of ventilation in cases in which conventional methods have failed. However, this is rare.

❍ **A previously healthy 68-year-old woman hospitalized for elective arthroplasty develops confusion and lethargy 48 hours postoperatively. Her blood pressure is 85/40 mm Hg, her heart rate is 125 beats per minute, her respiratory rate is 26 breaths per minute, and her temperature is 96°F. The skin is warm, and peripheral pulses are bounding. Chest, cardiac, and abdominal examinations produce normal results. The wound is clean and dry. A single peripheral IV site shows no signs of phlebitis. A Foley catheter is present, draining a scant amount of cloudy urine. Which of the following is the most appropriate initial management?**

A: Administration of nafcillin and gentamicin
B: Rapid infusion of intravenous 0.9% saline
C: Administration of 100% oxygen by facemask
D: Transfer patient to an intensive care unit (ICU)
E: All of the above

The correct answer is E. This patient has signs of distributive shock—hypotension with full peripheral pulses and a wide pulse pressure. The patient most likely has septic shock due to a urinary tract infection associated with the indwelling urinary catheter. Other likely sites of infection include the lung and the surgical site. Other potential, though less likely, causes of shock in light of her history might include anaphylaxis after administration of a drug, thromboembolic disease, cardiac disease, or a transfusion reaction. Shock due to bone marrow embolism associated with arthroplasty or the cardiodepressant effects of joint cement or general anesthetic agents would be unlikely this long after surgery. Nearly all patients with shock should be transferred to an ICU immediately. Oxygen should be administered routinely and adequate oxygenation confirmed. Hemodynamic resuscitation should begin immediately with rapid infusion of crystalloid, and dopamine or norepinephrine infusion should be considered if the hypotension is severe or if the circulation is not restored after infusion of 2-3 liters of intravenous fluid over 30-60 minutes. Patients with suspected septic shock should receive immediate empiric antibiotic therapy. Delay in administration of antibiotics is associated with increased mortality.

❍ **A 27-year-old man with a history of HIV infection is admitted to the intensive care unit (ICU) with respiratory failure, shock, and evidence of a lobar pneumonia on chest radiograph. The patient is intubated and mechanically ventilated. Ceftriaxone, erythromycin and trimethoprim-sulfamethoxazole, normal saline, and norepinephrine are administered intravenously. On the second hospital day, the patient's fever has resolved, gas exchange has improved, and blood culture results**

are positive for Streptococcus pneumoniae. However, the patient's blood pressure remains at 80/40 mm Hg despite fluid resuscitation and norepinephrine at a dose of 2 mcg/kg/min. Further examination reveals warm skin, full peripheral pulses, and otherwise normal examination results with the exception of the chest. Which of the choices listed below is the most appropriate next step?

A: Abdominal CT scan
B: Evaluation of the bacterial strain isolated from the blood for antibiotic susceptibility
C: Placement of a pulmonary artery (PA) catheter
D: Cosyntropin stimulation test followed by administration of hydrocortisone 100 mg IV q6h
E: Sinus CT scan

The correct answer is D. Adrenal insufficiency should always be considered in the differential for distributive shock, particularly when no other causes of distributive shock are present or when other clinical signs suggest that an original precipitating cause of shock (eg, infection) is being treated effectively. In this case, the patient with HIV infection and presumed pneumococcal pneumonia and septic shock remains hypotensive despite apparently effective therapy for pneumonia. Adrenal insufficiency is suggested by the refractory hypotension despite appropriate therapy and the presence of HIV infection, which is an independent risk factor for the disorder. Findings of hyponatremia, hyperkalemia, and hyperpigmentation of the skin or mucous membranes also may suggest adrenal insufficiency, but absence of these findings does not exclude the disorder. Placement of a PA catheter could help to determine whether this patient`s refractory shock is related to a low cardiac output, pulmonary vascular disease, or hypovolemia. The incidence of cardiomyopathy and pulmonary hypertension is increased in patients with HIV infection; thus, this intervention would not be inappropriate. However, the widened pulse pressure and peripheral examination results suggest a hyperdynamic circulation, which would not be expected with a decreased cardiac output. Multiple infections are common in patients with HIV infection. A search for a second source of infection is appropriate. However, transportation of an unstable patient to CT scan in the complete absence of findings suggesting disease in the sinuses or abdomen would not be the first course of action. The incidence of antibiotic resistance among strains of S pneumoniae is rising. However, clinical failure of ceftriaxone in the treatment of pneumococcal pneumonia remains uncommon.

❍ **(T/F): The blood pressure is a sensitive indicator of shock.**

The correct answer is False. Various mechanisms allow humans to compensate for loss of circulating volume. These mechanisms function to keep the blood pressure near normal in situations of blood loss. The blood pressure is one of the last vital signs to become abnormal in shock and, therefore, is not sensitive in judging the presence or severity of hypovolemia.

❍ **(T/F): The group of patients most commonly affected by staphylococcal toxic shock syndrome (TSS) is menstruating women.**

The correct answer is True. Staphylococcal TSS still is observed most commonly in women who are menstruating, but it also is associated with cutaneous infections, postpartum and cesarean section wound infections, and focal staphylococcal infections, such as abscess, empyema, pneumonia, and osteomyelitis.

❍ **3 (T/F): In severe distributive shock, only 10% of the cardiac output is consumed by the respiratory muscle system.**

The correct answer is False. As much as 40% is consumed by the respiratory muscle system due to increased work of breathing.

❍ **(T/F): The 2 physical findings that help to differentiate anaphylaxis from other forms of distributive shock are wheezing and urticaria.**

The correct answer is True. Wheezing and urticarial rash (hives) are found in anaphylaxis and are not found in other forms of distributive shock.

❍ **A 60-year-old man describes the onset of palpitations 8 hours ago that woke him from sleep. He has a history of hypertension and paroxysmal atrial fibrillation (AF). On presentation, he is noted to have a heart rate in the 140s with blood pressure of 110/60 mm Hg. Pertinent physical findings include mild basilar crackles in both lungs, an irregularly irregular rhythm, and a nondisplaced point of maximal intensity. His medications include aspirin and an ACE inhibitor. ECG confirms the presence of AF. Which of the following should be the next step?**

A: Perform synchronized cardioversion immediately.
B: Start Lopressor at 5 mg intravenously until the heart rate is 100 bpm, and follow this with oral Lopressor at 50 mg twice daily.
C: Begin heparin drip and cardiovert.
D: Perform transesophageal echo and cardiovert with 360 J synchronized to the R wave.
E: Start flecainide at 100 mg twice daily, heparin intravenously, and admit for anticoagulation with warfarin.

The correct answer is B. While the other answers can be part of the clinical options to restore sinus rhythm, the most important immediate step is to control the ventricular response and prevent possible hemodynamic compromise. Starting a type I-C agent without an atrioventricular nodal blocking agent can lead to an even faster ventricular response. If sinus rhythm can be restored within 48 hours of the onset of atrial fibrillation, then most patients do not need transesophageal echo or heparinization prior to cardioversion; however, if concern exists about the duration of AF and its frequency, start rate control and anticoagulation. The patient can be treated conservatively and cardioverted after 4 weeks of therapeutic International Normalized Ratio or have a transesophageal echo and cardioversion immediately. In both circumstances, anticoagulate the patient for 3-4 weeks after conversion to sinus rhythm.

❍ **Which of the following categories of medications is not indicated in treatment of patients with ST elevation in acute myocardial infarction (MI)?**

A: Thrombolytics
B: Beta-blockers
C: Calcium channel blockers
D: Angiotensive-converting enzyme (ACE) inhibitors
E: Nitrates

The correct answer is C. Calcium channel blockers have no role in the treatment of acute MI with ST elevation and actually may be harmful in this setting. Thrombolytics, beta-blockers, and ACE inhibitors have been shown to reduce mortality rates. Nitrates are useful for symptomatic relief and reducing preload.

❍ **Which of the following hemodynamic criteria is not associated with cardiogenic shock?**

A: Systolic blood pressure less than 90 mm Hg
B: Cardiac index less than 2.2 L/min/m^2
C: Pulmonary capillary occlusion pressure greater than 15 mm Hg
D: Arteriovenous oxygen content greater than 50 mL/L
E: Pulmonary capillary occlusion pressure less than 15 mm Hg

The correct answer is E. A pulmonary arterial occlusion pressure of greater than 15 mm Hg is required to make a diagnosis of cardiogenic shock.

❍ **(T/F): A patient with known aortic stenosis and hypertension presents to the emergency department with symptoms of decompensated heart failure. A recent radionuclide stress test**

revealed no reversible ischemia with a left ventricular ejection fraction of 58%. The emergency physician reports that this patient's ECG reveals atrial fibrillation with a ventricular rate of 120 beats per minute. He wants to start intravenous digoxin but wants to obtain approval of a heart specialist first. In this patient, digoxin would be the most appropriate agent to control the ventricular rate and to resolve the decompensated heart failure.

The correct answer is False. Patients with aortic stenosis and hypertension have dominant diastolic heart failure with ventricular hypertrophy and well-preserved systolic function. Beta-blockers and calcium channel blockers would be better in this particular patient. The role of digoxin in diastolic heart failure is unclear.

❍ **(T/F): Levels of B-type natriuretic peptide (BNP) are elevated when heart failure is due to systolic dysfunction but are within reference ranges in patients with heart failure due to diastolic dysfunction.**

The correct answer is False. BNP levels are strongly correlated with left ventricular filling pressure and are significantly increased in patients with decompensated heart failure, as evidenced by elevated pulmonary capillary wedge pressure, regardless of whether the patient has underlying systolic or diastolic dysfunction. BNP levels are highly useful in differentiating cardiac from noncardiac causes of dyspnea and pulmonary venous congestion.

❍ **(T/F): Intravenous glycoprotein IIb/IIIa inhibitors are only effective in conjunction with percutaneous coronary revascularization procedures in treating acute coronary syndromes.**

The correct answer is False. These intravenous antiplatelet agents, particularly tirofiban and eptifibatide, have been shown to be effective in reducing adverse events in patients who receive only medical therapy.

❍ **(T/F): The strategy of early routine cardiac catheterization with possible revascularization has not been shown to offer benefit over the conservative (selective angiography) approach to treating unstable angina.**

The correct answer is False. Using contemporary interventional techniques and adjunctive medications, 2 recent randomized clinical trials (Fragmin during Instability in Coronary Artery Disease [FRISC] II and Treat Angina with Aggrastat and Determine Cost of Therapy with an Invasive or Conservative Strategy [TACTICS/TIMI-18]) have shown a reduction in rates of death or myocardial infarction for patients who are managed aggressively. However, management still has to be individualized, and more data are necessary to refine patient selection for aggressive versus conservative approach based on a specific benefit-to-risk ratio.

❍ **Operative intervention for neurotrauma is indicated in which of the following instances?**

A: Significant mass effect from contusion or hemorrhage, resulting in a 5-mm shift of intracranial structures
B: Penetrating head injury with necrotic foreign body tracks
C: Significantly depressed skull fractures
D: Foreign body removal if compromising neurologic function
E: All of the above

The correct answer is E. Indications for operative treatment in patients with neurotrauma are indicated for all of the above situations and, additionally, in the instance of extra-axial collections.

❍ **Which of the following is the immediate treatment protocol for a patient with tension pneumothorax?**

A: Immediate drainage of blood from the chest
B: Immediate decompression of air from the affected side
C: Emergent endotracheal intubation with positive-pressure ventilation
D: Emergent thoracotomy on the affected side
E: Rapid infusion of isotonic fluid to maintain adequate cerebral perfusion pressure

The correct answer is B. Tension pneumothorax may prove fatal unless immediately diagnosed and managed. The clinical characteristics are respiratory distress, tracheal deviation (away from the affected side), absence of breath sounds (on the affected side), and distended neck veins. Treatment of patients with tension pneumothorax is immediate decompression followed by drainage. Decompression is achieved by inserting a large-bore cannula (eg, 14-gauge Angiocath) in the midclavicular line, second intercostal space, on the affected side. Drainage is begun by inserting a chest drain between the midclavicular line and the anterior axillary line, in the fourth or fifth intercostal space.

❍ **(T/F): The criterion standard procedure that is used to confirm the presence of an injury to the descending aorta is aortography.**

The correct answer is True. Diagnosis of an injury to the descending aorta typically is made based on clinical suspicion and plain chest x-ray findings and is confirmed by aortography, which is the criterion standard investigation to confirm this diagnosis. However, many centers effectively rely on transesophageal echocardiography and, increasingly commonly, contrast-enhanced thoracic CT scanning using a helical scanner.

❍ **(T/F): The spleen and liver are the most commonly injured organs following blunt trauma.**

The correct answer is True. Although all intra-abdominal organs are at risk of perforation or rupture, the solid organs (ie, spleen, liver) are the most commonly injured organs following blunt trauma.

❍ **(T/F): Pelvic fractures in trauma patients experiencing shock generally are benign incidental problems.**

The correct answer is False. Pelvic fractures often cause severe hemorrhage. In this circumstance, the patient presents with profound shock that frequently is unresponsive to aggressive resuscitation. Such fractures usually result from considerable force and often are accompanied by other injuries.

❍ **(T/F): In trauma patients with physiologic indications of significant injury, urinary catheters are mandatory, although precautions to avoid urethral injury should be taken in the setting of pelvic trauma and with the presence of blood at the urethral meatus.**

The correct answer is True. In all male patients, and especially in the setting of pelvic trauma and with the presence of blood at the urethral meatus, a digital rectal examination to identify a high-riding prostate should precede catheter insertion. If a urethral injury is suspected, a retrograde urethrogram should be performed. If such an injury is identified, a suprapubic catheter should be inserted and a urology consultation obtained.

❍ **A 20-year-old man was assaulted with a lead pipe and received a blow to the forehead. Upon arrival to the emergency department, his vital signs are stable and the patient is alert and oriented. He complains of severe pain to the forehead. Physical examination reveals swelling and crepitus over the supraorbital rims. Based on the CT scan, what is the most likely fracture?**

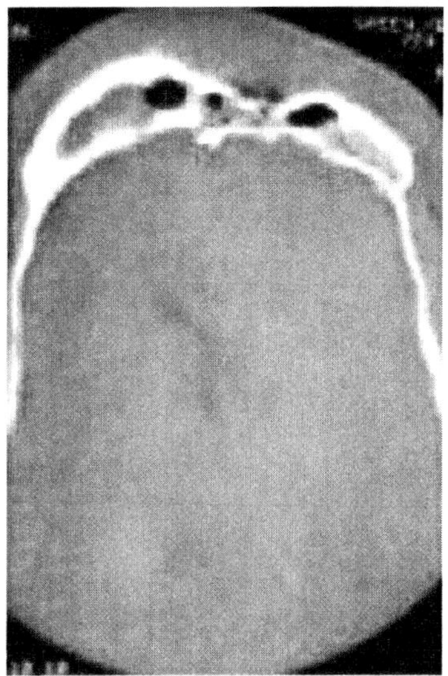

A: Frontal sinus fracture
B: Le Fort I fracture
C: Zygomaticomaxillary complex fracture
D: Le Fort III fracture
E: Mandibular fracture

The correct answer is A. In cases such as this, fractures of the anterior and posterior tables of the frontal sinus have occurred. The CT scan shows the fracture and fluid in the sinus. In this case, the posterior table was removed by the neurosurgeons, and the anterior table of the comminuted frontal bone was repaired by the oral and maxillofacial surgeons.

❍ **A passenger of a small automobile was not wearing a seatbelt and had a head-on collision with a tractor-trailer vehicle. The patient arrived at the emergency department unconscious and responsive only to pain. Once the patient was stabilized, a facial CT scan was obtained. Which of the following types of fracture did this patient sustain?**

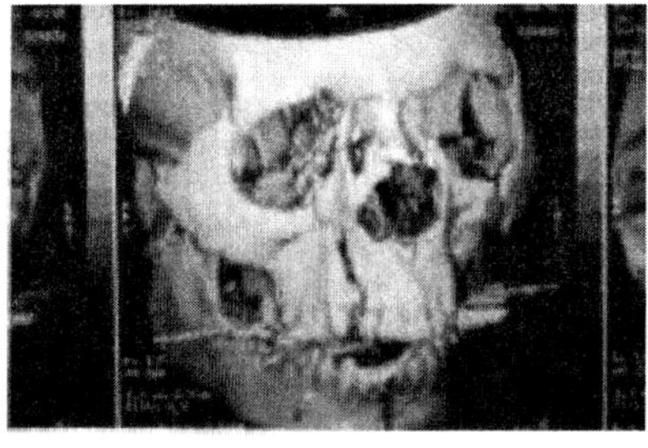

A: Le Fort I fracture
B: Mandibular fracture
C: Le Fort III fracture
D: Frontal bone fracture
E: Panfacial fracture

The correct answer is E. This patient had a combination of a Le Fort III and a mandibular fracture. The patient survived but was blind in both eyes.

❍ **(T/F): In head trauma, longitudinal fractures of the temporal bone are associated with a higher incidence of facial nerve dysfunction compared to transverse fractures of the temporal bone.**

The correct answer is False. Patients with transverse fractures of the temporal bone have a 30-50% incidence of facial nerve dysfunction. Those with longitudinal fractures of the temporal bone have an incidence of facial nerve dysfunction of 10-30%.

❍ **(T/F): An anterior open bite can be the result of a Le Fort III fracture.**

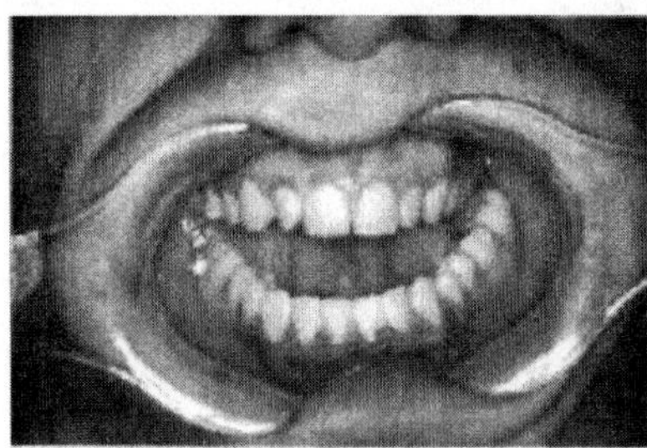

The correct answer is True. The anterior open bite results from the posterior and inferior displacement of the facial bones that occur in patients who sustain Le Fort III maxillary fractures. Patients with bilateral mandibular condyle or angle fractures also can present with this finding due to shortening of the vertical ramus of the mandible.

❍ **(T/F): A unilateral dilated pupil in a patient with head trauma is always a sign of transtentorial herniation.**

The correct answer is False. A unilateral dilated pupil can also result from a traumatic optic nerve injury. In the setting of a traumatic optic nerve injury, the pupil will be dilated and unresponsive to direct stimulation. However, it will constrict in response to stimulation of the contralateral pupil (ie, consensual response).

❍ **(T/F): Imaging of the spine in the initial evaluation of CNS injury should include at least plain x-ray films of the cervical spine (anteroposterior and lateral, a peg view, and with the C7-T1 junction visible).**

The correct answer is True. If a spinal injury is strongly suggested based on the mode of injury or because of suggestive findings on the x-ray film, a CT scan of the spine should be performed next.

❍ **Which of the following statements about pulmonary embolism (PE) is not accurate?**

A: PE is a common and lethal condition.
B: PE is not a disease but a complication of deep venous thrombosis (DVT).
C: The patients who die from PE do so within the first hour.
D: Further mortality occurs from recurrent embolism.
E: PE often resolves spontaneously.

The correct answer is E. PE does not resolve spontaneously; all of the other statements are accurate.

❍ **A 65-year-old man is seen for evaluation of progressive dyspnea. He has a 40-year smoking history. A spirometry is requested. Which of the following spirometric values is diagnostic of chronic obstructive pulmonary disease (COPD)?**

A: Forced vital capacity (FVC) 120% of predicted, forced expiratory volume in 1 second (FEV_1) 110% of predicted, and FEV_1/FVC 73%
B: FVC 90% of predicted, FEV_1 85% of predicted, and FEV_1/FVC 80%
C: FVC 75% of predicted, FEV_1/FVC 90%
D: FVC 85% of predicted, FEV_1/FVC 52%
E: FEV_1/FVC is 60% of predicted, improves to 75% post bronchodilator therapy

The correct answer is D. An obstructive spirometric pattern that does not normalize following bronchodilator administration is diagnostic of COPD (irreversible airflow obstruction).

❍ **(T/F): A comprehensive pulmonary rehabilitation program improves lung function and survival in patients with chronic obstructive pulmonary disease (COPD).**

The correct answer is False. A comprehensive pulmonary rehabilitation improves quality of life and walking distance but not lung function or survival.

❍ **(T/F): Pneumococcus is the most common cause of bacterial pneumonia.**

The correct answer is True. Streptococcus pneumoniae is the most common cause of bacterial pneumonia. Community-acquired pneumonia is caused most commonly by bacteria that traditionally have been divided into 2 groups, typical and atypical. Typical organisms include S pneumoniae (pneumococcus) and Haemophilus and Staphylococcus species. Atypical refers to pneumonia caused by Legionella, Mycoplasma, and Chlamydia species.

❍ **(T/F): A 62-year-old nonsmoking white male foundry worker presents with shortness of breath that has been gradually progressive over the past year. A chest radiograph (seen below) demonstrates multiple small (2-5 mm) nodules in all lung fields. Silicosis is the most likely pulmonary diagnosis.**

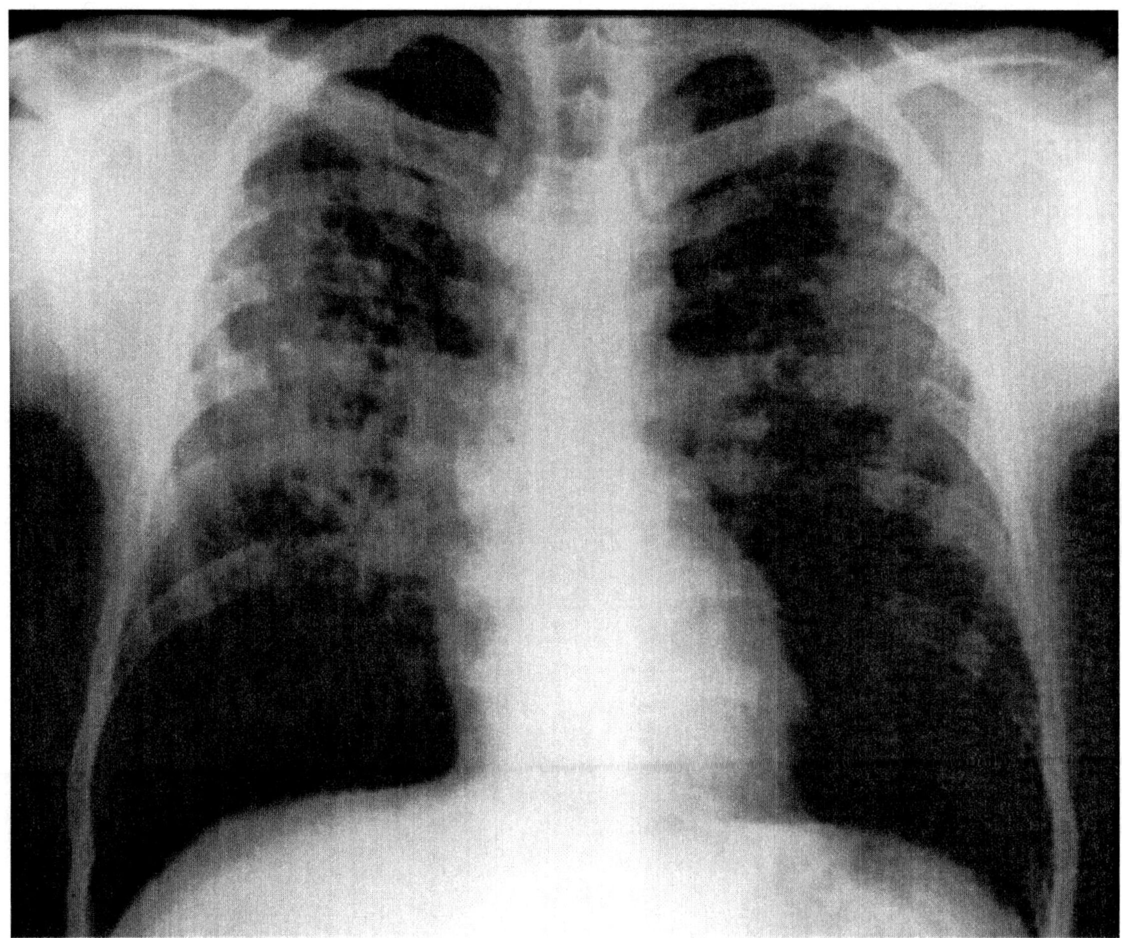

The correct answer is True. Foundry workers are at high risk to develop silicosis. Chest radiographs frequently demonstrate a diffuse pattern of small nodules.

❍ **(T/F): Of the list of conditions that include foreign body aspiration, allergic bronchopulmonary aspergillosis, cystic fibrosis, primary ciliary dyskinesia, and human immunodeficiency virus (HIV) disease, HIV disease is most commonly associated with central bronchiectasis.**

The correct answer is False. Bronchiectasis as a result of infection generally involves the lower lobes, the right middle lobe, and the lingula. Right middle lobe involvement alone suggests right middle lobe syndrome or a neoplastic cause. Bronchiectasis caused by cystic fibrosis, Mycobacterium tuberculosis, or chronic fungal infections tends to affect the upper lobe. Allergic bronchopulmonary aspergillosis also affects the upper lobes but usually involves the central bronchi, whereas most other forms of bronchiectasis involve distal bronchial segments.

❍ **Which of the following conditions is not an indication for dialytic therapy in acute renal failure?**

A: Serum potassium concentration of 7.2 mEq/L
B: Presence of a pericardial friction rub
C: Shortness of breath and orthopnea
D: Acidosis
E: Mental confusion and asterixis

The correct answer is D. Hyperkalemia, pulmonary edema, symptomatic uremia (especially pericarditis), and deterioration of cognitive function are indications for acute hemodialysis. In addition, refractory acidemia may be a rare indication if conservative measures fail.

❍ **Complete metabolic evaluation for urolithiasis is least indicated in which of the following situations?**

A: A 17-year-old male with a history of a single spontaneously passed stone
B: A 55-year-old woman with a history of 2 procedures for stones over the past 2 years and a current radiograph that indicates residual fragments still remaining in a kidney
C: A 65-year-old woman with a history of a single spontaneously passed stone
D: A 25-year-old man with a history of a single passed stone in his adolescence, another stone requiring ureteroscopy earlier this year, and both father and uncle with recurrent calculi
E: A 30-year-old man with a history of multiple bilateral stones who had some flank pain that spontaneously resolved several years ago

The correct answer is C: Indications for metabolic evaluation include residual calculi after surgical treatment, initial presentation with multiple calculi, family history of calculi, or more than a single stone in the past year. Additionally, it is advisable to aggressively treat patients who initially develop stones in their teens or twenties because this group is more likely to experience recurrent stone formation. Only the patient in situation C does not fit any of these criteria. However, even this patient must have her serum electrolytes, creatinine, calcium, uric acid, and phosphorus levels checked, as should all patients with nephrolithiasis.

❍ **(T/F): Urinalysis with microscopic sediment examination, particularly when conducted by a trained physician, is the crucial test in the evaluation of patients with acute nephritic syndrome.**

The correct answer is True. Dysmorphic RBCs and RBC casts found on microscopic examination of the urine sediment are the hallmark of acute nephritic syndrome, making this a crucial test in the evaluation of patients with acute nephritic syndrome.

❍ **(T/F): Hyperkalemia may be a sign of a uremic emergency and should be treated with glucose, insulin, bicarbonate, calcium, and dialysis if necessary.**

The correct answer is True. Hyperkalemia is an emergency, particularly in the setting of uremia. It should be treated emergently and aggressively. In the setting of significant ECG abnormalities, intensive care monitoring should be considered, as should dialysis if hyperkalemia is severe.

❍ **(T/F): The presence of mild eosinophilia, skin mottling, and hypocomplementemia in the setting of acute renal failure suggests atheroembolic renal disease, even in the absence of trauma or aortic manipulation.**

The correct answer is True: Spontaneous atheroembolization causing acute renal failure is common. In the clinical setting described here, atheroembolic renal disease is the most probable diagnosis, especially in patients who are elderly and have atherosclerotic disease elsewhere.

❍ **(T/F): Rate of decline of renal function can be slowed or possibly halted in patients with chronic renal insufficiency (CRI).**

The correct answer is True. In most circumstances, secondary prevention with angiotensin-converting enzyme (ACE) inhibition, aggressive blood pressure (BP) and glycemic control, and avoidance of nephrotoxins can delay progressive decline in renal function.

❍ **A 40-year-old man experiences head trauma in a bicycle accident. Upon arrival in the emergency department, he is alert and without evidence of skull fracture. CT scanning is performed before and after surgical evacuation of an intracranial epidural hematoma (EDH). Which of the following will influence the prognosis of this patient?**

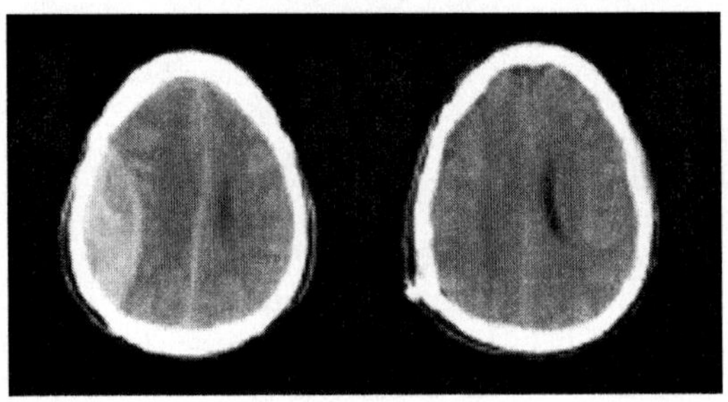

A: Age
B: Presence of other intracranial injuries
C: Initial level of consciousness
D: Time interval between injury and surgical evacuation
E: All of the above

The correct answer is E. The prognosis of EDH is dependent on the age of the patient, presence of other intracranial injuries, initial level of consciousness, and the time interval between injury and surgery.

❍ **A 62-year-old man complains of severe radiating pain in the lower back. MRI demonstrates spinal epidural hematoma (SEDH). Which of the following is not likely to be an associated finding on physical examination?**

A: Sensory deficits in the lower extremities
B: Decreased level of consciousness
C: Weakness
D: Alterations in reflexes
E: Bladder or anal sphincter dysfunction

The correct answer is B. Alterations in the level of consciousness are unlikely to occur in the context of SEDH. Variable physical examination findings, including sensory deficits, weakness, reflex abnormalities, and sphincter dysfunction, may be detected.

❍ **(T/F): A 27-year-old unhelmeted motorcyclist is brought to the trauma bay after being involved in a car accident. On admission, he is normotensive, has a fixed, dilated right pupil, and exhibits decorticate posturing on the left side (Glasgow Coma Scale score=5; eye opening=1, verbal=1, motor score=3). The hospital is rural, with no access to a CT scanner. After appropriate medical therapy has been given, the decision is made to place an emergent decompressive burr hole. The burr hole should be placed on the left side.**

The correct answer is False. The initial burr hole should be placed on the side of the dilated pupil—in this case, the right side. The majority of extraaxial hematomas are found on the side ipsilateral to the dilated pupil. Chesnut and colleagues have shown that 30% of comatose patients with anisocoria >1 mm harbor extraaxial hematomas. Of these, 73% are ipsilateral to the larger pupil.

❍ **(T/F): A 27-year-old unhelmeted motorcyclist is brought to the trauma bay after being involved in a car accident. On admission, he is normotensive, has a fixed, dilated right pupil, and exhibits decorticate posturing on the left side (Glasgow Coma Scale score=5; eye opening=1,**

verbal=1, motor score=3). The hospital is rural, with no access to a CT scanner. An emergency decompressive burr hole is placed on the right side. Appropriate medical therapy in this patient includes an intravenous injection of mannitol.

The correct answer is True. The patient should be given 1 g/kg of mannitol (if he is hemodynamically stable), because he exhibits signs of transtentorial herniation. Mannitol is an osmotic diuretic. Although some controversy exists concerning its mechanism of action on the brain, its ability to lower intracranial pressure has been proven.

❍ **(T/F): The most important prognostic indicator for patients with severe head injuries is the pupillary examination findings.**

The correct answer is False. Several studies have demonstrated that the score on the Glasgow Coma Scale, administered as part of the physical examination in hemodynamically stable patients, is one of the best prognostic indicators in head-injured patients.

❍ **(T/F): Vasospasm is the most feared and most devastating complication of subarachnoid hemorrhage.**

The correct answer is True. Vasospasm is the most feared and most devastating complication of SAH. It is responsible for 14-32% of deaths and permanent disability in SAH. A large amount of blood in the basal cisterns is a predictive factor for developing vasospasm. Once present, the mainstay of therapy is intravascular expansion (triple H therapy) to maintain perfusion in the narrowed vessel segments. Highly specialized centers offer intravascular interventions (eg, local papaverine injection, angioplasty) for the treatment of vasospasm. Hydrocephalus presents with headache, decline in mental status, and other signs of increased intracranial pressure. Focal neurological deficits are usually not a part of the presentation. Rebleeding is another major complication.

❍ **: A 70-year-old man with a history of chronic obstructive pulmonary disease is brought to the hospital with confusion, fever, chills, productive cough, and severe dyspnea. The patient is tachycardic, tachypneic, and hypotensive. His chest radiograph reveals bilateral infiltrates. The patient requires intubation and is monitored in the intensive care unit (ICU). His sputum is purulent (4+WBC, no epithelial cells), and sputum culture results are positive for *Pseudomonas aeruginosa.* Which of the following is appropriate antibiotic therapy at this point?**

A: Ceftriaxone and azithromycin
B: Levofloxacin and metronidazole
C: Cefuroxime
D: Cefuroxime and azithromycin
E: Amikacin and piperacillin/clavulanic acid

The correct answer is E. Pneumonia resulting from pseudomonal infection may develop in patients with chronic lung disease or congestive heart failure. Pneumonia results from the aspiration of upper tract secretions, which is more likely in patients with cardiovascular accident. Pneumonia may present as an acute life-threatening infection. Early antibiotic treatment should be instituted. When pseudomonal pneumonia is suspected, antibiotics with antipseudomonal activity are used, including aminoglycosides, select third-generation cephalosporins (eg, ceftazidime, cefoperazone), select extended-spectrum penicillins, carbapenems (imipenem, meropenem), aztreonam, and fluoroquinolones.

❍ **Which of the following is not commonly associated with sepsis?**

A: Cholecystitis
B: Diverticulitis

C: Tubo-ovarian abscess
D: Acute pyelonephritis
E: Community-acquired pneumonia

The correct answer is E. Community-acquired pneumonia in normal hosts virtually never presents as sepsis. Patients with impaired or absent splenic function may present with community-acquired pneumonia and sepsis.

❍ **(T/F): Vancomycin is the only alternative for treating staphylococcal infections in patients with serious penicillin/beta-lactam allergies.**

The correct answer is False. Clindamycin, trimethoprim-sulfamethoxazole, doxycycline, and vancomycin are all alternatives for patients with serious penicillin/beta-lactam allergies. Vancomycin should be reserved for isolates resistant to the other alternatives.

❍ **(T/F): Neutropenia is an important risk factor for staphylococci infections.**

The correct answer is True. Neutropenia or neutrophil dysfunction, diabetes, intravenous drug abuse, foreign bodies (including intravascular catheters), and trauma are all risk factors for staphylococci infections.

❍ **Ceftriaxone and vancomycin are the drug(s) of choice for the empiric treatment of pneumococcal meningitis (ie, cerebrospinal fluid Gram stain with gram-positive diplococci) occurring in a community where penicillin resistance is high.**

The correct answer is True. One of the most important developments during the past years has been the increasing incidence of penicillin resistance among the pneumococcal strains. Considering the grave consequences of meningitis, when pneumococcal meningitis is suspected in a community where resistance is a concern, empiric therapy should consist of a combination of ceftriaxone and vancomycin. The antimicrobial therapy should be modified once the antimicrobial susceptibilities are available.

❍ **(T/F): The most common cause of meningitis that complicates ventriculoperitoneal shunt infections is *Pseudomonas aeruginosa.***

The correct answer is False. Ventriculoperitoneal shunts are prone to infections by staphylococci, usually with the coagulase-negative strains. This foreign body device can also be contaminated and infected with *Staphylococcus aureus, P aeruginosa,* and other gram-negative bacillary organisms. However, coagulase-negative staphylococci account for the majority of cases.

❍ **A 45-year-old man has a hemoglobin level of 5 g/dL. Fragmented erythrocytes are present on the peripheral smear. Which one of the following tests could help establish the diagnosis?**

A: Direct Coombs test
B: Indirect Coombs test
C: Serum B12
D: Serum folate
E: Urine for hemosiderin

The correct answer is E. Fragmented erythrocytes suggest a microangiopathic hemolytic anemia. This form of anemia occurs in patients with cardiac valvular dysfunction or transfusion reactions. The only test that is helpful in this form of anemia is testing for urinary hemosiderin. The mechanism for a positive urine hemosiderin is that patients with this form of anemia can have hemoglobinemia and hemoglobinuria. The distal tubular renal cells reabsorb hemoglobin from the urine and convert it into hemosiderin. When the hemosiderin-laden renal tubules are sloughed, hemosiderin can be detected in the cellular component of the urinary sediment, and thus, urine is positive for hemosiderin. Fragmented RBCs do not suggest conditions in which a direct or indirect Coombs would be positive or conditions in which the serum folate and vitamin B-12 levels would be abnormal. A direct Coombs test is positive in autoimmune hemolytic anemia, and an indirect Coombs test is positive following transfusion reactions.

❍ **A 45-year-old woman presents with 4-month history of fatigue, early satiety, and left upper quadrant fullness and discomfort. Physical examination shows a massively enlarged spleen and pallor. Complete blood counts show elevated neutrophils of 60,000 with marked left shift. Which of the following studies will be most useful in confirming the diagnosis?**

A: Morphological and flow cytometric examination of the bone marrow aspirate and biopsy
B: Leukocyte alkaline phosphatase (LAP) score
C: Flow cytometric examination of the peripheral blood
D: Peripheral smear examination to detect *bcr-abl* gene rearrangement by fluorescent in-situ hybridization (FISH) or polymerase chain reaction (PCR)
E: CT scan of chest abdomen and pelvis

The correct answer is D. Determining the presence of *bcr-abl* gene rearrangement in the peripheral smear is a simple procedure and, when findings are positive, confirms the diagnosis of chronic myelogenous leukemia (CML). In some patients, when the peripheral blood count is not very high, the yield is lower. In this patient, leukocyte count is high. If she has CML, the likelihood of a positive test result is very high.

❍ **(T/F): CT scan of the brain should be included in the routine staging evaluation of patients with Hodgkin disease.**

The correct answer is False. Hodgkin disease almost never involves the brain; therefore, no role exists for routine brain imaging in the pretreatment evaluation.

❍ **(T/F): A quick way to exclude an acute immune-mediated (ABO) hemolytic reaction in a patient who had a severe generalized transfusion reaction 10 minutes previously is to examine a centrifuged tube of anticoagulated venous blood for hemoglobinemia or to examine a freshly collected urine sample for hemoglobinuria.**

The correct answer is True. Hemoglobinemia in a centrifuged tube of anticoagulated venous blood and hemoglobinuria in a freshly collected urine sample are both signs of acute (ABO) incompatibility

❍ **(T/F): Adenocarcinoma is the lung tumor most commonly associated with hypercalcemia.**

The correct answer is False. Hypercalcemia is a paraneoplastic manifestation most commonly associated with squamous cell carcinoma of the lung.

❍ **(T/F): A finding of malignant pleural effusion with lung cancer usually suggests unresectability of the lung cancer.**

The correct answer is True. Malignant pleural effusion with lung cancer signifies a T4 lesion. The stage of this cancer is IIIB, and it is considered unresectable.

❍ **A 67-year-old white woman with a history of chronic obstructive pulmonary disease (COPD) and diabetes mellitus presents to the emergency department (ED) with shortness of breath, weakness, and a 5-day history of diarrhea. On examination, she has orthostatic hypotension, tachycardia, and expiratory wheezing. Her initial laboratory results are significant for the following: sodium 137 mEq/L, potassium 2.0 mEq/L, chloride 111 mEq/L, total CO_2 15 mEq/L, glucose 359 mg/dL. On**

arterial blood gas (ABG) analysis, her serum pH is 7.15 and $PaCO_2$ is 50 mm Hg. Urinalysis shows a pH of 5.0 without ketones, urine sodium is 15 mEq/L, urine potassium is 15 mEq/L, and urine chloride is 75 mEq/L. Which of the following is the most likely etiology of the metabolic acidosis?

A: Diabetic ketoacidosis
B: GI loss
C: Proximal (type 2) renal tubular acidosis (RTA)
D: Distal (type 1) RTA
E: Type 4 RTA

The correct answer is B: The blood gas analysis reveals a mixed respiratory acidosis and metabolic acidosis. The metabolic acidosis is associated with a normal anion gap (ie, hyperchloremic acidosis). The most common etiologies for this are GI loss of HCO_3^- and RTA. The urine anion gap is -45, implying that the patient has increased NH_4^+ excretion in her urine, the response expected if she has extrarenal loss of HCO_3^-. This patient has a history of diarrhea, which is the likely source of her HCO_3^- and K^+ loss. Diabetic ketoacidosis is very unlikely with a normal anion gap and the absence of ketones in the urine. With type 1 RTA, the urine pH would be greater than 5.5; with type 4 RTA, the defect in ammoniagenesis would be revealed by a positive urine anion gap. Furthermore, type 4 RTA typically is associated with hyperkalemia.

❍ **A 50-year-old woman with a history of hypertension presents with a 2-week history of numbness and tingling in her extremities associated with progressive weakness. She is on amlodipine for blood pressure control. Her initial laboratory results show the following: sodium 144 mEq/L, potassium 1.9 mEq/L, bicarbonate 15 mEq/L, chloride 107 mEq/L, BUN 17 mEq/L, and creatinine 0.6 mg/dL. Her arterial blood gas (ABG) analysis on room air shows a pH of 7.38 and a $PaCO_2$ of 28 mm Hg. Her urinalysis shows a pH of 6.7 with no blood or ketones. Urine also shows sodium of 38 mEq/L, potassium of 24 mEq/L, and chloride of 62 mEq/L. Which of the following is the most likely associated feature in this clinical setting?**

A: Hypoaldosteronism
B: Fanconi syndrome
C: Nephrocalcinosis
D: Laxative abuse
E: Furosemide ingestion

The correct answer is C: The patient has a metabolic acidosis with a normal anion gap. She has no history of GI symptoms, and her urine anion gap is 0, which indicates no NH_4^+ excretion in the face of systemic acidosis. The high urine pH, low serum potassium, and normal renal function exclude type 4 renal tubular acidosis (RTA). Proximal RTA is unlikely because of the high urine pH. The most likely diagnosis in this setting is distal RTA, which is associated with nephrocalcinosis. Laxative abuse would produce a picture of extrarenal HCO_3^- loss, and furosemide use would produce metabolic alkalosis rather than acidosis.

❍ **(T/F): A 32-year-old woman with diabetes presents with weakness. She is not insulin dependent and admittedly is somewhat noncompliant with her diet and medications. Her physical examination results are remarkable only for the absence of deep tendon reflexes. She has a blood pressure of 150/100 mm Hg, a pulse of 52 beats per minute, a respiratory rate of 20 breaths per minute, and she is afebrile. Her laboratory evaluation shows a serum sodium level of 132 mEq/L, a potassium level of 7.2 mEq/L, a chloride level of 105 mEq/L, a bicarbonate level of 21 mEq/L, a BUN of 37 mg/dL, and a creatinine level of 2.0 mg/dL. She has a urine sodium level of 65 mEq/L, a potassium level of 18 mEq/L, and an osmolality of 400 mOsm/kg. Her ECG is remarkable only for first-degree atrioventricular (AV) block and sinus bradycardia. Adrenal insufficiency is the most likely cause of her hyperkalemia.**

The correct answer is False. Type IV or hyperkalemic renal tubular acidosis, secondary to Type II diabetes mellitus is the most likely cause of her hyperkalemia. Type II DM is the most common cause of type IV or hyperkalemic renal tubular acidosis and generally presents with mild renal insufficiency and hyperkalemia out of proportion to the degree of renal insufficiency, as in this case. Alone, excessive dietary potassium ingestion is an extraordinarily uncommon cause of hyperkalemia. A 32-year-old woman with a serum creatinine of 2 mg/dL likely has a glomerular filtration rate near 50 mL/min. At this level of kidney function, potassium homeostasis should be maintained, so renal failure alone also would not account for her hyperkalemia. The changes on her ECG are very suggestive of true hyperkalemia, causing doubt for a diagnosis of pseudohyperkalemia. Finally, although type IV renal tubular acidosis can appear similar to adrenal insufficiency from the standpoint of electrolyte abnormalities, individuals with adrenal insufficiency far more commonly are hypotensive, rather than hypertensive. Adrenal insufficiency is uncommon in younger individuals. Additionally, diabetes and adrenal insufficiency do not coexist commonly.

❍ **(T/F): A 55-year-old man with end-stage renal disease presents complaining of weakness and dyspnea. He has been on dialysis for several years and has been notoriously noncompliant with his dialysis regimen. He has known hypertension and coronary artery disease. His physical examination results show a blood pressure of 150/110 mm Hg and a pulse rate of 42 beats per minute that is regular, and he is afebrile. His general examination shows jugular venous distention, a grade II/VI systolic murmur, and 2^+ peripheral edema. His serum electrolytes show a sodium level of 132 mEq/L, a potassium level of 7.2 mEq/L, a chloride level of 105 mEq/L, and a bicarbonate level of 20 mEq/L. His BUN is 100 mg/dL, and his creatinine is 14.2 mg/dL. His ECG shows slightly peaked T waves, first-degree atrioventricular (AV) block, and a widened QRS not observed on a previous ECG. The most appropriate initial therapy is Calcium gluconate at 1 amp IV.**

The correct answer is True. Although patients with end-stage renal disease often show chronic degrees of hyperkalemia, they are not immune to the cardiotoxic effects as observed on this patient's ECG. This patient has evidence of at least bifascicular block, first-degree AV block, and a bundle branch block. This degree of cardiotoxicity might portend cardiac arrest. Although the calcium gluconate will not alter the potassium concentration, it will stabilize the cardiac membrane almost immediately and provide time to address the hyperkalemia more definitively. Loop diuretics and sodium bicarbonate are not effective hypokalemic agents in patients with renal failure. Glucose alone is far less effective than glucose with insulin in promoting cellular uptake of potassium. Intravenous isoproterenol is not a first-line therapy for hyperkalemia and is not the best choice in a patient who has underlying cardiac disease.

❍ **(T/F): Hyperkalemia often produces ventricular tachycardia.**

The correct answer is False: Hyperkalemia depolarizes the cardiac cell membranes, producing varying degrees of heart block, conduction delays, and bradycardia.

❍ **(T/F): Malignancy is the most common cause of life-threatening hypercalcemia.**

The correct answer is True. Malignancy accounts for 60-80% of the cases of hypercalcemia in hospitalized patients and always must be considered as a possible cause of hypercalcemia. Of the cases due to malignancy, approximately 80% are due to bony metastases. The other 20% are due to the effects of parathyroid hormone–related protein.

❍ **A 12-year-old boy is brought to the critical care department after being rescued from the water while learning to water ski. He is completely alert with no visible signs of trauma. His respiratory rate is 32 breaths per minute, his heart rate is 110 beats per minute, his blood pressure is 110/60 mm Hg, and his temperature is 37.5°C. His chest is clear to auscultation, with mild intercostal retractions. His pulse oximetry reads 98% on room air. How should this patient be managed?**

A: Discharge him home to follow up with his pediatrician in 24 hours.
B: Discharge him home after observing for 6 hours.
C: Admit him to the hospital while administering supplemental oxygen.
D: Intubate the patient and transfer him to the intensive care unit for mechanical ventilation.
E: His disposition depends on whether he was submerged in salt or fresh water.

The correct answer is C: Any patient with respiratory symptoms, altered oxygenation by pulse oximetry or blood gas analysis, or altered mental status or any child involved in a case of suspected child abuse must be admitted to the hospital.

❍ **Which of the following does not predict outcome in acute respiratory distress syndrome (ARDS)?**

A: Albumin level
B: Failure of chest radiographic findings to improve
C: Multiple organ failure
D: ARDS following bone marrow transplantation
E: Sex

The correct answer is E. The sex of the child provides no predictive information regarding prognosis. Mortality risk increases with an increasing number of organ failures. Recent data suggest that, in adults, a low albumin level correlates with increased mortality rate. Almost all series describing outcome (with the exception of a recent study from Toronto) in children with respiratory failure following bone marrow transplantation report a mortality rate approaching 90%.

❍ **(T/F): A 14-year-old adolescent boy with known asthma is seen in the emergency department (ED). He was well until the day of admission, when he played basketball with his friends in warm humid weather. When he returned home, he reported difficulty breathing and has since used his albuterol inhaler 10 times in the past 4 hours. His home medications include albuterol and inhaled steroids. His past medical history is significant for multiple ED visits, 4 ICU admissions in the past year (he was intubated 3 of the 4 times), and known noncompliance with medications.**

Physical examination reveals the following: heart rate (HR) is 120 beats per minute, respiratory rate (RR) is 45 breaths per minute, blood pressure (BP) is 140/98 mm Hg, and temperature is 37°C. He has difficulty speaking and is in severe distress. Auscultation reveals markedly decreased air entry, no wheezing, and no rales. The physician places place him on 100% nonrebreathing mask. If this patient deteriorates further and becomes somnolent, requiring intubation, he will most likely require a fast respiratory rate such as 30 breaths per minute to correct his significant respiratory acidosis.

The correct answer is False. Because people with asthma in status asthmaticus have severe airway obstruction and increased airway resistance, they develop a long time constant and should be ventilated at a lower rate (10-12 breaths per minute) with a longer inhalation-exhalation (I:E) ratio to allow complete emptying and exhalation. Ventilating them at a high rate such as 40-50 breaths per minute results in breath stacking (ie, delivery of the next breath before exhalation is completed) with the potential for even more carbon dioxide retention and the possibility of pneumothoraces.

❍ **(T/F): For patients with diabetic ketoacidosis (DKA), the insulin infusion should not be discontinued until subcutaneous insulin is administered.**

The correct answer is True. Insulin must be administered continuously to treat DKA. If blood sugar levels fall, glucose-containing solutions should be administered.

❍ **(T/F): Fever (ie, temperature >38.0°C or 100.4°F) should be avoided in traumatic brain injury.**

The correct answer is True. Elevated body temperature increases cerebral metabolic demand and oxygen consumption. Temperature control through the treatment of fever can aid in decreasing systemic and cerebral metabolic requirements. Control of metabolism may limit excitotoxicity and inflammation. Fever also decreases the seizure threshold. Efforts should be made to avoid hyperthermia with medications and cooling devices.

❍ **(T/F): Continuous infusion of IV barbiturate (eg, thiopental, pentobarbital) in infants and children with status epilepticus (SE) often causes hypertension, making pressor medications (eg, dopamine, dobutamine) contraindicated in these patients.**

The correct answer is False: Continuous infusion of IV barbiturate (eg, thiopental, pentobarbital) is the final step in the treatment of SE, which stops seizures in almost all patients. Nonetheless, continuous barbiturate infusion often causes hypotension, so pressor medications, such as dopamine and dobutamine, are commonly needed in these cases. Adequate hydration is important to treat patients with IV barbiturate treatment for SE. Continuous midazolam infusion is not a Food and Drug Administration (FDA)–approved alternative treatment of SE for infants and children; it has been associated with fewer blood pressure problems. Continuous IV barbiturate or midazolam infusion should preferably be performed in an intensive care unit. These patients have many needs, including careful ventilation, monitoring of fluids in and out, infection survey, and periodic changes in position in bed.

❍ **A 24-year-old woman with a history of seizure disorder is admitted to the ICU for observation because of lethargy. A suicide note was found at the bedside, along with an empty bottle of phenobarbital. Which of the following statements is most accurate regarding phenobarbital overdose?**

A: Phenobarbital is an ultra–short-acting barbiturate, and symptoms should be expected to resolve within 1 hour.
B: Flumazenil may be used to reverse phenobarbital toxicity.
C: Expected clinical findings include hypertension and tachycardia.
D: Alkalinization of the urine may be helpful in enhancing the elimination of phenobarbital.
E: Fever is a common finding in patients with barbiturate toxicity.

The correct answer is D. Phenobarbital is a long-acting barbiturate with duration of action exceeding 6 hours and a pKa of 7.2. Therefore, this agent is amenable to enhanced urinary excretion by manipulation of the pH. Phenobarbital and other barbiturates cause hypothermia and hypotension. Flumazenil is a benzodiazepine antidote.

❍ **Which patients with benzodiazepine overdoses should be treated with flumazenil?**

A: All patients, regardless of clinical stability
B: Only patients with respiratory depression
C: Patients who are known to have taken a benzodiazepine, with little chance of having taken other ingestants, and who are not addicted to benzodiazepines
D: Patients who have also ingested a cyclic antidepressant
E: None of these patients

The correct answer is C. Flumazenil use can cause seizures in patients who have also ingested other drugs or who are taking benzodiazepines on a long-term basis.

❍ **(T/F): Treatment of organophosphate (OP) poisoning with atropine should not begin until the patient's airway is secure.**

The correct answer is True. Atropine can precipitate ventricular fibrillation in patients who are hypoxic.

❍ **(T/F): Erythrocyte and plasma cholinesterase levels can be useful in diagnosing organophosphate (OP) poisoning.**

The correct answer is True. Erythrocyte and plasma cholinesterase levels can be useful in diagnosing OP poisoning. However, these tests are retrospective diagnostic modalities because testing requires approximately 5-7 weeks.

❍ **(T/F): Hemodialysis does not have a role in salicylate intoxication.**

The correct answer is False. The indications for hemodialysis of salicylate intoxication are severe manifestations, including encephalopathy, coma, seizure, cerebral edema, and acute respiratory distress syndrome (ARDS); renal failure; deteriorating condition despite adequate alkalinization of urine and/or serum; and deteriorating condition where alkalinization cannot be achieved.

❍ **(T/F): Hyperkalemia is commonly found in patients with a theophylline overdose.**

The correct answer is False. Hypokalemia is commonly found in patients with theophylline overdose. Monitor for hypokalemia, hyperglycemia, and hypercalcemia.

❍ **Which of the following would be the best choice for treatment of ventricular fibrillation in a patient with hypothermia?**

A: Procainamide
B: Lidocaine
C: Amiodarone
D: Atropine
E: Adenosine

The correct answer is C. Procainamide is arrhythmogenic in for patients with hypothermia and should not be used. Lidocaine is less effective in patients with hypothermia, and atropine is indicated for bradyarrhythmias. Adenosine is indicated for the treatment of supraventricular arrhythmias in children, but not ventricular fibrillation in hypothermia. Amiodarone is the drug of choice.

❍ **A 74-year-old woman is found in her apartment during a heat wave. She is stuporous and unresponsive. Her respirations appear superficial, her muscles are rigid, and her skin is warm to the touch. Which of the following is not a known complication of her condition?**

A: Generally benign condition without complications
B: Congestive heart failure
C: Rhabdomyolysis
D: Liver failure
E: Compartment syndrome

The correct answer is A. The patient exhibits signs of heatstroke, which is associated with multiple complications, including congestive heart failure, rhabdomyolysis, liver failure, and compartment syndrome.

❍ **(T/F): Mortality in heatstroke is related directly to duration of hyperthermia.**

The correct answer is True. When therapy is delayed, the mortality rate may be as high as 80%; however, with early diagnosis and immediate cooling, the mortality rate can be reduced to 10%.

❍ **(T/F): In frostbite, debride clear blisters but leave hemorrhagic blisters intact. Frostbite is a cold-related injury characterized by freezing of tissue.**

The correct answer is True. Clear blisters contain thromboxane, which can promote further tissue injury; therefore, they should be debrided. Hemorrhagic blisters lack thromboxane, and debridement can lead to infection. Most cases are encountered in soldiers, in those who work outdoors in the cold, and among winter outdoor enthusiasts. Mountain frostbite is a variation observed among mountain climbers and others exposed to extremely cold temperatures at high altitude. It combines tissue freezing with hypoxia and general body dehydration.

❍ **(T/F): While resuscitating a patient with hypothermia and a core temperature of 31°C, the rhythm shows ventricular fibrillation. Two attempts at defibrillation fail. The physician should defibrillate the patient repeatedly until a rhythm is restored or until the physician gives up.**

The correct answer is False. Cardiopulmonary resuscitation should be continued and the patient should be warmed as rapidly as possible. Defibrillation should then be repeated after every 1°C rise in core temperature.

❍ **(T/F): Cardiorespiratory arrest is the only immediate cause of death for lightning victims.**

The correct answer is True. Cardiorespiratory arrest is the only known direct cause of death, but it is still uncommon. Lightning acts as cosmic defibrillation, sending the heart into momentary asystole, which often spontaneously recovers.

❍ **An otherwise healthy 50-year-old man undergoes general anesthetic with isoflurane for an inguinal hernia repair. He develops fever, jaundice, and malaise 5 days after the operation. What is the most likely etiology?**

A: Halothane hepatitis
B: Preexisting viral hepatitis
C: Hypoxic liver injury
D: Sepsis
E: Prolonged hypotension

The correct answer is B. Halothane hepatitis after isoflurane has an incidence of less than 1 case per 1 million patients. Prolonged hypoxia or hypotension to a degree that would cause liver dysfunction is extremely unlikely in an uneventful instance of anesthetic use in minor surgery. Sepsis would likely be associated with hemodynamic instability. Preexisting viral hepatitis can have an incidence as high as 1 case per 700 surgical patients, with a third of these patients eventually developing jaundice.

❍ **A 22-year-old woman presents with the chief complaint of several days of nausea and vomiting. She has no significant medical history. Upon physical examination, her height is 5'7" with a weight of 100 pounds. Her supine blood pressure is 100/70 mm Hg, and her standing blood pressure is 70/50 mm Hg. Her supine pulse rate is 100 beats per minute (bpm), and her standing pulse rate is 130 bpm. She is afebrile and has significant tooth erosions. The results of her entire physical examination, including the abdominal examination, are benign.**

Laboratory studies upon admission provide the following results: hemoglobin/hematocrit, 12/35; WBC count, 8000; sodium, 135 mEq/L; potassium, 2.8 mEq/L; chloride, 80 mEq/L; bicarbonate, 32 mEq/L; BUN, 4 mg/dL; and serum creatinine, 0.6 mg/dL.

She is admitted with a diagnosis of gastroenteritis and dehydration and is started on parenteral

fluids, including 5% dextrose in isotonic sodium chloride solution with 40 mEq potassium chloride at 125 mL/h. Twenty-four hours later, she develops confusion and disorientation. She is still afebrile, and the rest of her examination findings are unchanged. She has no focal neurologic findings and no nuchal rigidity. Funduscopic examination findings are normal.

What is the most likely cause of her confusion?

A: Acute hyposmolar syndrome
B: Acute viral meningitis
C: Acute hypophosphatemic syndrome
D: Alcohol withdrawal
E: Acute hypokalemia

The correct answer is C. This young woman presents with some classic features of anorexia/bulimia, ie, a history of nausea and vomiting, markedly low body weight for height, and tooth erosions. Her electrolyte values are consistent with her history of nausea and vomiting. Most comprehensive biochemical panels do not routinely include serum phosphate determination, and it is likely that her phosphate concentration upon admission would have been in within reference ranges. However, treatment with dextrose should stimulate insulin secretion, driving phosphate into the cells.

In a normally nourished individual, the drop in serum phosphate would be mild and would result in no symptoms. However, in a chronically malnourished patient, the drop can be profound and can lead to delirium, heart failure, and rhabdomyolysis, ie, the acute hypophosphatemic syndrome. She was borderline hyponatremic upon admission, but treatment with isotonic sodium chloride solution would be expected to increase, not decrease, her serum sodium level. Thus, her osmolality would increase. The absence of fever, nuchal rigidity, or any neurologic signs or symptoms upon admission make the diagnosis of viral meningitis less likely. Alcohol withdrawal can also manifest as acute confusion, but it is not commonly observed in persons of this age group and this patient has no history of alcohol abuse. Acute hypokalemia generally does not produce confusion.

❍ **(T/F): Of the following conditions that include sprue, congestive heart failure, dextran infusion, cirrhosis and hypergammaglobulinemia, cirrhosis is not a condition that decreases albumin synthesis.**

The correct answer is False. In cirrhosis, synthesis is decreased because of loss of hepatic cell mass. In sprue, increased intestinal losses are present, which can actually result in a decrease in synthesis due to amino acid absorption. Conditions that increase other osmotically active substances in the serum tend to decrease the serum albumin concentration by decreasing synthesis. Examples include hypergammaglobulinemia and colloid (dextran) infusion. In congestive heart failure, albumin synthesis is normal. Hypoalbuminemia results from an increased volume of distribution.

❍ **(T/F): Riboflavin deficiency may cause cheilosis.**

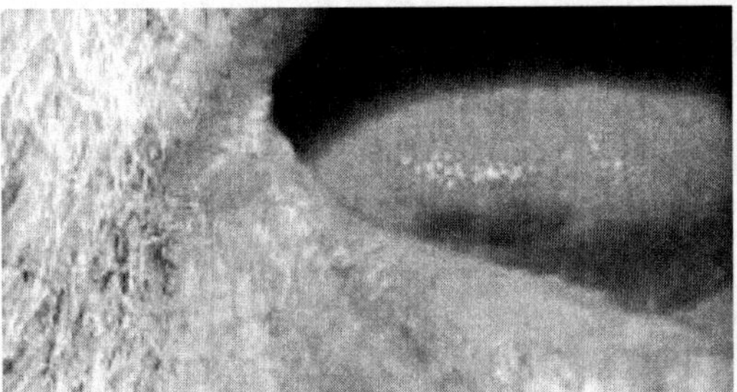

The correct answer is True. This effect of riboflavin deficiency on the skin is well established.

❍ **(T/F): The most likely cause of vitamin B-12 deficiency is small bowel bacterial overgrowth when stage 3 Schilling test results become normalized after antibiotic administration.**

The correct answer is True. Stage 3 of the Schilling test is designed to identify bacterial overgrowth in the intestine.

❍ **(T/F): In a critically ill patient with severe hypoalbuminemia, accurate determination of the active (ionized) fraction of serum calcium can be calculated.**

The correct answer is False. None of the various correction factors for determining the effects of hypoalbuminemia on the plasma calcium concentration has proven reliable. The only method of identifying true (ionized) hypocalcemia in the presence of hypoalbuminemia is to measure the ionized fraction directly.

❍ **Which of the following methods is most important in virtually eliminating the risk of developing transfusion-associated graft versus host disease (GVHD) in susceptible patients?**

A: Transfusion of blood products from close relatives
B: Leukodepletion of cellular blood products
C: Using cytomegalovirus (CMV)–negative blood products
D: Irradiation of blood products with approximately 2500 centigray (cGy)
E: Transfusion of human leukocyte antigen (HLA)–matched platelet products

The correct answer is D. Irradiation of blood products kills lymphocytes, the effector cells responsible for transfusion-associated GVHD. Leukocyte depletion and avoiding transfusions from close relatives who may have identical HLA decrease the incidence of transfusion-associated GVHD.

❍ **Which of the following is the type of rejection reaction that occurs within hours of the transplant and involves the presence of cytotoxic, preformed, antidonor antibodies?**

A: Chronic allograft rejection
B: Acute tubular interstitial rejection
C: Accelerated acute rejection
D: Hyperacute rejection
E: None of the above

The correct answer is D. Hyperacute rejection of the renal allograft occurs when there are circulating, preformed, cytotoxic, antidonor antibodies directed to the ABO blood group antigens or to donor HLA class I antigens. Antibodies bind to antigens expressed on the donor endothelium, resulting in activation of the complement system, platelet aggregation, and microvascular obstruction. Frequency is extremely low, being prevented by ruling out transplant recipients with a positive pretransplant crossmatch. Hyperacute rejection may occur within minutes of revascularization of the allograft and may be observed intraoperatively, or it may occur hours later. There is no ability to salvage the renal allograft. Pathological examination reveals significant interstitial hemorrhage, infiltration of neutrophils, and deposition of antibodies on the endothelium. Often, the diagnosis is obscured because of the severe degree of kidney destruction. Other considerations include arterial or venous thrombosis.

❍ **(T/F): 1.Asymptomatic candiduria should not be treated in renal transplant patients.**

The correct answer is False. Asymptomatic candiduria if untreated can cause ascending infection and fungal ball at ureteropelvic junction.

❍ **(T/F): Immunosuppression after kidney transplantation can be completely stopped if the patient's serum creatinine level has been stable for 5 years.**

The correct answer is False. Immunosuppressants must be continued for the life of the kidney. In certain patients whose renal function is stable, immunosuppressants may be gradually diminished, but never completely stopped. One of the most common reasons for rejection a few years from transplantation is noncompliance with medication regimens.

❍ **(T/F): Cyclosporine, azathioprine, and corticosteroids have been shown to result in a low rate of birth defects in renal transplantation patients who become pregnant.**

The correct answer is True. Azathioprine and corticosteroids have been used in pregnant renal transplantation patients for some time with good outcomes. More recent studies have demonstrated the relative safety of cyclosporine. All pregnant patients with renal allografts must be monitored as high-risk pregnancies.

❍ **(T/F): Allograft vascular disease is the main cause of late graft failure and patient death following heart transplantation.**

The correct answer is True. Allograft vascular disease is characterized by progressive myointimal hyperplasia of the coronary arteries in the allograft. The cause is unknown, and no treatment other than retransplantation exists. Allograft vascular disease is the main cause of late graft failure and patient death.

❍ **Which of the following is the usual cause of necrotizing fasciitis?**

A: Specific serotype of *Cryptococcus neoformans*
B: Variety of serotypes of *C neoformans*
C: The flesh-eating flagellate *protozoa Leishmania tropica*
D: *Leishmania tropica major*
E: A number of bacteria in isolation or as a polymicrobial infection

The correct answer is E. Necrotizing fasciitis can be caused by a number of bacteria in isolation or as a polymicrobial infection. The organisms most closely linked to necrotizing fasciitis are group A beta-hemolytic streptococci, though these bacteria may cause only a minority of the cases. Most cases are caused by other bacteria or different streptococcal serotypes.

❍ **A man presents 4 days after having a mild upper respiratory infection for which he has taken some antipyretics, decongestants, and vitamins. A symmetric eruption of mildly itching red macules, urticarial plaques, and 3 concentric rings develops on the extensor surfaces of the extremities and spreads to the trunk. He had herpes labialis 2 weeks ago and also had the same pattern of rash last year. What is the most appropriate therapy for this patient?**

A: Acyclovir prophylaxis
B: Antihistamine
C: Dapsone
D: Sulfonamide-containing ointment
E: Systemic glucocorticoid

The correct answer is B. Erythema multiforme (EM) is a self-limited condition. Supportive treatment is important. Acyclovir prophylaxis for recurrence of herpes-associated erythema multiforme should be considered in patients with more than 5 attacks per year.

❍ **(T/F): The most common cause of drug-induced linear immunoglobulin A (IgA) dermatosis is vancomycin.**

The correct answer is True: Drug-induced linear IgA dermatosis has been most commonly associated with vancomycin.

❍ **(T/F): An 18-year-old patient with dystrophic epidermolysis bullosa is admitted to the hospital with a wound infection. One of the common causative agents is *Staphylococcus aureus*.**

The correct answer is True: *Staphylococcus aureus* is the most common causative agent; however, *Streptococcus pyogenes* and *Pseudomonas aeruginosa* are other common infectious agents of epidermolysis bullosa wound infections.

❍ **(T/F): The single most diagnostic feature of atopic dermatitis is dry skin.**

The correct answer is False. Pruritus is the single most diagnostic feature of atopic dermatitis. Although skin lesions are eczematous, they vary in location and morphology. Most children have xerosis, but it is impossible to make the diagnosis (except in the first 3 months) without itch.

❍ **(T/F): Soft tissue infection is most commonly seen in staphylococcal toxic shock syndrome (TSS).**

The correct answer is False. It is most commonly seen in streptococcal toxic shock syndrome (STSS). The skin is often the portal of entry in STSS, with soft-tissue infections developing in 80% of patients. The initial presentation of STSS often is localized pain in an extremity, which rapidly progresses over 48-72 hours to manifest both local and systemic signs of STSS. Cutaneous signs may include localized edema and erythema, a bullous and hemorrhagic cellulitis, necrotizing fasciitis or myositis, and gangrene. Soft-tissue involvement of this nature is distinctly uncommon in staphylococcal TSS. STSS may uncommonly occur in the absence of cutaneous involvement; in these cases, differentiation from staphylococcal TSS becomes more difficult.

❍ **Which of the following radiologic methods is not preferred in identifying placenta previa?**

A: Transvaginal ultrasonography
B: CT scanning
C: Magnet resonance imaging
D: Transabdominal ultrasonography
E: Translabial ultrasonography

The correct answer is B. CT scanning does not identify soft tissue (placenta) as well as the other options provided. CT scanning places the fetus at increased risk. All other methods are safe and accurate for identifying placenta previa.

❍ **A 31-year-old woman, gravida 3, para 2, presents to the emergency department at 9 weeks' gestation with increasing lower abdominal pain and heavy vaginal bleeding, with 6 pads soaked in the last 1 hour. Upon examination, her pulse rate is 110 beats per minute and her blood pressure is 80/60 mm Hg. Her cervix is open, with products of conception protruding. What is the next most appropriate step?**

A: Order an immediate sonogram.
B: Administer methotrexate at 50 mg/m^2.
C: Order a serum progesterone test.
D: Monitor the patient with serial quantitative human chorionic gonadotropin titers.
E: Stabilize the patient and proceed with uterine evacuation, with appropriate anesthesia.

The correct answer is E. Patients with incomplete abortions can hemorrhage, and expectant

management has no place in emergent settings. The patient should be appropriately stabilized and undergo suction curettage of the uterus.

❍ **(T/F): All pregnant patients with a history of a seizure disorder should be weaned from their antiepileptic drug(s).**

The correct answer is False. Weaning to one medication or, occasionally, to no medications entirely, may be instituted preconceptually. However, this may not be possible for many patients, and concern for increased seizure frequency during pregnancy is greater than concern for long-term fetal exposure to the antiepileptic drugs during pregnancy.

❍ **(T/F): A 28-year-old woman developed a sudden onset of severe dyspnea, hypoxemia, and cardiovascular collapse while in labor. She most likely developed amniotic fluid embolism.**

The correct answer is True. During labor or delivery, a patient who presents with sudden dyspnea, hypoxemia, and cardiovascular collapse should be considered for a diagnosis of amniotic fluid embolism. The differential diagnosis includes septic shock, pulmonary thromboembolism, and placental abruption.

❍ **(T/F): The percentage of patients with a placental abruption presenting with vaginal bleeding is 80%.**

The correct answer is True. Vaginal bleeding is present in 80% of patients presenting with abruption. Importantly, realize that this means 20% of patients may have a concealed hemorrhage and may have their diagnosis confused with preterm labor due to the painful uterine contractions that occur. The recurrence rate of abruptio placentae in subsequent pregnancies is 4-12%.

❍ **(T/F): The first step in managing a patient with an eclamptic seizure is to deliver the fetus immediately.**

The correct answer is False. Management of an eclamptic seizure is similar to managing any patient with a seizure; the first step is to protect the patient from harm and to maintain an adequate airway. Once the mother is stabilized, delivery of the fetus should be initiated.

❍ **Which of the following symptoms is not a feature of dementia?**

A: Short-term memory
B: Personality
C: Sensory function
D: Language
E: Judgement

The correct answer is C. Disturbed cognitive function that results in impaired memory, personality, judgment or language. Dementia has an insidious onset, but it may present as acute worsened mental state when the patient is facing other physical or environmental stresses.

❍ **A 23-year-old white woman presents for a follow-up visit for major depressive disorder (MDD). She has been taking fluoxetine (Prozac) at a dose of 20 mg daily for 6 weeks, with a small improvement in her symptoms. She denies any significant adverse effects. Her Beck Depression Inventory score is improved, but it still shows depressive symptoms in the moderate range. She denies suicidal ideation or substance abuse. Which of the following is the best course of action?**

A: Change medication to another selective serotonin reuptake inhibitor (SSRI).
B: Augment the fluoxetine with lithium or buspirone (BuSpar).

C: Increase the dose of fluoxetine to 40 mg daily.
D: Discontinue fluoxetine and start a tricyclic antidepressant (TCA).
E: Discontinue fluoxetine and start venlafaxine.

The correct answer is C. In patients who have shown a partial response to an antidepressant, often the quickest and most effective intervention is to increase the dose to the upper safe and tolerable range, because a higher dose may produce further remission of symptoms.

❍ **(T/F): A patient who is fully coherent and is a Jehovah's Witness is having a massive lower GI hemorrhage. The patient is an adult and refuses blood products. The physician is legally bound to coerce the patient to receive blood because withholding it may result in the patient's death.**

The correct answer is False. The principle of autonomy dictates that this patient may refuse blood products even if it results in his/her death.

❍ **(T/F): A patient with stage I bronchogenic carcinoma has pulmonary edema requiring mechanical ventilation. You explain this to the patient and he agrees with proceeding with intubation and mechanical ventilation. His wife refuses. The physician should not intubate the patient.**

The correct answer is False. The principle of autonomy declares that each individual is the ultimate arbiter of his or her own health care.

❍ **(T/F): A physician is automatically liable for a child's reaction to a vaccine she or he administers.**

The correct answer is False. Only if a typical reasonable competent physician would not have acted as the physician did would the physician be held liable for an adverse reaction to an administered vaccine.

❍ **(T/F): There is no ethical difference between withholding and withdrawing life-support measures in patients with acute respiratory failure.**

The correct answer is False. Ethical principles underlying the decision to withhold intubation and mechanical ventilation apply equally when patients or proxies request discontinuance of care for patients who have no hope for an acceptable and meaningful recovery.

BIBLIOGRAPHY

ACCP Critical Care Board Reivew, 2004.

Advanced Cardiac Life Support. Dallas: American Heart Association; 2000.

Advanced Trauma Life Support. Chicago: American College of Surgeons; 1995.

Albert, DM. *Clinical Practice Principles and Practice of Ophthalmology,* Vol. 2. Philadelphia: W.B. Saunders Co.; 1994.

Anderson, JE. *Grant's Atlas of Anatomy,* 8th ed. Baltimore: Williams & Wilkins; 1983.

Arieff, A. & Defronzo, R. *Fluid, Electrolyte and Acid Base Disorders*, 2nd ed. New York: Churchill Livingstone; 1995.

Auerbach, PS. *Management of Wilderness and Environmental Emergencies,* 4th ed. St. Louis: CV Mosby Company; 2001.

Bakerman, S. *ABCs of Interpretive Laboratory Data,* 2nd ed. Greenville: Interpretive Laboratory Data, Inc; 1984.

Baum's Textbook of Pulmonary Diseases, Lippincott, 2003.

Barash PG, Cullen BF, Stoelting RK (eds): *Clinical Anesthesia*, 4th ed. Philadelphia: Lippincott-Raven; 2000.

Barie PS, Shires GT (eds): *Surgical Intensive Care*. Boston: Little, Brown and Co.; 1993.

Berkow, R. *The Merck Manual,* 15th ed. Rahway: Merck Sharp & Dohme Research Laboratories; 1987.

Blomquist, IK & Bayer, AS. Life-threatening deep fascial space infections of the head and neck. *Infect Dis Clin N America.* 1988; 2 (1):237.

Bone LB, Johnson KD, Weigelt J, et al: Early versus delayed stabilization of femoral fractures: a prospective randomized study. *J Bone Joint Surg.* 1989; 71;336.

Bone, RC (ed): *Pulmonary and Critical Care Medicine.* 1993.

Bouachour G, Tirot P, Varache N, Gouello JP, Harr P, Alquier P. Hemodynamic changes in acute adrenal insufficiency. *Intensive Care Med.* 1994; 20:138-41.

Bracken MB, Shepard MJ, Collins WF, et al: A randomized, controlled trial of methylprednisolone or naloxone in the treatment of acute spinal cord injury: results of the Second National Acute Spinal Cord Injury Study. *N Engl J Med.* 1990; 322:1405-11.

Bradley, WG. *Neurology in Clinical Practice,* 4th ed. Newtown: Butterworth-Heineman; 2003.

Braverman LE & Utiger RD, eds: *The Thyroid*, 7th ed. Philadelphia: Lippincott-Raven; 1996:286-296.

Cahill, BC & Ingbar, DH. Massive hemoptysis. *Clinics in Chest Medicine*. 1994; 15:147.

Calleja, GA & Barkin, JS. Acute Pancreatitis. *Med Clin North Am*. 1993; 77:1037-1056.

Civetta JM, Taylor RW, Kirby RR. *Critical Care,* 3rd ed. New York: Lippincott-Raven Publishers; 1997.

Claussen MS, Landercasper J, Cogbill THE. Acute adrenal insufficiency presenting as shock after trauma and surgery: Three cases and review of the literature. *J Trauma*. 1992; 32:94-100.

Current Diagnosis & Treatment in Pulmonary Medicine, McGraw-Hill/Appleton & Lange; 1 edition (October 17, 2003)

Chronic Obstructive Pulmonary Disease, Oxford University Press, 2003.

Critical Care Transport, Jones & Bartlett, 2003.

Cynober, L, *Nutrition and Critical Care*, Ag Med & Sci, 2003.

DeGowin, EL. *Bedside Diagnostic Examination,* 4th ed. New York: Macmillan Publishing Co. Inc; 1981.

Diepenbrock, Nancy, *Quick Reference to Critical Care*, Lippincott Williams and Wilkins, 2003.

Doods, Chris, *Anaesthesia and Critical Care*, Churchill Livingstone, 2003.

Edelstein, PH. Legionnaire's disease. *Clin Infect Dis*. 1993; 16:741.

Ellenhorn, MJ. *Ellenhorn's Medical Toxicology: Diagnosis and Treatment of Human Poisoning,* 2nd ed. Baltimore: Williams & Wilkins; 1997.

Farb, Daniel, *Basic Critical Care,* Atlasbooks, 2004.

Farwell, AP. Sick euthyroid syndrome. *J Intens Care Med*. vol. 12: 5:249-260.

Fauci, AS & Braunwald, E. *Harrison's Principles of Internal Medicine*, 14th ed. New York: McGraw-Hill; 1998.

Feliciano DV, Moore EE, Mattox KL (eds): *Trauma*, 3rd ed. Stamford: Appleton & Lange; 1996.

Fishman, AP. *Fishman's Pulmonary Diseases and Disorders*, 3rd ed. New York: McGraw-Hill; 1998.

Forrester JS, Diamond G, Chatterjee K, Swan JC. Medical therapy of acute myocardial infarction by application of hemodynamic subsets (parts 1 and 2). *N Engl J Med*. 1976; 295, 1356-1362 & 1204-1213.

Flomenbaum, N. *Emergency Diagnostic Testing,* 2nd ed. St. Louis: Mosby-Year Book, Inc.; 1995.

Goldfrank, LR, et al: *Goldfrank's Toxicologic Emergencies*, 6th ed. Stamford: Appleton & Lange; 1998.

Greenfield, LJ. *Surgery Scientific Principles and Practice*. Philadelphia: J.B. Lippincott Company; 1993.

Guyton, AC. *Textbook of Medical Physiology*. 10th ed. Philadelphia: W.B. Saunders Co.; 2000.

Hall JB, Schmidt GA, Wood LDH. *Principles of Critical Care*, 3rd ed. New York: McGraw Hill; 2005.

Harris, JH. *The Radiology of Emergency Medicine,* 2nd ed. Baltimore: Williams and Wilkins; 1981.

Harrison, TR. *Principles of Internal Medicine,* 16th ed. New York: McGraw-Hill Book Company; 2004.

Harwood-Nuss, A. *The Clinical Practice of Emergency Medicine,* 3rd ed. Philadelphia: JB Lippincott Company; 2001.

Holland, JF. *Cancer Medicine,* 6th ed. Baltimore: Williams & Wilkins; 2003.

Hoppenfeld, S. *Physical Examination of the Spine and Extremities.* Norwalk: Appleton-Century-Crofts; 1976.

International Consensus Conference: Clinical Investigation of Ventilator-Associated Pneumonia. *Chest.* Nov 1992; vol. 102; 5: 1.

International Study Group, The. In-hospital mortality and clinical course of 20,891 patients with suspected acute myocardial infarction randomized between alteplase and streptokinase with and without heparin. *Lancet.* 1990; 336: 71-75.

International Consensus Conference: Clinical Investigation of Ventilator-Associated Pneumonia. *Chest.* Nov 1992; vol. 102; 5: 1.

Ivatury, RR & Cayten, CG (eds): *The Textbook of Penetrating Trauma.* Philadelphia: Williams & Wilkins; 1996: 319-332.

Jenison, S & Hejelle, B. Hantavirus pulmonary syndrome; clinical, diagnostic and virologic aspects. *Seminars in Respiratory Infections.* December 1995; vol. 10; 4: 259 – 269.

Johnson D & Cunha, B. Drug Fever. *Infectious Disease Clinics of North America.* March 1996; vol 10; 1: 85-91.

Kelley, WN. *Textbook of Internal Medicine*, 3rd ed. Lippincott-Raven; 1997.

Kelly C, Pothoulakis C, LaMont J. Clostridium difficile colitis. *NEJM.* January 1994; vol. 330; 4: 257-261.

Koenig, K. *Clinical Emergency Medicine.* New York: McGraw-Hill; 1996.

Leach, Richard, *Critical Care Medicine at a Glance,* Blackwell, 2004.

Levin, DL & Morris, FC. *Essentials of Pediatric Intensive Care.* Quality Medical Publishing, Inc.; 1990.

Linden, BE & Aguilar, EA. Sinusitis in the nasotracheally intubated patient. *Arch Otolaryngol Head Neck Surg.* August 1988; vol. 114: 860-861.

Mandell, D & B. *Principles and Practice of Infectious Diseases*, 5th ed. WB Saunders; 2000.

Marino, P. *The ICU Book*, 2nd ed. Baltimore: Williams and Wilkins; 1998.

Marrie, TJ. Community-acquired pneumonia. *Clin Infect Dis.* 1994; 18:501.

Marriott, HJL. *Practical Electrocardiography,* 10th ed. Baltimore: Williams and Wilkins; 2001.

Marshall JB. Acute Pancreatitis. A review with an emphasis on new developments. *Arch Int Med.* 1993;153:1185-1198.

MayoSmith MF, Hirsch PJ, Wodzinski SF, Schiffman FP: Acute epiglottitis in adults. An eight-year experience in the state of Rhode Island. *N Engl J Med.* 1986; 314(18): 1133.

Meduri, GU. Diagnosis of ventilator-associated pneumonia. *Infect Dis clin North Am.* 1993; 7:295.

Miller, RD (ed): *Anesthesia*, 5th ed. New York: Churchill Livingstone; 2000.

Mittman, Bradley, *Frontrunner's Internal Medicine Board Revew*, Frontrunners, 2004.

Mirvis, Stuart, *Imaging in Trauma and Critical Care*, Elsevier Science Health, 2003.

Molitoris, Bruce, *Critical Care Nephrology,* Remedica, 2003.

Montaner JS, Lawson LM, Levitt N, Belzber A, Schechrer,MT, Ruedy J. Corticosteroids prevent early deterioration in patients with moderately sever Pneumocystitis carinii pneumonia and the acquired immunodeficiency syndrome. *Ann Intern Med.* 1990; 113:14-20.

Moore, KL. *Clinically Oriented Anatomy.* 4th ed. Baltimore: Williams & Wilkins; 1999.

Murray, JF and Nadel, JA (ed): *Textbook of Respiratory Medicine*, 3rd ed. Philadelphia: WB Saunders; 2004.

Musher, DM: Infections caused by Streptococcus pneumoniae: Clinical spectrum, pathogenesis, immunity and treatment. *Clin Infect Dis*. 1992;14:801.

Nelson, W.E. *Textbook of Pediatrics.* 17th ed. Philadelphia: W.B. Saunders Company; 2004.

Niederman MS et al.: Guidelines for the initial management of adults with community-acquired pneumonia: Diagnosis, assessment of severity and initial antimicrobial therapy. *Am Rev Respir Dis*. 1993; 148:1418.

Oelkers, W. Adrenal Insufficiency. *N Engl J Med.* 1996; 335:1206-1212.

Owings JT, Kennedy JP, Blaisdell. FW. *Injuries to the Extremities.* Surgery, Scientific American; 1997.

Peitzman AB, Rhodes M, Schwab CW, Yealy DM (eds): *The Trauma Manual.* 2nd ed. Philadelphia: Lippincott-Raven; 2002.

Physicians' Desk Reference, 50th ed. Oradell: Medical Economics Company Inc; 1996.

Plantz, SH. *Emergency Medicine PreTest, Self-Assessment and Review.* McGraw-Hill; 1990.

Plantz, SH. *Emergency Medicine.* Baltimore: Williams & Wilkins; 1998.

Plantz, SH. *Emergency Medicine Pearls of Wisdom,* 6th ed. McGraw-Hill, 2005.

Practical Pulmonary Pathology: A Diagnostic Approach, Churchill Livingstone, 2004.

Principles of Pulmonary Medicine, W.B. Saunders Company, 4th Edition, 2003.

Reddy PS, Curtiss EL, O'Toole JD, Shaver JA. Cardiac tamponade: hemodynamic observations in man. *Circulation.* 1978; 58: 265-272.

Reese, RE & Betts, RF (eds): *A Practical Approach to Infectious Diseases*, 4th ed. Boston: Little, Brown and Company.

Robbins, SL. *Pathologic Basis of Disease,* 3rd ed. Philadelphia: WB Saunders Company; 1984.

Roland, L. *Merritt's Textbook of Neurology.* Williams & Wilkins; 1995.

Rosen, P. *Emergency Medicine Concepts and Clinical Practice,* 4th ed. St. Louis: Mosby Year Book; 1998.

Rosenow EC, Myers JL, Swenson SJ & Pisani RJ: Drug-Induced Pulmonary Disease. *Chest.* 1992; 102:239-250.

Rowe, RC. *The Harriet Lane Handbook: A Manual for Pediatric House Officiers,* 16th ed. C.V Mosby; 2002.

Sabiston, DC. *Textbook of Surgery; The Biologic Basis of Modern Surgical Practice.* 17th ed, Philadelphia: W.B. Saunders Co.; 2004.

Salit, IE. Diagnostic approaches to head and neck infections. *Infect Dis Clin N America.* 1988; 2 (1):35.

Savage EB. *Essentials of Basic Science in Surgery.* Philadelphia: J.B. Lippincott Company; 1993.

Schrier, RW & Gottschalk, CW. *Diseases of the Kidney and Urinary Tract,* 7th ed. Williams & Wilkins; 2001.

Shapiro BA, Kacmarek RM, Cane RD, et al: *Clinical Application of Respiratory Care,* 4th.ed. St. Louis: Mosby-Year Book, Inc.; 1991.

Shapiro BA, Peruzzi WT, Templin R. *Clinical Application of Blood Gases,* 5th ed. St. Louis: Mosby-Year Book, Inc.; 1994.

Simon, RR. *Orthopedics in Emergency Medicine: The Extremities,* 2nd ed. Norwalk: Appleton & Lange; 1992.

Simon, RR. *Emergency Procedures and Techniques,* 2nd ed. Baltimore: Williams and Wilkins; 1987.

Squire, LF. *Fundamentals of Radiology,* 6th ed. Cambridge: Harvard University Press; 2004.

Stedman, TL. *Illustrated Stedman's Medical Dictionary,* 24th ed. Baltimore: Williams & Wilkins; 1982.

Stewart, CE. *Environmental Emergencies.* Baltimore: Williams and Wilkins; 1990.

Suarez, Jose, *Crtical Care Neurology and Neurosurgery,* Humana Press, 2003.

Tietjen PA, Kaner, RJ and Quinn CE: Aspiration Emergencies. *Clinics in Chest Medicine* 1994;15:117-135.

Tintinalli, JE. *Emergency Medicine A Comprehensive Study Guide,* 6th ed. New York: McGraw-Hill, Inc; 2003.

Urokinase Pulmonary Embolization Trial Study Group. Urokinase Pulmonary embolism trial- Phase I results. *JAMA.* 1970; 214: 2163-2172.

Vance, ML. Hypopituitarism. *N Engl J Med.* 1994; 330:1651-62 (Erratum, *N Engl J Med.* 1994; 331:487.)

Weigelt, JA & Lewis, FR (eds): *Surgical Critical Care.* Philadelphia: WB Saunders Co.; 1996.

Weiner, HL. *Neurology for the House Officer,* 7th ed. Baltimore: Williams & Wilkins; 2004.

Werber, SS & Ober, KP. Acute adrenal insufficiency. *Endocrinol Metab Clin North Am.* 1993; 22:303-28.

West, JB. *Respiratory Physiology: The Essentials,* 6th ed. Baltimore: Williams & Wilkins; 2000.

Whitley, RJ. Viral Encephalitis. *NEJM.* July 1990; 242 – 248.

Williams, RD & Larsen, PR. *Williams Textbook of Endocrinology*, 10th ed. Philadelphia: W.B. Saunders; 2002.

Wilson, R & Walt, A. *Management of Trauma: Pitfalls and Practice*, 2nd ed. Philadelphia: Williams & Wilkins; 1996.

Yoshikawa, TT & Quinn, W. The aching head: intracranial suppuration due to head and neck infections. *Infect Dis Clin N America.* 1988; 2 (1):265,

Youmans, JR. *Neurological Surgery,* 5th ed. Philadelphia: W.B. Saunders; 2003.

Zevitz, M. *Cardiovascular Pearls of Wisdom*. McGraw-Hill, 2005.

Zevitz, M. *Internal Medicine Pearls of Wisdom*. McGraw-Hill, 2005.